Therapeutic Strategies

ASTHMA: MODERN THERAPEUTIC TARGETS

Therapeutic Strategies

ASTHMA: MODERN THERAPEUTIC TARGETS

Edited by

Riccardo Polosa
Stephen T. Holgate

CLINICAL PUBLISHING

OXFORD

Clinical Publishing
an imprint of Atlas Medical Publishing Ltd

Oxford Centre for Innovation
Mill Street, Oxford OX2 0JX, UK

Tel: +44 1865 811116
Fax: +44 1865 251550
Web: www.clinicalpublishing.co.uk

Distributed in USA and Canada by:

Clinical Publishing
30 Amberwood Parkway
Ashland OH 44805 USA

Tel: 800-247-6553 (toll free within U.S. and Canada)
Fax: 419-281-6883
E-mail: order@bookmasters.com

Distributed in UK and Rest of World by:

Marston Book Services Ltd
PO Box 269
Abingdon
Oxon OX14 4YN, UK

Tel: +44 1235 465500
Fax: +44 1235 465555
E-mail: trade.orders@marston.co.uk

A catalogue record for this book is available from the British Library

ISBN-10 1 904392 70 9
ISBN-13 978 1 904392 70 5

The publisher makes no representation, express or implied, that the dosages in this
book are correct. Readers must therefore always check the product information and
clinical procedures with the most up-to-date published product information and data
sheets provided by the manufacturers and the most recent codes of conduct and safety
regulations. The authors and the publisher do not accept any liability for any errors in
the text or for the misuse or misapplication of material in this work.

Project manager: Gavin Smith, GPS Publishing Solutions, Hitchin, Hertfordshire, UK
Typeset by Mizpah Publishing Services Private Limited, Chennai, India
Printed in Spain by T G Hostench s.a., Barcelona, Spain

Contents

Editors

STEPHEN T. HOLGATE, DSc, FRCP, MRC Clinical Professor of Immunopharmacology, Allergy and Inflammation Research, School of Medicine, University of Southampton, Southampton, UK

RICCARDO POLOSA, MD, PhD, Professor of Internal and Respiratory Medicine, Department of Internal Medicine, University of Catania, Catania, Italy

Contributors

YASSINE AMRANI, PhD, Research Assistant and Professor of Medicine, Pulmonary, Allergy and Critical Care Division, University of Pennsylvania, Philadelphia, Pennsylvania, USA

LUIZ BELARDINELLI, MD, Senior Vice President, Pharmacology and Translational Biomedical Research, Department of Pharmacology, CV Therapeutics, Inc., Palo Alto, California, USA

PATRICK BERGER, MD, PhD, Laboratory of Cell Physiology (INSERM 356), University of Bordeaux 2, Department of Respiratory Medicine, Bordeaux Teaching Hospital, Bordeaux, France

MIKE A. BERRY, MRCP, Research Fellow, Institute for Lung Health, Department of Respiratory Medicine, Thoracic Surgery and Allergy, University Hospitals of Leicester NHS Trust, Glenfield Hospital, Leicester, UK

ITALO BIAGGIONI, MD, Professor, Medicine and Pharmacology, Vanderbilt University, Nashville, Tennessee, USA

JUDITH L. BLACK, MBBS, PhD, FRACP, Professor, Discipline of Pharmacology, Faculty of Medicine, Woolcock Institute of Medical Research, University of Sydney, NSW, Australia

KIAN FAN CHUNG, MD, DSc, FRCP, Professor of Respiratory Medicine and Honorary Consultant Physician, Section of Experimental Medicine, National Heart and Lung Institute, Imperial College, London, UK

ANUK M. DAS, PhD, Assistant Director, Department of Immunobiology, Centocor Research and Development, Radnor, Pennsylvania, USA

GERT FOLKERTS, PhD, Department of Pharmacology and Pathophysiology, Faculty of Pharmaceutical Sciences, Utrecht University, Utrecht, The Netherlands

PIERANGELO GEPPETTI, MD, Professor of Clinical Pharmacology, Department of Critical Care Medicine and Surgery, Florence, Italy

GUY JOOS, MD, PhD, Pulmonologist, Professor of Medicine, Director, Department of Respiratory Diseases, Ghent University Hospital, Ghent, Belgium

ROBIN J. MCANULTY, PhD, Reader in Lung Pathobiology, Head of Lung Pathobiology Group, Centre for Respiratory Research, University College London, London, UK

LYNNE A. MURRAY, PhD, Research Scientist, Department of Immunobiology, Centocor Research and Development, Radnor, Pennsylvania, USA

ROMINA NASSINI, BSc, Assistant Pharmacologist, Department of Critical Care Medicine and Surgery, Florence, Italy

IAN D. PAVORD, DM, FRCP, Consultant Physician and Honorary Professor of Medicine, Institute for Lung Health, Department of Respiratory Medicine, Thoracic Surgery and Alllergy, University Hospitals of Leicester NHS Trust, Glenfield Hospital, Leicester, UK

JAMES EDWARD PEASE, BSc, PhD, Reader in Leukocyte Biology, Leukocyte Biology Section, National Heart and Lung Institute, Faculty of Medicine, Imperial College London, UK

RICCARDO POLOSA, MD, PhD, Professor of Internal and Respiratory Medicine, Department of Internal Medicine, University of Catania, Catania, Italy

FABIO L.M. RICCIARDOLO, MD, PhD, Consultant Pneumologist, Unit of Pneumology, IRCCS Gaslini Institute, Genoa, Italy

MICHAEL ROTH, PhD, Research Group Leader, Molecular Medicine, The Woolcock Institute for Medical Research, University of Sydney, Camperdown, NSW, Australia

ROZSA SCHLENKER-HERCEG, MD, Senior Director, Clinical Research, General Medicine, Centocor Research and Development, Radnor, Pennsylvania, USA

PAUL S. THOMAS, MD, FRCP, FRACP, Associate Professor and Consultant Physician, Faculty of Medicine, UNSW and Respiratory Medicine, Prince of Wales' Hospital, Sydney, Australia

MARCELLO TREVISANI, PhD, Assistant Pharmacologist, Department of Critical Care Medicine and Surgery, Florence, Italy

J. MANUEL TUNON DE LARA, MD, PhD, Professor of Respiratory Medicine, Laboratory of Cell Physiology (INSERM 356), University of Bordeaux 2, Department of Respiratory Medicine, Bordeaux Teaching Hospital, Bordeaux, France

EMMA WISE, BSc, PhD, Research Associate, Leukocyte Biology Section, National Heart and Lung Institute, Faculty of Medicine, Imperial College London, UK

DEWAN ZENG, PhD, Director, Translational Biomedical Research, CV Therapeutics, Inc., Palo Alto, California, USA

Preface

The discovery of adrenergic agonists and corticosteroids at the start of the 20th century has provided the basis for much of the treatment of asthma. The last 50 years has witnessed major advances in our understanding of asthma and significant improvement in these therapeutic agents with respect to safety, efficacy and duration of action. Inhaled corticosteroids (ICS), short and long acting β_2-agonists (SABAs and LABAs) are now the mainstay of asthma treatment as advocated by disease management guidelines. When used regularly, ICS reduce both morbidity and the addition of LABAs to the management plan appears to improve control of moderate-to-severe asthma. Yet, despite the undoubted efficacy of this combination for most patients, there remains ~10% of the asthmatic population in whom symptoms persist with considerable impact on quality of life and disproportionate use of health care resources.

While ICS are highly effective in suppressing airway inflammation in asthma, they do not influence the natural history of the disease even when started in early childhood and are largely ineffective in virus-induced exacerbations and in those asthmatics who smoke. There is also heterogeneous group of asthma patients who are genuinely refractory to corticosteroids. A few additional therapies are available and include methlyxanthines, anticholinergics, cromones and leukotriene modifiers, but these are of variable efficacy. The introduction of a monoclonal antibody that is able to block IgE effects in severe allergic asthma is a breakthrough in asthma management but only for a limited number of patients. It should also be remembered that 'reagin', the biological activity of IgE was first discovered in 1922 by Prausnitz and Kustner and the biological activity of the leukotrienes, slow reacting substance (SRS), was recognised by Trethewie and Kellaway in 1938 and yet for both of these "activities" a further 40–45 years elapsed before their molecular basis was discovered and a another 15–40 years before the development of therapies that target these. One could legitimately ask why progress has been so slow in the development of new therapeutic agents in this field. Part of the difficulty may be in the high dependency that the pharmaceutical and biotechnology industries have placed on antigen challenge models both in animals and humans to screen for anti-asthma activity whereas allergen/antigen driven responses represent only part of the asthmatic paradigm: diet, air pollutants, tobacco smoke, drugs and viruses are all known to impact on the origins and progression of asthma. Much of the testing of novel chemical activities has also been undertaken on "acute" models, whereas asthma is often a chronic, albeit relapsing disease that often spreads across a lifetime. Some of the therapeutic targets identified in these models such as neuropeptide antagonists, PAF antagonists, bradykinin inhibitors, adhesion molecule antagonists, mast cell "stabilising" agents and some cytokine blockers (e.g. anti-IL5) have all shown great promise in animal models but have failed when tested in humans with asthma. The time has therefore arrived to take a fresh look at asthma and at the novel therapeutic agents that are appearing on the horizon, including biologicals that have proven so successful in other chronic inflammatory diseases such as rheumatoid arthritis, inflammatory bowel diseases and psoriasis.

Looking into the future, *Asthma – Modern Therapeutic Targets* provides readers with an overview of possible new therapeutics in a field in need of innovation. The book is divided into four sections, each covering a particular theme. The first section provides a series of contributions on a number of approaches targeted towards specific autocoid mediators (including newly identified mediators such as adenosine), and transcription factors. Increasingly, tissue injury and disordered repair is being recognised as important in asthma, with the airways behaving like a 'chronic wound'. Thus, the second section of the book focuses on proteases and their inhibitors as novel therapeutic targets. Although simple neuropeptide receptor antagonists have been proven to lack efficacy, the next section underscores the fact that there is a resurgence of interest in modulating neural pathways. Given that asthma is an inflammatory disorder with a strong immunological basis, the book ends with a section focusing on some exciting new immunological molecular targets, including cytokines (with a particular focus on a newly identified target in corticosteroid refractory asthma – TNFα), chemokines, and IgE.

The range of subjects covered and the level of imagination required to make each section a stimulating and educational read has called for remarkable commitment from a large number of leading experts from the pharmaceutical industry and academic world. We would like to acknowledge their considerable contributions to this book without whose help, this collection of informative and up-to-date reviews would not have been possible.

We hope that you will find this book interesting and helpful, and that it will give as much enjoyment to you, the reader, as we have had in its design and editing. Finally, and most importantly of all, our hope is that this new publication shows that the field of novel asthma therapies has a most promising future and that it may be of assistance in the process of finding better therapies for our patients with asthma both now and in the future.

Riccardo Polosa
Stephen T. Holgate

Section I

Autocoids and their receptors in airway diseases

1

Adenosine receptors: novel molecular targets in asthma

D. Zeng, R. Polosa, I. Biaggioni, L. Belardinelli

INTRODUCTION

Adenosine is proposed to play a pro-inflammatory and immunomodulatory role in the pathogenic mechanisms of chronic inflammatory disorders of the airways such as asthma and chronic obstructive pulmonary disease (COPD) [1, 2]. Elevated levels of adenosine are present in chronically inflamed airways [3, 4]. Inhaled adenosine causes dose-dependent bronchoconstriction in subjects with asthma [5] and COPD [6]. Mice with genetic deletion of the adenosine deaminase (ADA) gene [7] or over-expression of interleukin (IL)-13 cytokine [8] in the lung develop features of pulmonary inflammation and airway remodelling with concurrent increases in tissue levels of adenosine in the lung. This and other evidence summarized in this article suggest that adenosine plays an important role in the initiation and progression of inflammatory disorders of the airways. Because adenosine exerts its multiple biological activities by activating four adenosine receptor subtypes, selective activation or blockade of these receptors may lead to therapeutic benefit in the management of pulmonary diseases. Several agonists and antagonists to the adenosine receptors are currently in pre-clinical and clinical development for the treatment of asthma and COPD. In this chapter, we review the rationale of targeting adenosine receptors and the current status of adenosine ligands in development.

ROLE OF ADENOSINE IN PULMONARY DISEASES

Adenosine modulates numerous cardiovascular functions [9] and is currently used clinically as a rapid intravenous bolus for the acute termination of re-entrant supraventricular tachyarrhythmias (Adenocard) and used with radionuclide imaging of the heart to detect under-perfused areas of myocardium as a diagnostic test to detect coronary artery disease in patients unable to exercise (Adenoscan). In the last two decades, it has been recognized that adenosine may also play a critical role in the pathogenesis of chronic inflammatory disorders of the airways such as asthma and COPD. Elevated levels of adenosine are present in chronically inflamed airways; they have been observed both in the bronchoalveolar

Dewan Zeng, PhD, Director, Translational Biomedical Research, CV Therapeutics, Inc., Palo Alto, California, USA

Riccardo Polosa, MD, PhD, Professor of Internal and Respiratory Medicine, Department of Internal Medicine, University of Catania, Catania, Italy

Italo Biaggioni, MD, Professor, Medicine and Pharmacology, Vanderbilt University, Nashville, Tennessee, USA

Luiz Belardinelli, MD, Senior Vice President, Pharmacology and Translational Biomedical Research, Department of Pharmacology, CV Therapeutics, Inc., Palo Alto, California, USA

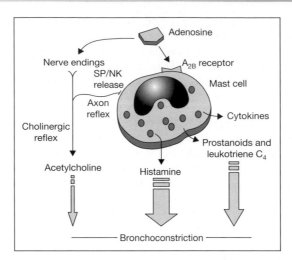

Figure 1.1   Proposed mechanisms for adenosine-induced bronchoconstriction. Stimulation of specific adenosine A_{2B} receptors by adenosine activates airway mast cells to release pro-inflammatory mediators some of which (e.g. histamine, prostaglandins and leukotrienes) act as potent bronchoconstrictors *in vivo* (modified from reference [79]). Note that mast-cell derived mediators are largely implicated in the airway response to adenosine (largest arrow), whereas the role of neural pathways is negligible (smallest arrow). NK = neurokinins; SP = substance P.

lavage fluid (BALF) [3] and the exhaled breath condensate [4] of patients with asthma. Adenosine levels are also increased after allergen exposure [10] and during exercise in atopic individuals [11]. The observed increases in adenosine concentrations suggest that adenosine signalling may regulate aspects of acute and chronic airway disease.

The acute effect of adenosine on bronchoconstriction is well-established by now. Adenosine administration by inhalation was shown to elicit concentration-dependent bronchoconstriction in subjects with asthma whereas the nucleoside had no discernible effect on airway calibre of normal individuals [5]. Since this initial observation, a considerable effort has been directed at revealing the cellular and molecular mechanisms of adenosine-induced bronchoconstriction [1, 2]. One of the proposed mechanisms involves an interaction between adenosine and activated airway mast cells with subsequent release of preformed and newly formed mediators [12] (Figure 1.1). In addition to mast cells, other cells may also play a role in adenosine-mediated bronchial hyperresponsiveness (BHR). The observation that adenosine-mediated BHR is reduced but persistent in mast cell-deficient mice supports the existence of a mast cell independent mechanism [13].

Consistent with the hypothesis of adenosine playing a critical role in the pathogenesis of chronic inflammatory disorders, mice deficient in ADA develop features of severe pulmonary inflammation and airway remodelling in association with increases in adenosine concentrations in the lung [7]. Features of the pulmonary phenotype noted include the following: (1) the accumulation of eosinophils and activated macrophages in the airways, (2) mast cell degranulation, (3) mucus metaplasia in the bronchial airways, and (4) emphysema-like injury of the lung parenchyma. Although the histological observation in ADA-deficient mice does not completely resemble that of human asthma due to the lack of epithelial shedding, subepithelial fibrosis, or muscle/submucosal gland hypertrophy, the ADA-deficient mouse model is a useful tool to study the pathogenic role of adenosine in chronic airway inflammation. The central role of adenosine in chronic lung inflammation is also supported by studies carried out in mice that have increased levels of IL-13 in the lung. These mice develop inflammation, fibrosis, and alveolar destruction concurrently with increases in adenosine concentrations in the lung [8]. Treatment with polyethylene glycol adenosine deaminase (PEG-ADA) to prevent the increases in adenosine concentrations result in a marked decrease in the pulmonary phenotypes suggesting that adenosine mediates IL-13-induced inflammation and tissue remodelling in this experimental model.

An important clinical development in this research area is the use of an adenosine (or AMP) inhalation challenge as a diagnostic test for asthma and COPD [14, 15]. Unlike BHR to methacholine, which is related to the changes in airway calibre, BHR to inhaled AMP seems to be more sensitive to treatment with inhaled corticosteroids (ICS) [16]. In addition, AMP provocation also increases the release of serum neutrophil chemotactic factor [17] and induces sputum eosinophilia [18]. Moreover, inhalation challenge with AMP appears to be useful at establishing the appropriate dose of ICS needed to control airway inflammation, or at predicting safe dose reductions of ICS in patients with mild-to-moderate asthma [19]. The growing body of evidence supports the hypothesis that BHR to inhaled AMP may reflect the inflammatory status of allergic patients and could be useful in evaluating the effectiveness of different treatment regimens with ICS and monitoring corticosteroid requirements and dose selection in asthma treatment [20].

ADENOSINE RECEPTOR SUBTYPES

Extracellular adenosine elicits its biological effects by interacting with four cell surface G protein-coupled receptors designated as A_1, A_{2A}, A_{2B}, and A_3 adenosine receptors [21]. The genes for these receptors have been cloned from human and several animal species. Tissue distributions of these receptors have been determined at the mRNA level using Northern blot or *in situ* hybridization techniques, or at the protein level using subtype-selective radioligands or antibodies. In general, these receptors are widely expressed. For example, high levels of A_1 receptors are found in brain, adipose tissue and atria, whereas high levels of A_{2A} receptors are found in spleen, thymus, striatum, and blood vessels [22, 23]. In addition, these receptor subtypes are often found to co-express in the same tissues or even on the same cell types. The relative expression levels of these receptors have been found to be modulated by physiological and/or pathological tissue environments [24–29]. It remains challenging to attribute the actions of adenosine to specific receptor subtypes based on the distribution of these receptors.

The four adenosine receptors also differ in their coupling to G proteins and the intracellular signalling pathways they activate [21]. In most cells, A_1 and A_3 receptors couple to $G_{i/o}$ and inhibit the adenylate cyclase (AC), whereas A_{2A} and A_{2B} receptors couple to G_s proteins and increase AC activity and intracellular cyclic AMP (cAMP) levels (Figure 1.2). While the AC–cAMP-protein kinase A axis is the most well-studied second messenger system involved in adenosine receptor function, it is clear that adenosine receptors utilize other signalling pathways as well. These include members of the mitogen-activated protein kinase (MAPk) family, such as p38, p42/p44 (ERK 1/2), and c-Jun terminal kinase, as well as various phospholipases, protein phosphatases, and ion channels.

Although adenosine is the natural agonist for these four receptor subtypes, its ability to activate these receptor subtypes varies. In many tissues, A_1 and A_{2A} receptors have relatively higher receptor reserves for adenosine, and can be activated by the physiological levels of adenosine, and thus mediate the tonic actions of adenosine [27–29]. On the other hand, A_{2B} and A_3 receptors appear to have relatively lower affinities and/or receptor reserves for adenosine and require higher concentrations of adenosine for their activation. However, it is hypothesized that the tissue adenosine levels in many pathological conditions are increased to sufficiently high levels to activate the A_{2B} and A_3 receptors.

Numerous subtype-selective agonists and antagonists of adenosine receptors have been synthesized and are used as pharmacological tools [21]. Although these ligands were classified as selective ligands based on their differential binding affinities for the four adenosine receptors, these compounds are often not well characterized functionally in biological sys-

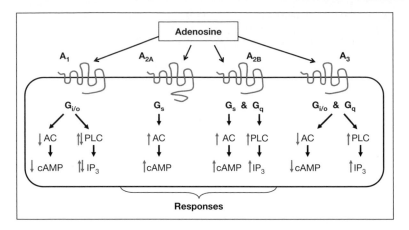

Figure 1.2 Adenosine signalling pathways. In most cell systems, adenosine binding to A_1 and A_3 receptors results in the inhibition of AC with overall reduction of cAMP levels. On the other hand, the canonical signalling mechanism of adenosine A_{2A} and A_{2B} receptors is the stimulation of AC with increase in cAMP levels *via* coupling to stimulatory G proteins (G_s). However, adenosine A_{2B} and A_3 receptors can, in addition, elevate inositol (1,4,5)-trisphosphate (IP_3) levels *via* G_q activation.

tems and many have been found not to be as selective as originally suggested. There are pharmacological reasons for the lack of functional selectivity. For example, potencies of an agonist for a given receptor subtype could vary from one tissue (or cell) to another depending on receptor reserve, receptor expression levels and coupling efficiencies. As mentioned above, adenosine receptors are widely distributed and their expression levels are often modified during disease processes. This certainly adds complexity in predicting functional selectivity of agonists. In the case of antagonists, the functional blocking effects of competitive antagonists are related to the tissue adenosine levels. If the adenosine levels are too low to activate a given receptor, antagonists for this receptor would not have any functional effects, regardless of their binding affinities. In addition to these pharmacological issues, the pharmacokinetic properties of these compounds need to be considered when using them as 'selective' ligands *in vivo*. In many cases, the half-life and tissue distributions of these compounds are poorly understood, making it difficult to draw conclusions on the role of receptor subtypes based on the absence of effects of 'selective ligands' in animal models (Table 1.1). In spite of these limitations, selective agonists and antagonists are commonly utilized to establish the functions mediated by adenosine receptor subtypes.

RATIONALES OF TARGETING ADENOSINE RECEPTOR SUBTYPES

Asthma and COPD are complex diseases sharing clinical heterogeneity and a number of pathogenic traits, which include variable degree of airflow obstruction, BHR, and chronic airway inflammation [30–32]. Many cell types that play important roles in the pathogenesis of chronic inflammatory airway diseases are known to express adenosine receptors. These cell types include various inflammatory cells, such as mast cells, eosinophils, lymphocytes, neutrophils, and macrophages, and the structural cells in the lung, such as bronchial epithelial cells, smooth muscle cells, lung fibroblasts, and endothelial cells. In addition, numerous animal models have been used to assess the contribution of adenosine and its receptor subtypes in the pathology of pulmonary diseases. The most commonly used models are allergic animal models and genetically modified models including receptor knockout mouse models and the ADA-deficient mouse model.

Table 1.1 Effect of adenosine ligands in animal models

Class of compounds	Compounds (route of administration)	Animal model	Biological effects	Reference
A_1 antagonist	L-97-1 (intragastric)	Allergic rabbit model	Blocked BHR to allergen or adenosine	[36]
A_{2A} agonist	CGS21680 (intratracheal)	Ovalbumin-sensitized Brown Norway rat	Reduced eosinophils and neutrophils and inflammatory markers in BALF	[48]
A_{2B} antagonist	CVT-6883 (i.p.)	Allergic mouse model	Inhibited adenosine-induced BHR	[75]
		ADA KO	Inhibited pulmonary inflammation, fibrosis, airway enlargement	[76]
A_3 antagonist	MRS 1523 (osmotic pump)	ADA KO	Reduced eosinophils and mucus production	[66]
A_1, A_{2B}, A_3 antagonist and p38 α, β and PDE4D inhibitor	CGH2466 (intranasal or oral)	Allergic mouse challenged by ovalbumin	Reduced eosinophils in BALF	[78]
		LPS-induced neutrophilic lung inflammation	Reduced neutrophils in BALF	

BALF = bronchoalveolar lavage fluid; KO = Knockout; LPS = lipopolysaccharide

A_1 ADENOSINE RECEPTOR

The early evidence suggesting a role of the A_1 receptor in asthma came from experimental work using an allergic rabbit model [33]. In this model, aerosolized adenosine caused dose-dependent bronchoconstriction in rabbits sensitized with allergens but not in non-immunized animals. In addition, adenosine produced contractions of tracheal and bronchial smooth muscles isolated from the sensitized animals [34]. Pharmacological studies using selective agonists and antagonists revealed that this effect of adenosine was mediated by the A_1 subtype [33]. Furthermore, the expression of the A_1 receptor was increased in smooth muscles of the allergic rabbits suggesting that the acute bronchoconstriction effect of adenosine in this model was mediated by the A_1 receptors on bronchial smooth muscles. Two potential therapeutic agents were tested in this allergic rabbit model; EPI-2010, which is a 21-mer antisense oligodeoxynucleotide targeting the adenosine A_1 receptor [35], and L-97-1, which is a small molecule A_1 receptor antagonist [36]. As expected, both agents blocked the BHR to allergen or adenosine. The relevance of these observations to human asthma has been questioned due to the fundamental mechanistic difference between adenosine-induced bronchoconstriction in allergic rabbits, which appears to be due to activation of A_1 receptor on the bronchial smooth muscle, and that in man, which appears to be dependent on activation of mast cells [37].

The A_1 receptor has also been implicated in both pro- and anti-inflammatory aspects of disease processes. For example, it has been shown that activation of A_1 receptor promotes activation of human neutrophils and enhances neutrophil adhesion to the endothelium suggesting a pro-inflammatory role of the A_1 receptor [38, 39]. In contrast, in ADA/A_1

double knockout mice, the lack of A_1 receptors results in enhanced pulmonary inflammation, mucus metaplasia, alveolar destruction and earlier death possibly due to the respiratory distress [40]. These later findings suggest that A_1 receptors may play an anti-inflammatory and/or tissue-protective role in the regulation of pulmonary disorders triggered by adenosine.

A_{2A} ADENOSINE RECEPTOR

It is now well known that activation of A_{2A} receptors on lymphoid cells by adenosine causes inhibition of an inflammatory response and this response is largely due to its effect of inducing accumulation of intracellular cAMP in activated immune cells [41, 42]. The actions of A_{2A} receptors on these inflammatory cells are numerous. For example, in human neutrophils, stimulation of A_{2A} receptors reduces neutrophil adherence to the endothelium [39], inhibits formyl-Met-Leu-Phe (fMLP)-induced oxidative burst and inhibits superoxide anion generation [38]. In monocytes and macrophages, activation of A_{2A} receptors inhibits lipopolysaccharide (LPS)-induced tumour necrosis factor α (TNFα) expression [43, 44]. Therefore, A_{2A} agonist may have an anti-inflammatory effect in diseases such as COPD where neutrophil/monocyte-mediated tissue injury is implicated [32]. Activation of lymphocytes, which plays a key role in the recruitment of leukocytes to the lung in clinical asthma, is also suppressed by activation of A_{2A} receptors [45]. Thus, there are a multitude of mechanisms by which activation at A_{2A} receptors could suppress inflammation.

Results from studies in animal models have confirmed the anti-inflammatory effects of A_{2A} receptors. Perhaps the strongest evidence for the critical role of A_{2A} receptors in the regulation of inflammation *in vivo* comes from studies using mice deficient in A_{2A} receptors. In this model, the absence of the A_{2A} receptors resulted in enhanced tissue inflammation and damage [46] and increased levels of pro-inflammatory cytokines associated with enhanced activity of nuclear factor-κB (NF-κB) transcription factor [47] confirming an anti-inflammatory role of A_{2A} receptor. As for airway inflammation, the effect of a selective A_{2A} agonist, CGS 21680, on allergen-induced airway inflammation was tested in the ovalbumin-sensitized Brown Norway rat model [48]. CGS 21680 (administered intratracheally) significantly reduced the numbers of eosinophils and neutrophils, it also reduced the activities of myeloperoxidase and eosinophil peroxidase, and protein concentrations in BALF. These anti-inflammatory effects of CGS 21680 were comparable to the effect of budesonide in the same model. However, similar doses of CGS 21680 also caused marked decreases in blood pressure. Thus, it is difficult to separate the anti-inflammatory effect of CGS 21680 from its cardiovascular effects.

A_{2B} ADENOSINE RECEPTOR

The initial evidence for the role of A_{2B} receptors in asthma and COPD came from pharmacological studies of enprofylline, a methylxanthine structurally closely related to theophylline [49]. It was shown that enprofylline is a selective antagonist for the A_{2B} receptors whereas theophylline has similar binding affinities for A_1, A_{2A} and A_{2B} receptors. Importantly, the therapeutic concentrations of theophylline and enprofylline are in the range of their affinities for A_{2B} receptors. Thus, it was proposed that A_{2B} receptor might be the therapeutic target for the long-term clinical benefit achieved with relatively low doses of theophylline and enprofylline [50].

Recently, A_{2B} receptors have been shown to mediate several pro-inflammatory effects of adenosine in mast cells and lung structural cells. For example, functional human adenosine A_{2B} receptors have been identified in mast cells [49, 51–53], endothelial cells [24, 54, 55], bronchial smooth muscle cells [56, 57], lung fibroblasts [58], and bronchial epithelium. In these cells, adenosine, *via* activation of A_{2B} receptors, increases the release of various inflammatory cytokines, which induce IgE synthesis from human B lymphocytes [53], and promote differentiation of lung fibroblasts into myofibroblasts [58]. Such findings provide support for the hypothesis that adenosine, *via* activation of A_{2B} receptors, could enhance the inflammatory responses associated with asthma. Thus, an A_{2B} antagonist could potentially be beneficial in the treatment of asthma and other pulmonary inflammatory diseases.

A_3 ADENOSINE RECEPTOR

The functional significance of the A_3 receptor in the pathogenesis of chronic inflammatory airway diseases remains controversial largely due to major species differences in the expression and function of A_3 receptor subtype [59]. Studies performed in rodents have revealed that the effects of adenosine on mast cell degranulation and/or enhancement of mast degranulation in response to allergen are dependent on the activation of A_3 receptor [60–62]. Perhaps the strongest evidence came from studies using genetic knockout mice. While the A_3 receptor knockout mouse appears to reproduce and develop well and has normal cardiovascular functions, it does exhibit altered mast cell functions [63, 64]. Unlike mast cells from wild type mice, adenosine could no longer potentiate antigen-induced release of hexosaminidase from bone marrow-derived mast cells [63] nor could adenosine induce histamine release from lung mast cells of A_3 knockout mice [65]. Interestingly, adenosine-induced airway hyperresponsiveness was markedly reduced but not completely blunted in the A_3 knockout mice (C57BL/6), suggesting the existence of both A_3-dependent and -independent mechanisms in mice [13].

Besides the effects on mast cells, A_3 receptors have been shown to play an important role in eosinophilia and mucus production in animal models [66]. The effects of a selective A_3 antagonist, MRS 1523, on pulmonary inflammation and remodelling were tested in ADA- deficient mice. While MRS 1523 had no significant effects in wild type mice, treatment with MRS 1523 reduced the numbers of eosinophils in BALF and mucus production by airway epithelium in the ADA-deficient mice. Consistent with this finding, in ADA/A_3 double knockout, lack of A_3 receptors resulted in marked reduction in eosinophils and mucus production suggesting an important role of A_3 receptors mediating the lung eosinophilia and mucus hyperplasia in the pulmonary disorders triggered by elevated adenosine levels.

In man, there is not yet convincing evidence to support the role of A_3 receptor in promoting degranulation of lung mast cells [67]. On the other hand, A_3 receptors are found in human eosinophils [67, 68] and transcript levels for the A_3 receptor are elevated in lung biopsies of patients with asthma or COPD [67]. Activation of A_3 receptors inhibited eosinophil chemotaxis and migration [67, 69], eosinophil degranulation, and superoxide anion (O^{2-}) release [70]. Because inflammation in asthmatic patients is characterized by extensive infiltration of the airways by activated eosinophils, it is possible that the elevated adenosine concentrations associated with asthma contribute to the inhibition of eosinophil activation *via* activation of A_3 receptors in human. If this is the case, A_3 agonists would potentially be useful in the management of asthma. Hence, there is conflicting evidence between animal and human data on the possible role(s) of A_3 receptors in the pathophysiology of asthma. Therefore, the role of A_3 receptor in the lung of asthmatics remains to be established.

ADENOSINE LIGANDS IN CLINICAL DEVELOPMENT FOR ASTHMA AND COPD

All four adenosine receptor subtypes are expressed in the lung and in inflammatory cells involved in asthma. It is not surprising, therefore, that selective agonists or antagonists to these receptor subtypes are being exploited by the pharmaceutical industry in an attempt to generate novel therapies for asthma and COPD (Table 1.2).

Table 1.2   Adenosine ligands in clinical development for asthma and/or COPD

Drug name	Molecular targets	Proposed mechanisms of action	Status
EPI-2010	Antisense oligonucleotide of A_1 receptor	Inhibition of BHR	Discontinued
UK-432097	A_{2A} agonist	Anti-inflammation	Phase 2
GW328267	A_{2A} agonist	Anti-inflammation	Phase 2
CVT-6883	A_{2B} antagonist	Inhibition of BHR and anti-inflammation	Phase 1

EPI-2010

EPI-2010 is a 21-mer antisense oligodeoxynucleotide of the A_1 receptor [35]. In an allergic rabbit model, it was shown that intratracheal administration of aerosolized EPI-2010 (twice daily for 2 days) inhibited the BHR triggered by either adenosine or allergen [35]. In the same model, EPI-2010 also caused approximately 75% reduction in the numbers of A_1 receptor in airway smooth muscle. In a placebo-controlled phase 2 trial in asthmatics with moderate-to-severe persistent disease who were already on ICS, inhaled EPI-2010 (once or twice weekly for 4 weeks) did not cause any significant improvement in indices of bronchoconstriction, such as baseline forced expiratory volume at one second (FEV_1), peak expiratory flow rate (PEFR), forced expiratory flow $(FEF)_{25-75}$, symptoms of nocturnal wakening, or rescue β-agonist use [71]. Based on this disappointing clinical result, the development of EPI-2010 has been reported to have been discontinued.

GW328267

GW328267 is an agonist to the A_{2A} receptor. In a randomized, double-blind, placebo-controlled three-way crossover study, the effects of inhaled GW328267 (25 μg, twice daily for 6 days and once on the seventh day), inhaled fluticasone propionate (FP, 250 μg, twice daily), or placebo on allergen-induced early and late asthmatic responses, sputum cell differential counts, inflammatory markers in sputum and blood, and exhaled nitrc oxide (NO) were compared in 14 asthmatics without concurrent steroid treatment. Inhaled fluticasone significantly inhibited both early and late asthmatic responses accompanied by inhibitory effects on sputum eosinophils, eosinophil cationic protein and exhaled NO. In contrast, no protective effect of GW328267 was found [72]. In addition, GW328267 did not cause significant changes in baseline FEV_1. This dose of GW328267 was chosen based on the findings in previous studies in healthy non-asthmatic subjects that higher doses of GW328267 may cause decreases in blood pressure and increases in heart rate.

UK-432,097

UK-432,097 is a potent and selective agonist to the A_{2A} receptor. The selectivity of UK-432,097 for the recombinant adenosine receptors was determined using cAMP assays, and the potencies (EC_{50} values) for stimulation of cAMP mediated by A_{2A} and A_{2B} receptors were 0.46 and 67.5 nM, respectively, whereas the potencies (IC_{50} values) for the inhibition of cAMP mediated by A_1 and A_3 receptors were >300 and 66.5 nM, respectively [73]. UK-432,097 inhibited the fMLP-induced release of elastase, superoxide and LTB4 in human neutrophil and also inhibited the LPS-induced release of MIP1β and TNFα in human peripheral blood mononuclear cell (PBMC) with IC_{50} values of approximately 2–3 nM [74]. In a randomized, double-blind, placebo-controlled two-way crossover study, the effect of inhaled UK-432,097 or placebo on lung functions were compared in 16 non-smoking, mild asthmatic subjects [73]. Inhaled UK-432,097 had no effect on baseline FEV_1/FVC and PC_{20}-AMP, suggesting that adenosine-induced bronchoconstriction in humans is unlikely to be mediated by the A_{2A} receptor. It would need to be determined whether chronic use of this A_{2A} agonist would provide a beneficial anti-inflammatory effect in the lung without eliciting cardiovascular side-effects.

CVT-6883

CVT-6883 is an antagonist to the A_{2B} receptors. In an allergic mouse model, CVT-6883 (1 mg/kg, i.p.) inhibited AMP-induced airway hyperreactivity [75]. In the ADA-deficient mouse model, CVT-6883 attenuated pulmonary inflammation, fibrosis, airway enlargement, production of cytokines and chemokines in the lung tissues [76]. CVT-6883 is currently being developed as an oral treatment for asthma.

OTHER APPROACHES AND CHALLENGES

NON-SELECTIVE ADENOSINE LIGANDS

Several compounds that have multiple mechanisms of action have been described in the literature [77, 78]. Among these, CGH2466 has combined activities for multiple targets of asthma. CGH2466 is not only an antagonist for A_1, A_{2B} and A_3 adenosine receptors but also an inhibitor of the p38 mitogen-activated protein (MAP) kinase α and β and PDE4D isoenzyme [78]. In human neutrophils and monocytes, CGH2466 is a more potent anti-inflammatory compound than selective inhibitors of MAP kinase or PDE4, or non-selective adenosine antagonist alone. In two mouse models of lung inflammation, CGH2466 (administered intranasally or orally) inhibited the allergen-induced increase in eosinophils and LPS-induced increases in neutrophils. Thus, CGH2466 is a powerful anti-inflammatory agent due to the multiple mechanisms of action. However, it is possible that CGH2466 would be more likely to have side-effects due to its effects on multiple targets.

CURRENT CHALLENGES IN THE DEVELOPMENT OF THERAPEUTIC AGENTS TARGETING ADENOSINE RECEPTORS

One of the most formidable challenges is the lack of animal models that mimic the clinical features of asthma and predict the therapeutic efficacy in human. The endpoints measured in animal models are often different from those in the clinical studies. While monitoring the changes in lung physiology in humans is a routine test in clinics, measuring bronchoconstriction in animal models is neither easy nor routinely done. On the other hand, while invasive procedures such as BAL collection and histological examination of the lung to monitor pulmonary inflammation and remodelling are routinely performed in animal models, these procedures could not easily be carried out in large-scale clinical studies. Thus, it remains challenging to translate pre-clinical results into the clinical setting.

Given that adenosine receptors are widely distributed in different organs, another critical challenge is to develop agonists or antagonists to adenosine receptors that are devoid of side-effects due to the possible actions of adenosine receptors in other organ systems. Disturbances in cardiac and renal functions, in metabolic homeostasis and in activities of the central nervous system may be potential problems especially for systemically-delivered agents targeting A_1 and A_{2A} receptors.

SUMMARY

It has been 20 years since the first demonstration that adenosine is a bronchoconstrictor in asthmatics [5]. Since then, a large body of literature supports the hypothesis that adenosine plays an important role in airway hyperresponsiveness. In addition, BHR to adenosine has been shown to correlate well with the inflammatory status of the lungs of asthmatic patients. While adenosine has been convincingly shown to be implicated in the inflammatory and remodelling processes of the lungs in numerous animal models, the exact role of adenosine in the inflammatory processes of asthmatic patients is yet to be clearly defined. Due to the multiple and sometimes opposing functions of adenosine receptor subtypes, selective antagonists for the A_1, A_{2B}, A_3 receptors as well as A_{2A} agonist have been proposed to inhibit bronchial hyperresponsiveness and/or airway inflammation. A number of compounds targeting adenosine receptors have been in pre-clinical and clinical development in recent years. We eagerly await proof of the efficacy of these compounds in clinical asthma and other pulmonary diseases.

REFERENCES

1. Spicuzza L, Bonfiglio C, Polosa R. Research applications and implications of adenosine in diseased airways. *Trends Pharmacol Sci* 2003; 24:409–413.
2. Rorke S, Holgate ST. Targeting adenosine receptors: novel therapeutic targets in asthma and chronic obstructive pulmonary disease. *Am J Respir Med* 2002; 1:99–105.
3. Driver AG, Kukoly CA, Ali S, Mustafa SJ. Adenosine in bronchoalveolar lavage fluid in asthma. *Am Rev Respir Dis* 1993; 148:91–97.
4. Huszar E, Vass G, Vizi E *et al*. Adenosine in exhaled breath condensate in healthy volunteers and in patients with asthma. *Eur Respir J* 2002; 20:1393–1398.
5. Cushley MJ, Tattersfield AE, Holgate ST. Inhaled adenosine and guanosine on airway resistance in normal and asthmatic subjects. *Br J Clin Pharmacol* 1983; 15:161–165.
6. Rutgers SR, Kerstjens HA, Timens W, Tzanakis N, Kauffman HF, Postma DS. Airway inflammation and hyperresponsiveness to adenosine 5'-monophosphate in COPD. *Chest* 2000; 117:285S.
7. Blackburn MR, Volmer JB, Thrasher JL *et al*. Metabolic consequences of adenosine deaminase deficiency in mice are associated with defects in alveogenesis, pulmonary inflammation, and airway obstruction. *J Exp Med* 2000; 192:159–170.
8. Blackburn MR, Lee CG, Young HW *et al*. Adenosine mediates IL-13-induced inflammation and remodeling in the lung and interacts in an IL-13-adenosine amplification pathway. *J Clin Invest* 2003; 112:332–344.
9. Shryock JC, Belardinelli L. Adenosine and adenosine receptors in the cardiovascular system: biochemistry, physiology, and pharmacology. *Am J Cardiol* 1997; 79:2–10.
10. Mann JS, Holgate ST, Renwick AG, Cushley MJ. Airway effects of purine nucleosides and nucleotides and release with bronchial provocation in asthma. *J Appl Physiol* 1986; 61:1667–1676.
11. Csoma Z, Huszar E, Vizi E *et al*. Adenosine level in exhaled breath increases during exercise-induced bronchoconstriction. *Eur Respir J* 2005; 25:873–878.
12. Polosa R, Ng WH, Crimi N *et al*. Release of mast-cell-derived mediators after endobronchial adenosine challenge in asthma. *Am J Respir Crit Care Med* 1995; 151:624–629.
13. Tilley SL, Tsai M, Williams CM *et al*. Identification of A3 receptor- and mast cell-dependent and -independent components of adenosine-mediated airway responsiveness in mice. *J Immunol* 2003; 171:331–337.
14. Spicuzza L, Polosa R. The role of adenosine as a novel bronchoprovocant in asthma. *Curr Opin Allergy Clin Immunol* 2003; 3:65–69.
15. van den Berge M, Kerstjens HA, Postma DS. Provocation with adenosine 5'-monophosphate as a marker of inflammation in asthma, allergic rhinitis and chronic obstructive pulmonary disease. *Clin Exp Allergy* 2002; 32:824–830.
16. van den Berge M, Kerstjens HA, Meijer RJ *et al*. Corticosteroid-induced improvement in the PC20 of adenosine monophosphate is more closely associated with reduction in airway inflammation than improvement in the PC20 of methacholine. *Am J Respir Crit Care Med* 2001; 164:1127–1132.
17. Driver AG, Kukoly CA, Metzger WJ, Mustafa SJ. Bronchial challenge with adenosine causes the release of serum neutrophil chemotactic factor in asthma. *Am Rev Respir Dis* 1991; 143:1002–1007.
18. van den Berge M, Kerstjens HA, de Reus DM, Koeter GH, Kauffman HF, Postma DS. Provocation with adenosine 5'-monophosphate, but not methacholine, induces sputum eosinophilia. *Clin Exp Allergy* 2004; 34:71–76.

19. Prieto L, Bruno L, Gutierrez V *et al*. Airway responsiveness to adenosine 5'-monophosphate and exhaled nitric oxide measurements: predictive value as markers for reducing the dose of inhaled corticosteroids in asthmatic subjects. *Chest* 2003; 124:1325–1333.

20. Proietti L, Di Maria A, Polosa R. Monitoring the adjustment of antiasthma medications with adenosine monophosphate bronchoprovocation. *Chest* 2004; 126:1384–1385; author reply 1385.

21. Fredholm BB, Ijzerman AP, Jacobson KA, Klotz KN, Linden J. International Union of Pharmacology. XXV. Nomenclature and classification of adenosine receptors. *Pharmacol Rev* 2001, 53:527-552.

22. Dixon AK, Gubitz AK, Sirinathsinghji DJ, Richardson PJ, Freeman TC. Tissue distribution of adenosine receptor mRNAs in the rat. *Br J Pharmacol* 1996; 118:1461–1468.

23. Fozard JR, McCarthy C. Adenosine receptor ligands as potential therapeutics in asthma. *Curr Opin Investig Drugs* 2002; 3:69–77.

24. Feoktistov I, Ryzhov S, Zhong H *et al*. Hypoxia modulates adenosine receptors in human endothelial and smooth muscle cells toward an A2B angiogenic phenotype. *Hypertension* 2004; 44:649–654.

25. Khoa ND, Montesinos MC, Reiss AB, Delano D, Awadallah N, Cronstein BN. Inflammatory cytokines regulate function and expression of adenosine A(2A) receptors in human monocytic THP-1 cells. *J Immunol* 2001; 167:4026–4032.

26. Nguyen DK, Montesinos MC, Williams AJ, Kelly M, Cronstein BN. Th1 cytokines regulate adenosine receptors and their downstream signaling elements in human microvascular endothelial cells. *J Immunol* 2003; 171:3991–3998.

27. Srinivas M, Shryock JC, Dennis DM, Baker SP, Belardinelli L. Differential A1 adenosine receptor reserve for two actions of adenosine on guinea pig atrial myocytes. *Mol Pharmacol* 1997; 52:683–691.

28. Shryock JC, Snowdy S, Baraldi PG *et al*. A2A-adenosine receptor reserve for coronary vasodilation. *Circulation* 1998; 98:711–718.

29. Liang HX, Belardinelli L, Ozeck MJ, Shryock JC. Tonic activity of the rat adipocyte A1-adenosine receptor. *Br J Pharmacol* 2002; 135:1457–1466.

30. Busse WW, Lemanske RF Jr. Asthma. *N Engl J Med* 2001; 344:350–362.

31. Barnes PJ. Chronic obstructive pulmonary disease. *N Engl J Med* 2000; 343:269–280.

32. Barnes PJ. Mechanisms in COPD: differences from asthma. *Chest* 2000; 117:10S–14S.

33. Ali S, Mustafa SJ, Metzger WJ. Adenosine receptor-mediated bronchoconstriction and bronchial hyperresponsiveness in allergic rabbit model. *Am J Physiol* 1994; 266:L271–L277.

34. Ali S, Mustafa SJ, Metzger WJ. Adenosine-induced bronchoconstriction and contraction of airway smooth muscle from allergic rabbits with late-phase airway obstruction: evidence for an inducible adenosine A1 receptor. *J Pharmacol Exp Ther* 1994; 268:1328–1334.

35. Nyce JW, Metzger WJ. DNA antisense therapy for asthma in an animal model. *Nature* 1997; 385:721–725.

36. Obiefuna PC, Batra VK, Nadeem A, Borron P, Wilson CN, Mustafa SJ. A novel A1 adenosine receptor antagonist, L-97-1 [3-[2-(4-aminophenyl)-ethyl]-8-benzyl-7-{2-ethyl-(2-hydroxy-ethyl)-amino]-ethyl}-1-propyl-3,7-dihydro-purine-2,6-dione], reduces allergic responses to house dust mite in an allergic rabbit model of asthma. *J Pharmacol Exp Ther* 2005; 315:329–336.

37. Fozard JR, Hannon JP. Species differences in adenosine receptor-mediated bronchoconstrictor responses. *Clin Exp Allergy* 2000; 30:1213–1220.

38. Cronstein BN, Daguma L, Nichols D, Hutchison AJ, Williams M. The adenosine/neutrophil paradox resolved: human neutrophils possess both A1 and A2 receptors that promote chemotaxis and inhibit O2 generation, respectively. *J Clin Invest* 1990; 85:1150–1157.

39. Cronstein BN, Levin RI, Philips M, Hirschhorn R, Abramson SB, Weissmann G. Neutrophil adherence to endothelium is enhanced via adenosine A1 receptors and inhibited via adenosine A2 receptors. *J Immunol* 1992; 148:2201–2206.

40. Sun CX, Young HW, Molina JG, Volmer JB, Schnermann J, Blackburn MR. A protective role for the A1 adenosine receptor in adenosine-dependent pulmonary injury. *J Clin Invest* 2005; 115:35–43.

41. Sullivan GW. Adenosine A2A receptor agonists as anti-inflammatory agents. *Curr Opin Investig Drugs* 2003; 4:1313–1319.

42. Sitkovsky MV, Lukashev D, Apasov S *et al*. Physiological control of immune response and inflammatory tissue damage by hypoxia-inducible factors and adenosine A2A receptors. *Annu Rev Immunol* 2004; 22:657–682.

43. Pinhal-Enfield G, Ramanathan M, Hasko G *et al*. An angiogenic switch in macrophages involving synergy between Toll-like receptors 2, 4, 7, and 9 and adenosine A(2A) receptors. *Am J Pathol* 2003; 163:711–721.

44. Zhang JG, Hepburn L, Cruz G, Borman RA, Clark KL. The role of adenosine A2A and A2B receptors in the regulation of TNF-alpha production by human monocytes. *Biochem Pharmacol* 2005; 69:883–889.

45. Huang S, Apasov S, Koshiba M, Sitkovsky M. Role of A2a extracellular adenosine receptor-mediated signaling in adenosine-mediated inhibition of T-cell activation and expansion. *Blood* 1997; 90:1600–1610.

46. Ohta A, Sitkovsky M. Role of G-protein-coupled adenosine receptors in downregulation of inflammation and protection from tissue damage. *Nature* 2001; 414:916–920.

47. Lukashev D, Ohta A, Apasov S, Chen JF, Sitkovsky M. Cutting edge: physiologic attenuation of proinflammatory transcription by the Gs protein-coupled A2A adenosine receptor in vivo. *J Immunol* 2004; 173:21–24.

48. Fozard JR, Ellis KM, Villela Dantas MF, Tigani B, Mazzoni L. Effects of CGS 21680, a selective adenosine A2A receptor agonist, on allergic airways inflammation in the rat. *Eur J Pharmacol* 2002; 438:183–188.

49. Feoktistov I, Biaggioni I. Adenosine A2b receptors evoke interleukin-8 secretion in human mast cells. An enprofylline-sensitive mechanism with implications for asthma. *J Clin Invest* 1995; 96:1979–1986.

50. Feoktistov I, Polosa R, Holgate ST, Biaggioni I. Adenosine A2B receptors: a novel therapeutic target in asthma? *Trends Pharmacol Sci* 1998; 19:148–153.

51. Feoktistov I, Biaggioni I. Pharmacological characterization of adenosine A2B receptors: studies in human mast cells co-expressing A2A and A2B adenosine receptor subtypes. *Biochem Pharmacol* 1998; 55:627–633.

52. Feoktistov I, Ryzhov S, Goldstein AE, Biaggioni I. Mast cell-mediated stimulation of angiogenesis: cooperative interaction between A2B and A3 adenosine receptors. *Circ Res* 2003; 92:485–492.

53. Ryzhov S, Goldstein AE, Matafonov A, Zeng D, Biaggioni I, Feoktistov I. Adenosine-activated mast cells induce IgE synthesis by B lymphocytes: an A2B-mediated process involving Th2 cytokines IL-4 and IL-13 with implications for asthma. *J Immunol* 2004; 172:7726–7733.

54. Grant MB, Tarnuzzer RW, Caballero S *et al*. Adenosine receptor activation induces vascular endothelial growth factor in human retinal endothelial cells. *Circ Res* 1999; 85:699–706.

55. Grant MB, Davis MI, Caballero S, Feoktistov I, Biaggioni I, Belardinelli L. Proliferation, migration, and ERK activation in human retinal endothelial cells through A(2B) adenosine receptor stimulation. *Invest Ophthalmol Vis Sci* 2001; 42:2068–2073.

56. Zhong H, Belardinelli L, Maa T, Feoktistov I, Biaggioni I, Zeng D. A(2B) adenosine receptors increase cytokine release by bronchial smooth muscle cells. *Am J Respir Cell Mol Biol* 2004; 30:118–125.

57. Mundell SJ, Olah ME, Panettieri RA, Benovic JL, Penn RB. Regulation of G protein-coupled receptor-adenylyl cyclase responsiveness in human airway smooth muscle by exogenous and autocrine adenosine. *Am J Respir Cell Mol Biol* 2001; 24:155–163.

58. Zhong H, Belardinelli L, Maa T, Zeng D. Synergy between A2B adenosine receptors and hypoxia in activating human lung fibroblasts. *Am J Respir Cell Mol Biol* 2005; 32:2–8.

59. Linden J. Cloned adenosine A3 receptors: pharmacological properties, species differences and receptor functions. *Trends Pharmacol Sci* 1994; 15:298–306.

60. Ramkumar V, Stiles GL, Beaven MA, Ali H. The A3 adenosine receptor is the unique adenosine receptor which facilitates release of allergic mediators in mast cells. *J Biol Chem* 1993; 268:16887–16890.

61. Thorne JR, Danahay H, Broadley KJ. Analysis of the bronchoconstrictor responses to adenosine receptor agonists in sensitized guinea-pig lungs and trachea. *Eur J Pharmacol* 1996; 316:263–271.

62. Fozard JR, Pfannkuche HJ, Schuurman HJ. Mast cell degranulation following adenosine A3 receptor activation in rats. *Eur J Pharmacol* 1996; 298:293–297.

63. Salvatore CA, Tilley SL, Latour AM, Fletcher DS, Koller BH, Jacobson MA. Disruption of the A(3) adenosine receptor gene in mice and its effect on stimulated inflammatory cells. *J Biol Chem* 2000; 275:4429–4434.

64. Tilley SL, Wagoner VA, Salvatore CA, Jacobson MA, Koller BH. Adenosine and inosine increase cutaneous vasopermeability by activating A(3) receptors on mast cells. *J Clin Invest* 2000; 105:361–367.

65. Zhong H, Shlykov SG, Molina JG *et al*. Activation of murine lung mast cells by the adenosine A3 receptor. *J Immunol* 2003; 171:338–345.

66. Young HW, Molina JG, Dimina D *et al*. A3 adenosine receptor signaling contributes to airway inflammation and mucus production in adenosine deaminase-deficient mice. *J Immunol* 2004; 173:1380–1389.

67. Walker BA, Jacobson MA, Knight DA *et al*. Adenosine A3 receptor expression and function in eosinophils. *Am J Respir Cell Mol Biol* 1997; 16:531–537.

68. Kohno Y, Ji X, Mawhorter SD, Koshiba M, Jacobson KA. Activation of A3 adenosine receptors on human eosinophils elevates intracellular calcium. *Blood* 1996; 88:3569–3574.
69. Knight D, Zheng X, Rocchini C, Jacobson M, Bai T, Walker B. Adenosine A3 receptor stimulation inhibits migration of human eosinophils. *J Leukoc Biol* 1997; 62:465–468.
70. Ezeamuzie CI, Philips E. Adenosine A3 receptors on human eosinophils mediate inhibition of degranulation and superoxide anion release. *Br J Pharmacol* 1999; 127:188–194.
71. Langley SJ, Allen DJ, Houghton C, Woodcock A. Efficacy of EPI-2010 (an inhaled respirable anti sense oligonucleotide: RASON) in moderate/severe persistent asthma. *Proc Am Thorac Soc* 2005.
72. Luijk B, Cass L, Lammers J-W. The adenosine A2A-Receptor is not involved in adenosine induced bronchoconstriction in asthmatics. *Eur Respir J* 2003; 22(suppl 45):P718.
73. Luijk B, Bruijnzeel P, Tan EF, Ward JK, Lammers J-WJ. The effects of the adenosine A2a agonist UK-432,097 on lung function and AMP airway hyperresponsiveness in mild asthmatic patients. *Proc Am Thorac Soc* 2005; 2(suppl):A512.
74. Trevethick MA, Salmon G, Banner K *et al*. UK-432,097 a novel adenosine A2a receptor agonist: comparison of in vitro anti-inflammatory properties with the phosphodiesterase 4 (PDE4) inhibitor, Ariflo. *Proc Am Thorac Soc* 2005; 2(suppl):A73.
75. Fan M, Zeng D, Belardinelli L, Mustafa SJ. A2B adenosine receptor antagonist and montelukast prevent AMP-induced bronchoconstriction in an allergic mouse model. *Proc Am Thorac Soc* 2005; 2(suppl):A784.
76. Sun C, Zhong H, Molina JG, Belardinelli L, Zeng D, Blackburn MR. A2B adenosine receptor antagonist attenuates pulmonary inflammation and injury in adenosine deaminase deficient mice. *Proc Am Thorac Soc* 2005; 2(suppl):A96.
77. Press NJ, Taylor RJ, Fullerton JD *et al*. A new orally bioavailable dual adenosine A2B/A3 receptor antagonist with therapeutic potential. *Bioorg Med Chem Lett* 2005; 15:3081–3085.
78. Trifilieff A, Keller TH, Press NJ *et al*. CGH2466, a combined adenosine receptor antagonist, p38 mitogen-activated protein kinase and phosphodiesterase type 4 inhibitor with potent in vitro and in vivo anti-inflammatory activities. *Br J Pharmacol* 2005; 144:1002–1010.

2

The role of transforming growth factor βs in asthma and their potential as a target for therapy

R. J. McAnulty

INTRODUCTION

Asthma is a chronic disease of the airways that affects approximately 10% of individuals in the western world [1–3]. Symptoms are well-controlled in the majority of asthmatics, primarily by the use of inhaled β_2 adrenergic agonists and glucocorticoids to relieve bronchoconstriction and control the underlying chronic inflammation, respectively. However, approximately 10% of all asthmatics have severe disease which is refractory to current therapies [3]. In the UK and USA alone, this subgroup consists of approximately 2.5 million individuals [3, 4]. Furthermore, currently used therapeutic agents target the symptoms of asthma and not the underlying pathology. There is therefore a significant unmet clinical need for improved symptomatic and disease-modifying treatments for asthma.

The pathophysiological features of asthma include airways hyperresponsiveness, eosinophilic inflammation, together with structural remodelling of the airways. This includes epithelial disruption, mucous cell hyperplasia and mucus production. Within the airway wall there is increased smooth muscle mass and subepithelial deposition of extracellular matrix (ECM) proteins, which correlate with airway hyperresponsiveness, reduced lung function and an increase in fibroblast/myofibroblast numbers. The mechanisms involved in the development of airway remodelling are incompletely understood, but are thought to involve one or more isoforms of transforming growth factor β (TGFβ).

The TGFβs are pleiotropic mediators which have important roles in development, immunoregulation, cell growth and differentiation, cell migration and ECM metabolism. There are three mammalian isoforms of TGFβ, $TGF\beta_{1-3}$, all of which are present in the airways. They are synthesized by many cells in the normal or asthmatic airway including, epithelial cells, macrophages, eosinophils, lymphocytes, mast cells, endothelial cells, smooth muscle cells and fibroblasts. $TGF\beta_1$ and $-\beta_2$ have thus far been shown to be increased in asthmatic airways and cells, together with evidence of increased TGFβ signalling. Effects of TGFβ including epithelial disruption, recruitment of inflammatory cells and induction of ECM deposition likely contribute to asthma pathophysiology and evidence from animal models suggests that airway remodelling may be prevented or reversed using agents which target TGFβ. Therefore, modulation of TGFβs or their activity represent a potential therapeutic target for asthma.

Robin J. McAnulty, PhD, Reader in Lung Pathobiology, Head of Lung Pathobiology Group, Centre for Respiratory Research, University College London, London, UK

This chapter provides an extensive review of the current knowledge of TGFβ$_{1-3}$, their role in normal and asthmatic airways, as well as the potential for modulating the TGFβs and their effects as a therapeutic approach to asthma.

TGFβ: SYNTHESIS TO INTRACELLULAR SIGNALLING

The section provides a brief overview of the synthesis and regulation of TGFβ necessary for an understanding of the role and potential modes of modulation of TGFβ in asthma (for a recent full review see [5]).

SYNTHESIS AND SECRETION OF LATENT INACTIVE TGFβ

TGFβ mRNAs, transcribed from genes located on separate chromosomes [6–9], are translated into precursor proteins of 390–412 amino acids which form disulphide bonded dimers that are cleaved by a furin-like endopeptidase to generate the mature C-terminal 112 amino acid peptides and N-terminal latency associated peptides (LAP). The mature peptide and LAP form an inactive small latent complex through non-covalent interactions [10] (Figure 2.1). The N-terminal LAP of the small latent complex may bind to one of four latent TGFβ binding proteins (LTBP-1–4) to form a large latent complex (LLC), which facilitates secretion from the cell and targets the complex to the ECM through transglutaminase mediated crosslinking [11, 12]. The mature peptides of TGFβ$_{1-3}$ are highly conserved with 71–76% amino acid sequence homology between isoforms [8, 9]. However, the genes for each isoform possess distinct 5′ and 3′ untranslated regions [13–15] which may contribute to differential isoform expression patterns.

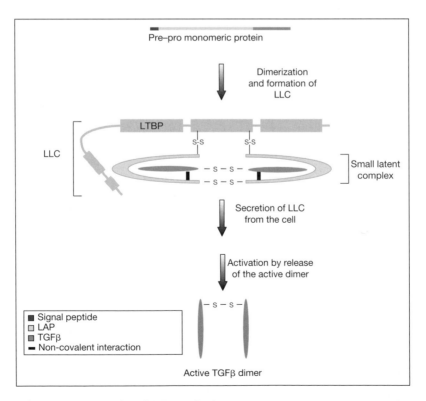

Figure 2.1   Schematic representation of TGFβ production.

TGFβ ACTIVATION

The potent and diverse actions of TGFβ isoforms in development, homeostatic regulation and response to injury necessitate tight regulation of their activity. Thus activation, through the release of mature 25 kDa TGFβ dimers from their non-covalent interactions with LAP, forms a major regulatory mechanism of TGFβ function. There are several diverse mechanisms which provide site- and isoform specific activation of TGFβ. In addition, sequence differences between the LAPs of each isoform [13–15] may provide further specificity in binding and activation. Mechanisms of release and/or activation include proteolysis, thrombospondin and integrin-mediated mechanisms, generation of reactive oxygen species and acidic microenvironments.

Proteases capable of releasing and/or activating TGFβ include plasmin, mast cell chymase and leucocyte elastase [16, 17], which are often present at sites of inflammation, including the asthmatic airway. Enzymatic release of small latent TGFβ from LTBP exposes a mannose 6-phosphate binding site on the small latent complex [18, 19], targeting it to the cell membrane where enzymes or other cell-specific processes can release active TGFβ from LAP [20, 21].

Glycosidases such as sialidase and neuraminidase cause stress in carbohydrate structures allowing non-covalent bonds between LAP and the mature peptide to be broken [22]. Sialidases are present on many cell surfaces including activated T cells, monocytes and viruses (neuraminidase) and have been shown to activate TGFβ [23, 24]. Thus sialidases could activate TGFβ in asthmatic airways where there is chronic inflammation and during exacerbations related to viral infection.

Thrombospondin-1 (TSP-1) activates TGFβ *via* interaction with the LAP [25, 26]. It is produced by many cell types and is also present in the α-granules of platelets together with TGFβ [27]. A major *in vivo* role for TSP-1 mediated TGFβ$_1$ activation in several tissues, including the bronchial epithelium, has been inferred from TSP-1 knockout mice [28]. Additionally, antisense oligonucleotides to TSP-1 inhibit TSP-1 synthesis with a subsequent reduction in TGFβ activation, and cell signalling [29]. Although less well-characterized, thrombospondin-2 is an equally potent activator of latent TGFβ [30].

Binding of latent TGFβ to epithelial cell restricted integrins, αvβ$_6$/αvβ$_8$, represents a major pathway of TGFβ$_1$ and -β$_3$ activation by epithelial cells [31–33], but not for TGFβ$_2$ as this isoform lacks the necessary RGD integrin binding motif. αvβ$_6$ is upregulated by injury and inflammation and mice deficient in the β$_6$ subunit are protected from lung fibrosis [31].

Additionally, reactive oxygen species are capable of generating active TGFβ from the LLC [34], a mechanism that may be physiologically relevant since oxidative stress is associated with a range of inflammatory diseases including asthma.

Further investigation is required to determine the major mechanism(s) of TGFβ activation in asthmatic airways. *In vivo* evidence supports a major role for TGFβ$_1$ activation by TSP-1 and by integrin interactions in the lung but enzymes including plasmin, mast cell chymase, neutrophil elastase, thrombin and glycosidases, as well as reactive oxygen species present in the asthmatic airway, are also good candidates.

TGFβ LIGAND RECEPTOR INTERACTION

Active TGFβs bind a number of cell surface serine threonine kinase signalling receptors [35]. There are two types of signalling receptor, type I receptors are distinguished from type II receptors by the presence of a glycine-serine (GS) rich juxtamembrane domain which is critical for their transactivation by type II receptors [36, 37]. Type I TGFβ receptors are members of the ALK receptor family. TGFβs interact predominantly with the ALK5 (TβRI) receptor but also bind ALK1 and 2 [38, 39]. One TGFβ type II receptor has been identified (TβRII) which binds TGFβ$_1$ and -β$_3$ with high affinity but only binds TGFβ$_2$ with low affinity [40]. Signalling is regulated by several other transmembrane proteins. Betaglycan, also called the TGFβ type III receptor (TβRIII) binds TGFβ$_1$ and -β$_2$ [41], whilst endoglin binds TGFβ$_1$ and -β$_3$ [42]. These are thought to be primarily involved in the presentation of ligand to TβRII but, in addition, the cytoplasmic tails of TβRII and TβRIII interact to enhance signalling, and in the case of TGFβ$_2$ this overcomes the low affinity binding to TβRII [43].

Active TGFβs bind other soluble, cell membrane and matrix associated proteins including soluble forms of betaglycan and endoglin, fibronectin, collagen IV, fibromodulin, decorin, and biglycan [44–48] which generally inhibit their activity or provide reservoirs of growth factor. Non-metastatic gene A protein, present on the cell membrane, has sequence similarity to type I receptors and acts as a pseudo or decoy receptor [49, 50].

The range of ligand–receptor interactions and differences in affinity for the three TGFβ isoforms provide potential explanations for the different responses observed in different cell types, as well as the existence of distinct and varying cellular responses within cell types.

INTRACELLULAR SIGNALLING

In order to signal, TGFβ binds the constitutively active TβRII, inducing a conformational change in the extracellular domain, which allows recruitment of type I receptors to form a tetrameric complex leading to serine phosphorylation of the type I receptor by TβRII (Figure 2.2). This results in a conformational change in the GS box, enabling ATP binding and phosphorylation of receptor R-Smads 2 and 3, followed by subsequent association of

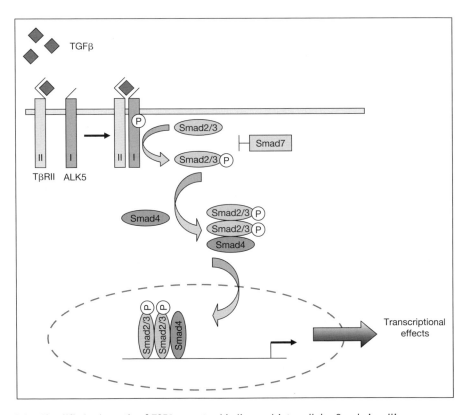

Figure 2.2 Simplified schematic of TGFβ receptor binding and intracellular Smad signalling.

R-Smads with the common co-Smad 4 to form a heterotrimeric complex which translocates to the nucleus and regulates transcriptional responses (for recent reviews see [51, 52]). Recruitment of alternative type I receptors (ALK1 and 2) to the complex lead to signalling through Smad1/5 and different functional outcomes. In addition, there is increasing evidence for alternative signalling pathways *via* MAPK, PI3 kinase, and protein kinase C (reviewed in [53]). One of the genes that TGFβ induces is the inhibitory Smad7 (I-Smad7), which competes with R-Smads for binding of type I receptors inhibiting signalling [54, 55].

Receptor internalization plays roles in signalling as well as turnover of receptors. Internalization of receptor/R-Smad/SARA complexes to endosomes containing the early endosomal protein, EEA1, has been shown to be necessary to propagate Smad phosphorylation [56–58] whereas Smad7–Smurf–receptor complex formation targets it for caveolin-dependent endocytosis, ubiquitination and degradation [58]. In addition, Smad7 can recruit GADD34 and the catalytic subunit of protein phosphatase I to the activated type I receptor leading to dephosphorylation and inactivation [59]. Furthermore, in the absence of TGFβ, receptors are constitutively internalized and recycled to the cell surface [60].

TGFβ ISOFORM EXPRESSION IN THE NORMAL AND ASTHMATIC AIRWAY

In the adult lung TGFβ$_1$ mRNA has been localized predominantly to the bronchial epithelium including Clara cells and macrophages but is also expressed in the vascular endothelium, smooth muscle and fibroblast-like cells of the airway wall [61–63]. TGFβ$_3$ expression is also predominantly associated with the bronchial epithelium and macrophages, but not endothelial or mesenchymal cells [61, 62]. TGFβ$_1$ immunostaining shows a similar cellular localization to that of mRNA [63–65] with the exception of fibroblasts [64]. In addition, immunostaining for TGFβ$_1$ has been localized to the subepithelial ECM [63–65]. There is little information on the localization of mRNA and protein for other isoforms in human airways. However, in mice, similar patterns of mRNA and protein expression have been observed [61, 66] and immunostaining for TGFβ$_2$ also appears to be predominantly associated with the bronchial epithelium of the large conducting airways [66].

In the asthmatic airway, immunohistochemical localization using TGFβ$_1$ or pan-specific antibodies show that TGFβ is increased and associated predominantly with submucosal and inflammatory cells, including fibroblasts, smooth muscle cells, eosinophils, macrophages and the ECM, with variable expression reported in epithelial cells [63–65, 67–71]. *In situ* hybridization shows a similar pattern of TGFβ$_1$ mRNA localization [63, 68, 72]. Increased TGFβ in asthmatic airways has been attributed to increases in the number of eosinophils [68, 71, 72] and macrophages [73]. Elevated levels of TGFβ$_1$ have been detected in asthmatic lavage fluid [74] and levels of TGFβ$_1$ and -β$_2$ increase following allergen challenge [74, 75]. Consistent with this, increased phosphorylated Smad2 immunoreactivity demonstrates increased TGFβ signalling [76]. In addition, a TGFβ$_1$ promoter polymorphism (C-509T), which associates functionally with increased plasma TGFβ$_1$ [77] and elevated immunoglobulin E (IgE) titre [78], correlates with asthma severity in some populations [79, 80]. Further studies are required to fully characterize the expression and localization of TGFβ isoforms in the normal and asthmatic airway.

ROLE OF TGFβ IN THE NORMAL AND ASTHMATIC AIRWAY

The TGFβs play critical roles in regulating inflammation, cell proliferation, differentiation and wound healing. Targeted deletion of individual isoforms has demonstrated distinct developmental roles for each isoform in the lung. TGFβ$_1$-deficient mice die within the first few weeks of life due to development of a progressive multifocal inflammation which is most severe in the lungs [81, 82]. Interestingly, TGFβ$_1$-null mice backcrossed onto a SCID background do not develop this inflammation and survive to adulthood, demonstrating that lack of TGFβ$_1$ causes death directly through lymphocyte-mediated inflammation [83]. TGFβ$_2$ knockout mice die perinatally with evidence of collapsed distal and dilated conducting airways [84] whereas TGFβ$_3$-deficient mice exhibit delayed pulmonary development with alveolar hypoplasia, loss of alveolar septal formation, mesenchymal thickening and hypercellularity, together with haemorrhage associated with fragile capillaries and veins and die within 24h of birth [85, 86]. Thus, studies of knockout mice demonstrate that the three isoforms have distinct non-redundant roles in the developing lung, TGFβ$_1$ appearing to play particularly important roles in the regulation of inflammation, whilst TGFβ$_2$ and -β$_3$ play distinct roles in regulating epithelial–mesenchymal interactions. The roles of each isoform in normal and asthmatic growing and adult lung have not been fully characterized, however there is considerable evidence indicating that they play potentially critical roles in homeostasis and asthma pathogenesis.

EPITHELIUM

The bronchial epithelium is the first line of defence against inhaled environmental agents and pathogens. Bronchial epithelial cells are capable of synthesizing all three TGFβ isoforms [63, 69, 71, 74, 87] and are considered to be a major source of TGFβ in the asthmatic airway, with TGFβ$_2$ possibly being the most abundant [87]. Altered compartmentalization and staining intensity in asthmatic airways [67] indicate changes in TGFβ expression and secretion by these cells. The primacy of TGFβ$_2$ is supported by *in vitro* studies demonstrating that human bronchial epithelial cells (HBEC) predominantly release TGFβ$_2$ [88]. Stimulation of HBECs with IL-4 or IL-13 [89, 90] or by mechanical stress/injury [88, 91–93] induces release of TGFβ$_2$ but not TGFβ$_1$ or -β$_3$. However, another major role of epithelial cells in relation to TGFβ is their ability to bind and activate TGFβ$_1$ and -β$_3$ through integrin-mediated mechanisms [31–33]. Thus, although TGFβ$_2$ may be the main isoform released, production of TGFβ$_1$ and -β$_3$ with subsequent autocrine cell surface binding and activation may also be important responses of the epithelial cell. The *in vivo* effects of TGFβ isoforms on epithelial cells in asthma are poorly understood although *in vitro* effects include inhibition of proliferation, induction of epithelial motility, squamous differentiation, apoptosis, induction of epithelial–mesenchymal transition (EMT) and induction of mucin expression [87, 94–97]. Thus, TGFβ production by, and effects on, epithelial cells may contribute to many of the characteristic pathologic features of asthma including limited epithelial regeneration, disruption of the pseudostratified epithelial structure, mucus hypersecretion and increased numbers of subepithelial fibroblasts through EMT.

THE FIBROBLAST AND SUBEPITHELIAL FIBROSIS

Fibroblasts and myofibroblasts are capable of synthesizing [98] and responding to TGFβs. TGFβ is a chemoattractant for fibroblasts, modulates proliferation, induces fibroblast–myofibroblast differentiation and regulates the synthesis and degradation of numerous ECM proteins including collagens, proteoglycans, elastin, fibronectin, and tenascin (for a recent review see [5]). In asthmatics there is a 2–3-fold increase in the thickness of the region just below the basement membrane, called the *lamina reticularis*, due to increased deposition of ECM proteins [70, 99–108] and this is often referred to as subepithelial fibrosis. Thickening of the *lamina reticularis* correlates with increases in fibroblast/myofibroblast number [102, 105, 109], airway hyperresponsiveness [110, 111] and reduced lung function [68] suggesting that these cells and the excessive subepithelial deposition of ECM proteins play important roles in asthma pathogenesis. TGFβ is further implicated in this process as its expression also correlates with fibroblast/myofibroblast number, subepithelial thickening and severity of asthma [63, 68, 102].

Although the fibroblast is capable of synthesizing TGFβ, it does not appear to be a major producer. However, fibroblasts and myofibroblasts are often closely associated with TGFβ positive eosinophils in the thickened *lamina reticularis* and mounting evidence suggests that eosinophil-derived TGFβ plays an important role in modulating fibroblast function and airway remodelling. Measurement of procollagen type I C-terminal peptide, a marker of collagen synthesis, in induced sputum from asthmatics, correlates with numbers of TGFβ$_1$ positive eosinophils [112]. In addition, TGFβ$_1$ or -β$_2$ in combination with IL-13 can stimulate fibroblast eotaxin expression and biopsies from severe asthmatics contain greater numbers of eotaxin positive fibroblasts which promote eosinophil recruitment [113]. More importantly, treatment of asthmatics with anti-IL-5 reduced numbers of TGFβ$_1$ positive airway eosinophils and lavage TGFβ$_1$ levels with a concomitant reduction in tenascin, lumican and collagen type III expression in the *lamina reticularis* [114]. Thus, it is likely that increased numbers of fibroblasts in the lamina reticularis potentially derived from expansion of the normal airway fibroblast pool, EMT or from circulating bone marrow-derived fibrocytes, interacting with TGFβ derived from eosinophils and possibly epithelial cells and macrophages, produce excessive amounts of subepithelial ECM proteins leading to reduced lung function.

AIRWAY SMOOTH MUSCLE

In conjunction with the increased subepithelial deposition of ECM proteins, there is also a significant increase in smooth muscle mass in fatal asthma [115, 116] and to a lesser extent in non-fatal asthma [115, 117], due to hyperplasia and hypertrophy of airway smooth muscle cells (ASMC). Human ASMC can synthesize all three TGFβ isoforms and express TGFβ receptors [118]. In addition, bovine ASMC are capable of secreting plasmin at levels sufficient to activate the latent TGFβ they produce and induce autocrine collagen synthesis [119]. Apart from increasing ECM protein synthesis by ASMC, TGFβ also induces hypertrophy [120] and, depending on the presence and concentration of other mediators, stimulates or inhibits proliferation [120–123]. It may also induce eotaxin release [124] further contributing to eosinophil recruitment.

INFLAMMATORY CELLS

Another characteristic feature of asthma pathology is the presence of chronic airway inflammation. Many inflammatory cells are capable of producing and/or responding to TGFβ. Large numbers of T lymphocytes are found in the airway wall of asthmatics with and without provocation [125, 126]. TGFβ$_1$ induces T lymphocyte chemotaxis [127], modulates proliferation [128, 129] and enhances survival [130] by inhibiting apoptosis [128, 131]. In addition, TGFβ may also be involved in the generation of regulatory T cells (Treg) which express TGFβ$_1$ [132]. Several studies in animals suggest that TGFβ$_1$ expression by T helper (Th2) cells or their response to TGFβ$_1$ may be important in limiting allergen-induced airways reactivity and inflammation [133–136]. However, suppression of Th2 cells by DNA vaccines has been shown to reduce allergen-induced inflammation with a concomitant reduction in TGFβ$_1$ levels [137], suggesting that it may be more beneficial to prevent the influx of Th2 cells.

Macrophages represent approximately 80% of bronchoalveolar lavage (BAL) cells recovered from asthmatics and numbers increase following antigen challenge [138]. TGFβ is a chemoattractant for monocytes [127, 139, 140], from which macrophages are derived, and macrophages have also been identified as a major source of TGFβ$_1$ [73].

Eosinophils are characteristic of the Th2 response and eosinophilic inflammation is a prominent feature of asthma [141, 142]. As described above, they have been shown to be a major source of TGFβ$_1$ [68] and more recently TGFβ$_2$ [71], and appear to be important in eosinophil/fibroblast interactions inducing excess subepithelial deposition of ECM proteins [114].

Neutrophils are present in the lung tissue of asthmatics [143] and become more prominent in severe asthma and during the late allergic reaction [144–146]. TGFβ$_1$ is a chemoattractant for neutrophils and they have been shown to express mRNA for and release TGFβ$_1$ [143]. TGFβ$_1$ can also stimulate degranulation and H$_2$O$_2$ release [147]. TGFβ is chemotactic for mast cells [148, 149] which are prominent in the asthmatic airway [150]. TGFβ may also aid recruitment of inflammatory cells through its effects on endothelial permeability [151]. Thus TGFβ may be involved in the recruitment and activation of inflammatory cells in the asthmatic airway. This in turn leads to further production of TGFβ by several of these cells including eosinophils, macrophages and Treg cells thus potentially contributing to the vicious cycle of chronic inflammation and airway remodelling.

TGFβ AS A NOVEL THERAPEUTIC TARGET IN THE TREATMENT OF ASTHMA

The available evidence suggests that TGFβ plays potentially deleterious roles in many aspects of asthma pathophysiology (Figure 2.3). It appears to contribute to the recruitment and activation of inflammatory cells as well as maintenance of chronic inflammation. In addition, it is produced by structural cells of the airway, and in particular epithelial cells, potentially contributing to impaired repair of the epithelium, increased numbers of subepithelial fibroblast/myofibroblasts, excess deposition of ECM proteins and expansion of smooth muscle mass. Inhibition of TGFβ therefore represents a strong candidate for novel therapeutic strategies in asthma although TGFβ also has important roles in immunoregulation and wound healing which, if inhibited could have potentially adverse effects. However, most studies to date have not identified any major adverse effects of TGFβ inhibition in animals [152–154] or man [155, 156]. Furthermore, life-long exposure to soluble type II TGFβ receptor in animals did not induce any major inflammatory or histopathologic effects [153]. Together, these studies suggest there may be potential for long-term inhibition of TGFβ in the treatment of diseases such as asthma.

POTENTIAL APPROACHES TO THE MODULATION OF TGFβ

There are a number of potential approaches to regulate TGFβ including inhibition of its synthesis, activation, ligand–receptor interaction and intracellular signalling (for a recent review see [5]).

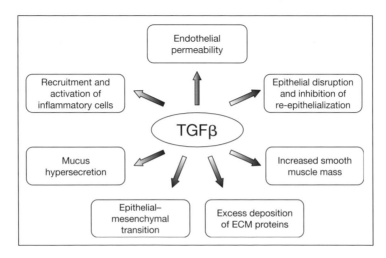

Figure 2.3   Potentially deleterious effects of TGFβ in asthma.

INHIBITION OF SYNTHESIS

Inhibition of TGFβ synthesis is appealing due to the potential for isoform selectivity. There are currently no reports utilizing this approach in asthma or animal models of asthma. However, antisense oligonucleotides which inhibit transcription and siRNA which inhibits translation of TGFβ$_1$ have been used in animal models to inhibit glomerulonephritis and diabetic renal hypertrophy [157–159]. Furthermore, this approach is being pursued as a target for the treatment of cancer. NovaRx has an antisense TGFβ$_2$ vaccine [160, 161], which has successfully completed phase I and II trials and is due to go into phase III trials for the treatment of non-small cell lung cancer. In addition, Antisense Pharma have two antisense oligonucleotides, AP-12009 against TGFβ$_2$ and AP-11014 against TGFβ$_1$, in phase I/II and pre-clinical development respectively, also for the treatment of cancers [162, 163]. The development of such compounds, if successful, could have potential for future applications in other settings including asthma.

INHIBITION OF ACTIVATION

A major means of regulating TGFβ physiologically is through its activation. A number of experimental approaches have been found to effectively inhibit TGFβ activation including inhibition of thrombospondin synthesis [29] or thrombospondin-induced activation [164], inhibition of plasmin [165] and peptide inhibitors derived from LAP [166]. However, as far as I am aware, none of these approaches are being developed for use in man.

INHIBITION OF LIGAND–RECEPTOR INTERACTION

The majority of approaches to inhibit TGFβ have been targeted towards disruption of ligand–receptor interactions. These include TGFβ isoform selective and pan-specific neutralizing antibodies, small molecule receptor antagonists, antisense gene transfer and siRNA against the receptors, dominant negative receptor expression [167], soluble receptors [168, 169], upregulation or administration of natural inhibitors such as decorin [170, 171], LAP [172] and betaglycan or peptides derived from natural inhibitors [173]. Of these approaches, TGFβ antibodies and receptor antagonists are currently in various stages of pre-clinical and clinical development.

It has been known for some time that neutralizing antibodies to various TGFβ isoforms can inhibit fibrotic responses in animals [174, 175]. More recently, it has been shown that pan-specific TGFβ antibodies reduce peribronchial ECM deposition following ovalbumin sensitization and challenge without inducing any adverse effects on airway inflammation or hyperreactivity [176]. In addition, antibodies to TGFβ$_1$ have been shown to promote re-epithelialization in injured corneal organ cultures [177]. Human monoclonal antibodies to TGFβ$_1$ (CAT-192, Metelimumab) TGFβ$_2$ (CAT-152, Lerdelimumab) and TGFβ$_{1–3}$ (GC-1008) have been developed jointly by Cambridge Antibody Technology and Genzyme. CAT-152 and CAT-192 have both been found to be generally safe and well-tolerated in phase I/II trials [155, 156] and GC-1008 is undergoing phase I trials in idiopathic pulmonary fibrosis. In addition, preliminary reports from our laboratory suggest that CAT-192 and CAT-152 inhibit ovalbumin-induced subepithelial deposition of collagens in mice but only CAT-192 prevented the increased deposition of decorin [178, 179]. This suggests there may be TGFβ isoform specific regulation of different ECM proteins in the airway wall and that further investigation of TGFβ isoform selective inhibition for the potential treatment of asthma is warranted.

Another area where there is pharmaceutical interest is in the development of small molecule inhibitors of the ALK5, TβRI kinase. These include SB431542, SB505124, SB525334, GW6604, GW788388 and SD208 [180–185], of which SD208 has been shown to inhibit lung fibrosis induced by overexpression of TGFβ$_1$ [180]. GW6604, GW788388 and SB525334 have also been shown to reduce liver [184, 185] and renal [183] fibrosis, respectively.

However, there are currently no reports on the use of TGFβ receptor antagonists in models of asthma.

INHIBITION OF INTRACELLULAR SIGNALLING

TGFβ signals primarily through the ALK5 Smad2/3 pathway and Smad2/3 signalling is increased in asthma [76] and animal models of asthma [186], thus making it an attractive target for inhibition. Experimental approaches to inhibit Smad signalling have included use of siRNA against Smad3, dominant negative expression of Smad4 [187, 188] and upregulation of I-Smad7 [189–192]. TGFβ also interacts with the MAPK cascade and inhibitors of p38 MAPK are currently in phase I and II trials for various chronic inflammatory disorders. Inhibition of p38, p42/44, or JNK MAPKs reduce airway inflammation, Th2 cytokine release and hyperresponsiveness in ovalbumin-induced models of asthma [193–196]. However, the degree to which this reflects inhibition of TGFβ signalling is unknown. It is also unknown whether these inhibitors reduce airway remodelling, although p38 inhibitors are able to limit renal and lung fibrosis [197–199].

SUMMARY

TGFβ is a pleiotropic cytokine which is increased and plays potentially deleterious roles in many aspects of asthma pathophysiology. It appears to contribute to the recruitment and activation of inflammatory cells as well as the maintenance of chronic inflammation. It is also likely to contribute to impaired repair of the epithelium, increased numbers of fibroblast/myofibroblasts in the subepithelium, the excess deposition of ECM proteins and expansion of smooth muscle mass. Inhibition of TGFβ therefore represents a strong target for novel therapeutic strategies in asthma. This is tempered by the possibility that inhibition of TGFβ may have potentially adverse effects on immunoregulation and wound healing, although evidence available to date suggest these concerns may be unfounded. Thus, further investigation of TGFβ inhibition as a potential novel treatment for asthma is warranted. The relatively large number of products currently in development for other conditions make this eminently feasible.

REFERENCES

1. Chung F, Barnes N, Allen M *et al*. Assessing the burden of respiratory disease in the UK. *Respir Med* 2002; 96:963–975.
2. NHLBI/WHO. Global Initiative for Asthma: Global Strategy for Asthma Management and Prevention. 2003; available at http://www.ginasthma.com.
3. Asthma UK. Living on a Knife Edge. 2004; available at http://www.asthma.org.uk/document.rm?id=98.
4. American Lung Association. Trends in Asthma Morbidity and Mortality. 2005; available at http://www.lungusa.org/site/pp.asp?c=dvLUK9O0E&b=33347.
5. Howell JE, McAnulty RJ. TGF-β: Its role in asthma and therapeutic potential. *Curr Drug Targets* 2006; 7:547–565.
6. Derynck R, Jarrett JA, Chen EY *et al*. Human transforming growth factor-β complementary DNA sequence and expression in normal and transformed cells. *Nature* 1985; 316:701–705.
7. de Martin R, Haendler B, Hofer-Warbinek R *et al*. Complementary DNA for human glioblastoma-derived T cell suppressor factor, a novel member of the transforming growth factor-β gene family. *EMBO J* 1987; 6:3673–3677.
8. Derynck R, Lindquist PB, Lee A *et al*. A new type of transforming growth factor-β, TGF-β 3. *EMBO J* 1988; 7:3737–3743.
9. Ten Dijke P, Geurts van Kessel AH, Foulkes JG, Le Beau MM. Transforming growth factor type β 3 maps to human chromosome 14, region q23-q24. *Oncogene* 1988; 3:721–724.
10. Wakefield LM, Smith DM, Flanders KC, Sporn MB. Latent transforming growth factor-β from human platelets. A high molecular weight complex containing precursor sequences. *J Biol Chem* 1988; 263:7646–7654.

11. Taipale J, Miyazono K, Heldin CH, Keski-Oja J. Latent transforming growth factor-β 1 associates to fibroblast extracellular matrix via latent TGF-β binding protein. *J Cell Biol* 1994; 124:171–181.

12. Nunes I, Gleizes PE, Metz CN, Rifkin DB. Latent transforming growth factor-β binding protein domains involved in activation and transglutaminase-dependent cross-linking of latent transforming growth factor-β. *J Cell Biol* 1997; 136:1151–1163.

13. Kim SJ, Glick A, Sporn MB, Roberts AB. Characterization of the promoter region of the human transforming growth factor β 1 gene. *J Biol Chem* 1989; 264:402–408.

14. Lafyatis R, Lechleider R, Kim SJ, Jakowlew S, Roberts AB, Sporn MB. Structural and functional characterization of the transforming growth factor β 3 promoter. A cAMP-responsive element regulates basal and induced transcription. *J Biol Chem* 1990; 265:19128–19136.

15. Noma T, Glick AB, Geiser AG *et al.* Molecular cloning and structure of the human transforming growth factor-β 2 gene promoter. *Growth Factors* 1991; 4:247–255.

16. Lyons RM, Keski-Oja J, Moses HL. Proteolytic activation of latent transforming growth factor-β from fibroblast-conditioned medium. *J Cell Biol* 1988; 106:1659–1665.

17. Taipale J, Koli K, Keski-Oja J. Release of transforming growth factor-β 1 from the pericellular matrix of cultured fibroblasts and fibrosarcoma cells by plasmin and thrombin. *J Biol Chem* 1992; 267:25378–25384.

18. Kovacina KS, Steele-Perkins G, Purchio AF *et al.* Interactions of recombinant and platelet transforming growth factor-β 1 precursor with the insulin-like growth factor II/mannose 6-phosphate receptor. *Biochem Biophys Res Commun* 1989; 160:393–403.

19. Gleizes PE, Munger JS, Nunes I *et al.* TGF-β latency: biological significance and mechanisms of activation. *Stem Cells* 1997; 15:190–197.

20. Ghahary A, Tredget EE, Shen Q, Kilani RT, Scott PG, Houle Y. Mannose-6-phosphate/IGF-II receptors mediate the effects of IGF-1-induced latent transforming growth factor β 1 on expression of type I collagen and collagenase in dermal fibroblasts. *Growth Factors* 2000; 17:167–176.

21. Yang L, Tredget EE, Ghahary A. Activation of latent transforming growth factor-β1 is induced by mannose 6-phosphate/insulin-like growth factor-II receptor. *Wound Repair Regen* 2000; 8:538–546.

22. Miyazono K, Heldin CH. Role for carbohydrate structures in TGF-β 1 latency. *Nature* 1989; 338:158–160.

23. Schultz-Cherry S, Hinshaw VS. Influenza virus neuraminidase activates latent transforming growth factor β. *J Virol* 1996; 70:8624–8629.

24. Oh S, McCaffery JM, Eichelberger MC. Dose-dependent changes in influenza virus-infected dendritic cells result in increased allogeneic T-cell proliferation at low, but not high, doses of virus. *J Virol* 2000; 74:5460–5469.

25. Schultz-Cherry S, Ribeiro S, Gentry L, Murphy-Ullrich JE. Thrombospondin binds and activates the small and large forms of latent transforming growth factor-β in a chemically defined system. *J Biol Chem* 1994; 269:26775–26782.

26. Ribeiro SM, Poczatek M, Schultz-Cherry S, Villain M, Murphy-Ullrich JE. The activation sequence of thrombospondin-1 interacts with the latency-associated peptide to regulate activation of latent transforming growth factor-β. *J Biol Chem* 1999; 274:13586–13593.

27. Adams JC. Thrombospondin-1. *Int J Biochem Cell Biol* 1997; 29:861–865.

28. Crawford SE, Stellmach V, Murphy-Ullrich JE *et al.* Thrombospondin-1 is a major activator of TGF-β1 in vivo. *Cell* 1998; 93:1159–1170.

29. Daniel C, Takabatake Y, Mizui M *et al.* Antisense oligonucleotides against thrombospondin-1 inhibit activation of TGF-β in fibrotic renal disease in the rat in vivo. *Am J Pathol* 2003; 163:1185–1192.

30. Souchelnitskiy S, Chambaz EM, Feige JJ. Thrombospondins selectively activate one of the two latent forms of transforming growth factor-β present in adrenocortical cell-conditioned medium. *Endocrinology* 1995; 136:5118–5126.

31. Munger JS, Huang X, Kawakatsu H *et al.* The integrin α v β 6 binds and activates latent TGF β 1: a mechanism for regulating pulmonary inflammation and fibrosis. *Cell* 1999; 96:319–328.

32. Annes JP, Rifkin DB, Munger JS. The integrin αVβ6 binds and activates latent TGFβ3. *FEBS Lett* 2002; 511:65–68.

33. Fjellbirkeland L, Cambier S, Broaddus VC *et al.* Integrin αvβ8-mediated activation of transforming growth factor-β inhibits human airway epithelial proliferation in intact bronchial tissue. *Am J Pathol* 2003; 163:533–542.

34. Barcellos-Hoff MH, Dix TA. Redox-mediated activation of latent transforming growth factor-β 1. *Mol Endocrinol* 1996; 10:1077–1083.

35. de Caestecker M. The transforming growth factor-β superfamily of receptors. *Cytokine Growth Factor Rev* 2004; 15:1–11.

36. Wrana JL, Attisano L, Wieser R, Ventura F, Massague J. Mechanism of activation of the TGF-β receptor. *Nature* 1994; 370:341–347.
37. Huse M, Muir TW, Xu L, Chen YG, Kuriyan J, Massague J. The TGF β receptor activation process: an inhibitor- to substrate-binding switch. *Mol Cell* 2001; 8:671–682.
38. Oh SP, Seki T, Goss KA *et al.* Activin receptor-like kinase 1 modulates transforming growth factor-β 1 signaling in the regulation of angiogenesis. *Proc Natl Acad Sci USA* 2000; 97:2626–2631.
39. Goumans MJ, Valdimarsdottir G, Itoh S, Rosendahl A, Sideras P, Ten Dijke P. Balancing the activation state of the endothelium via two distinct TGF-β type I receptors. *EMBO J* 2002; 21:1743–1753.
40. Qian SW, Burmester JK, Tsang ML *et al.* Binding affinity of transforming growth factor-β for its type II receptor is determined by the C-terminal region of the molecule. *J Biol Chem* 1996; 271:30656–30662.
41. Andres JL, Ronnstrand L, Cheifetz S, Massague J. Purification of the transforming growth factor-β (TGF-β) binding proteoglycan βglycan. *J Biol Chem* 1991; 266:23282–23287.
42. Cheifetz S, Bellon T, Cales C *et al.* Endoglin is a component of the transforming growth factor-β receptor system in human endothelial cells. *J Biol Chem* 1992; 267:19027–19030.
43. Blobe GC, Schiemann WP, Pepin MC *et al.* Functional roles for the cytoplasmic domain of the type III transforming growth factor β receptor in regulating transforming growth factor β signaling. *J Biol Chem* 2001; 276:24627–24637.
44. Andres JL, Stanley K, Cheifetz S, Massague J. Membrane-anchored and soluble forms of βglycan, a polymorphic proteoglycan that binds transforming growth factor-β. *J Cell Biol* 1989; 109:3137–3145.
45. Venkatesha S, Toporsian M, Lam C *et al.* Soluble endoglin contributes to the pathogenesis of preeclampsia. *Nat Med* 2006; 12:642–649.
46. Hildebrand A, Romaris M, Rasmussen LM *et al.* Interaction of the small interstitial proteoglycans biglycan, decorin and fibromodulin with transforming growth factor β. *Biochem J* 1994; 302:527–534.
47. Mooradian DL, Lucas RC, Weatherbee JA, Furcht LT. Transforming growth factor-β 1 binds to immobilized fibronectin. *J Cell Biochem* 1989; 41:189–200.
48. Paralkar VM, Vukicevic S, Reddi AH. Transforming growth factor β type 1 binds to collagen IV of basement membrane matrix: implications for development. *Dev Biol* 1991; 143:303–308.
49. Tsang M, Kim R, de Caestecker MP, Kudoh T, Roberts AB, Dawid IB. Zebrafish nma is involved in TGFβ family signaling. *Genesis* 2000; 28:47–57.
50. Onichtchouk D, Chen YG, Dosch R *et al.* Silencing of TGF-β signalling by the pseudoreceptor BAMBI. *Nature* 1999; 401:480–485.
51. Shi Y, Massague J. Mechanisms of TGF-β signaling from cell membrane to the nucleus. *Cell* 2003; 113:685–700.
52. Ten Dijke P, Hill CS. New insights into TGF-β-Smad signalling. *Trends Biochem Sci* 2004; 29:265–273.
53. Derynck R, Zhang YE. Smad-dependent and Smad-independent pathways in TGF-β family signalling. *Nature* 2003; 425:577–584.
54. Hayashi H, Abdollah S, Qiu Y *et al.* The MAD-related protein Smad7 associates with the TGFβ receptor and functions as an antagonist of TGFβ signaling. *Cell* 1997; 89:1165–1173.
55. Nakao A, Afrakhte M, Moren A *et al.* Identification of Smad7, a TGFβ-inducible antagonist of TGF-β signalling. *Nature* 1997; 389:631–635.
56. Penheiter SG, Mitchell H, Garamszegi N, Edens M, Dore JJ Jr, Leof EB. Internalization-dependent and -independent requirements for transforming growth factor β receptor signaling via the Smad pathway. *Mol Cell Biol* 2002; 22:4750–4759.
57. Hayes S, Chawla A, Corvera S. TGF β receptor internalization into EEA1-enriched early endosomes: role in signaling to Smad2. *J Cell Biol* 2002; 158:1239–1249.
58. Di Guglielmo GM, Le Roy C, Goodfellow AF, Wrana JL. Distinct endocytic pathways regulate TGF-β receptor signalling and turnover. *Nat Cell Biol* 2003; 5:410–421.
59. Shi W, Sun C, He B *et al.* GADD34-PP1c recruited by Smad7 dephosphorylates TGFβ type I receptor. *J Cell Biol* 2004; 164:291–300.
60. Dore JJ Jr, Yao D, Edens M, Garamszegi N, Sholl EL, Leof EB. Mechanisms of transforming growth factor-β receptor endocytosis and intracellular sorting differ between fibroblasts and epithelial cells. *Mol Biol Cell* 2001; 12:675–684.
61. Coker RK, Laurent GJ, Shahzeidi S *et al.* Diverse cellular TGF-β 1 and TGF-β 3 gene expression in normal human and murine lung. *Eur Respir J* 1996; 9:2501–2507.
62. Coker RK, Laurent GJ, Jeffery PK, du Bois RM, Black CM, McAnulty RJ. Localisation of transforming growth factor β1 and β3 mRNA transcripts in normal and fibrotic human lung. *Thorax* 2001; 56:549–556.

63. Vignola AM, Chanez P, Chiappara G et al. Transforming growth factor-β expression in mucosal biopsies in asthma and chronic bronchitis. *Am J Respir Crit Care Med* 1997; 156:591–599.

64. Aubert JD, Dalal BI, Bai TR, Roberts CR, Hayashi S, Hogg JC. Transforming growth factor β 1 gene expression in human airways. *Thorax* 1994; 49:225–232.

65. Redington AE, Roche WR, Holgate ST, Howarth PH. Co-localization of immunoreactive transforming growth factor-β 1 and decorin in bronchial biopsies from asthmatic and normal subjects. *J Pathol* 1998; 186:410–415.

66. Pelton RW, Johnson MD, Perkett EA, Gold LI, Moses HL. Expression of transforming growth factor-β 1, -β 2, and -β 3 mRNA and protein in the murine lung. *Am J Respir Cell Mol Biol* 1991; 5:522–530.

67. Magnan A, Retornaz F, Tsicopoulos A et al. Altered compartmentalization of transforming growth factor-β in asthmatic airways. *Clin Exp Allergy* 1997; 27:389–395.

68. Minshall EM, Leung DY, Martin RJ et al. Eosinophil-associated TGF-β1 mRNA expression and airways fibrosis in bronchial asthma. *Am J Respir Cell Mol Biol* 1997; 17:326–333.

69. Hoshino M, Nakamura Y, Sim JJ. Expression of growth factors and remodelling of the airway wall in bronchial asthma. *Thorax* 1998; 53:21–27.

70. Chakir J, Shannon J, Molet S et al. Airway remodeling-associated mediators in moderate to severe asthma: effect of steroids on TGF-β, IL-11, IL-17, and type I and type III collagen expression. *J Allergy Clin Immunol* 2003; 111:1293–1298.

71. Balzar S, Chu HW, Silkoff P et al. Increased TGF-β2 in severe asthma with eosinophilia. *J Allergy Clin Immunol* 2005; 115:110–117.

72. Ohno I, Nitta Y, Yamauchi K et al. Transforming growth factor β 1 (TGF β 1) gene expression by eosinophils in asthmatic airway inflammation. *Am J Respir Cell Mol Biol* 1996; 15:404–409.

73. Vignola AM, Chanez P, Chiappara G et al. Release of transforming growth factor-β (TGF-β) and fibronectin by alveolar macrophages in airway diseases. *Clin Exp Immunol* 1996; 106:114–119.

74. Redington AE, Madden J, Frew AJ et al. Transforming growth factor-β 1 in asthma. Measurement in bronchoalveolar lavage fluid. *Am J Respir Crit Care Med* 1997; 156:642–647.

75. Batra V, Musani AI, Hastie AT et al. Bronchoalveolar lavage fluid concentrations of transforming growth factor (TGF)-β1, TGF-β2, interleukin (IL)-4 and IL-13 after segmental allergen challenge and their effects on α-smooth muscle actin and collagen III synthesis by primary human lung fibroblasts. *Clin Exp Allergy* 2004; 34:437–444.

76. Sagara H, Okada T, Okumura K et al. Activation of TGF-β/Smad2 signaling is associated with airway remodeling in asthma. *J Allergy Clin Immunol* 2002; 110:249–254.

77. Grainger DJ, Heathcote K, Chiano M et al. Genetic control of the circulating concentration of transforming growth factor type β1. *Hum Mol Genet* 1999; 8:93–97.

78. Hobbs K, Negri J, Klinnert M, Rosenwasser LJ, Borish L. Interleukin-10 and transforming growth factor-β promoter polymorphisms in allergies and asthma. *Am J Respir Crit Care Med* 1998; 158:1958–1962.

79. Pulleyn LJ, Newton R, Adcock IM, Barnes PJ. TGFβ1 allele association with asthma severity. *Hum Genet* 2001; 109:623–627.

80. Silverman ES, Palmer LJ, Subramaniam V et al. Transforming growth factor-β1 promoter polymorphism C-509T is associated with asthma. *Am J Respir Crit Care Med* 2004; 169:214–219.

81. Shull MM, Ormsby I, Kier AB et al. Targeted disruption of the mouse transforming growth factor-β 1 gene results in multifocal inflammatory disease. *Nature* 1992; 359:693–699.

82. Kulkarni AB, Huh CG, Becker D et al. Transforming growth factor β 1 null mutation in mice causes excessive inflammatory response and early death. *Proc Natl Acad Sci USA* 1993; 90:770–774.

83. Diebold RJ, Eis MJ, Yin M et al. Early-onset multifocal inflammation in the transforming growth factor β 1-null mouse is lymphocyte mediated. *Proc Natl Acad Sci USA* 1995; 92:12215–12219.

84. Sanford LP, Ormsby I, Gittenberger-de Groot AC et al. TGFβ2 knockout mice have multiple developmental defects that are non-overlapping with other TGFβ knockout phenotypes. *Development* 1997; 124:2659–2670.

85. Kaartinen V, Voncken JW, Shuler C et al. Abnormal lung development and cleft palate in mice lacking TGF-β 3 indicates defects of epithelial-mesenchymal interaction. *Nat Genet* 1995; 11:415–421.

86. Proetzel G, Pawlowski SA, Wiles MV et al. Transforming growth factor-β 3 is required for secondary palate fusion. *Nat Genet* 1995; 11:409–414.

87. Chu HW, Balzar S, Seedorf GJ et al. Transforming growth factor-β2 induces bronchial epithelial mucin expression in asthma. *Am J Pathol* 2004; 165:1097–1106.

88. Zhang S, Smartt H, Holgate ST, Roche WR. Growth factors secreted by bronchial epithelial cells control myofibroblast proliferation: an in vitro co-culture model of airway remodeling in asthma. *Lab Invest* 1999; 79:395–405.

89. Wen FQ, Kohyama T, Liu X *et al*. Interleukin-4- and interleukin-13-enhanced transforming growth factor-β2 production in cultured human bronchial epithelial cells is attenuated by interferon-gamma. *Am J Respir Cell Mol Biol* 2002; 26:484–490.

90. Richter A, Puddicombe SM, Lordan JL *et al*. The contribution of interleukin (IL)-4 and IL-13 to the epithelial-mesenchymal trophic unit in asthma. *Am J Respir Cell Mol Biol* 2001; 25:385–391.

91. Puddicombe SM, Polosa R, Richter A *et al*. Involvement of the epidermal growth factor receptor in epithelial repair in asthma. *FASEBJ* 2000; 14:1362–1374.

92. Howat WJ, Holgate ST, Lackie PM. TGF-β isoform release and activation during in vitro bronchial epithelial wound repair. *Am J Physiol Lung Cell Mol Physiol* 2002; 282:115–123.

93. Tschumperlin DJ, Shively JD, Kikuchi T, Drazen JM. Mechanical stress triggers selective release of fibrotic mediators from bronchial epithelium. *Am J Respir Cell Mol Biol* 2003; 28:142–149.

94. Sacco O, Romberger D, Rizzino A, Beckmann JD, Rennard SI, Spurzem JR. Spontaneous production of transforming growth factor-β 2 by primary cultures of bronchial epithelial cells. Effects on cell behavior in vitro. *J Clin Invest* 1992; 90:1379–1385.

95. Boland S, Boisvieux-Ulrich E, Houcine O *et al*. TGF β 1 promotes actin cytoskeleton reorganization and migratory phenotype in epithelial tracheal cells in primary culture. *J Cell Sci* 1996; 109:2207–2219.

96. Pelaia G, Cuda G, Vatrella A *et al*. Effects of transforming growth factor-[β] and budesonide on mitogen-activated protein kinase activation and apoptosis in airway epithelial cells. *Am J Respir Cell Mol Biol* 2003; 29:12–18.

97. Willis BC, Liebler JM, Luby-Phelps K *et al*. Induction of epithelial-mesenchymal transition in alveolar epithelial cells by transforming growth factor-β1: potential role in idiopathic pulmonary fibrosis. *Am J Pathol* 2005; 166:1321–1332.

98. Zhang K, Flanders KC, Phan SH. Cellular localization of transforming growth factor-β expression in bleomycin-induced pulmonary fibrosis. *Am J Pathol* 1995; 147:352–361.

99. Roche WR, Beasley R, Williams JH, Holgate ST. Subepithelial fibrosis in the bronchi of asthmatics. *Lancet* 1989; 1:520–524.

100. Wilson JW, Li X. The measurement of reticular basement membrane and submucosal collagen in the asthmatic airway. *Clin Exp Allergy* 1997; 27:363–371.

101. Chu HW, Halliday JL, Martin RJ, Leung DY, Szefler SJ, Wenzel SE. Collagen deposition in large airways may not differentiate severe asthma from milder forms of the disease. *Am J Respir Crit Care Med* 1998; 158:1936–1944.

102. Hoshino M, Nakamura Y, Sim J, Shimojo J, Isogai S. Bronchial subepithelial fibrosis and expression of matrix metalloproteinase-9 in asthmatic airway inflammation. *J Allergy Clin Immunol* 1998; 102:783–788.

103. Jeffery PK, Godfrey RW, Adelroth E, Nelson F, Rogers A, Johansson SA. Effects of treatment on airway inflammation and thickening of basement membrane reticular collagen in asthma. A quantitative light and electron microscopic study. *Am Rev Respir Dis* 1992; 145:890–899.

104. Cho SH, Seo JY, Choi DC *et al*. Pathological changes according to the severity of asthma. *Clin Exp Allergy* 1996; 26:1210–1219.

105. Gabbrielli S, Di Lollo S, Stanflin N, Romagnoli P. Myofibroblast and elastic and collagen fiber hyperplasia in the bronchial mucosa: a possible basis for the progressive irreversibility of airway obstruction in chronic asthma. *Pathologica* 1994; 86:157–160.

106. Laitinen A, Altraja A, Kampe M, Linden M, Virtanen I, Laitinen LA. Tenascin is increased in airway basement membrane of asthmatics and decreased by an inhaled steroid. *Am J Respir Crit Care Med* 1997; 156:951–958.

107. Huang J, Olivenstein R, Taha R, Hamid Q, Ludwig M. Enhanced proteoglycan deposition in the airway wall of atopic asthmatics. *Am J Respir Crit Care Med* 1999; 160:725–729.

108. Roberts CR. Is asthma a fibrotic disease? *Chest* 1995; 107(suppl):111S–117S.

109. Brewster CE, Howarth PH, Djukanovic R, Wilson J, Holgate ST, Roche WR. Myofibroblasts and subepithelial fibrosis in bronchial asthma. *Am J Respir Cell Mol Biol* 1990; 3:507–511.

110. Boulet L, Belanger M, Carrier G. Airway responsiveness and bronchial-wall thickness in asthma with or without fixed airflow obstruction. *Am J Respir Crit Care Med* 1995; 152:865–871.

111. Chetta A, Foresi A, Del Donno M *et al*. Bronchial responsiveness to distilled water and methacholine and its relationship to inflammation and remodeling of the airways in asthma. *Am J Respir Crit Care Med* 1996; 153:910–917.

112. Nomura A, Uchida Y, Sakamoto T et al. Increases in collagen type I synthesis in asthma: the role of eosinophils and transforming growth factor-β. Clin Exp Allergy 2002; 32:860–865.

113. Wenzel SE, Trudeau JB, Barnes S et al. TGF-β and IL-13 synergistically increase eotaxin-1 production in human airway fibroblasts. J Immunol 2002; 169:4613–4619.

114. Flood-Page P, Menzies-Gow A, Phipps S et al. Anti-IL-5 treatment reduces deposition of ECM proteins in the bronchial subepithelial basement membrane of mild atopic asthmatics. J Clin Invest 2003; 112:1029–1036.

115. Dunnill MS, Massarella GR, Anderson JA. A comparison of the quantitative anatomy of the bronchi in normal subjects, in status asthmaticus, in chronic bronchitis, and in emphysema. Thorax 1969; 24:176–179.

116. Carroll N, Elliot J, Morton A, James A. The structure of large and small airways in nonfatal and fatal asthma. Am Rev Respir Dis 1993; 147:405–410.

117. Jeffery PK. Structural and inflammatory changes in COPD: a comparison with asthma. Thorax 1998; 53:129–136.

118. Khalil N, O'Connor RN, Flanders KC, Unruh H. TGF-β 1, but not TGF-β 2 or TGF-β 3, is differentially present in epithelial cells of advanced pulmonary fibrosis: an immunohistochemical study. Am J Respir Cell Mol Biol 1996; 14:131–138.

119. Coutts A, Chen G, Stephens N et al. Release of biologically active TGF-β from airway smooth muscle cells induces autocrine synthesis of collagen. Am J Physiol Lung Cell Mol Physiol 2001; 280:L999–L1008.

120. Black PN, Young PG, Skinner SJ. Response of airway smooth muscle cells to TGF-β 1: effects on growth and synthesis of glycosaminoglycans. Am J Physiol 1996; 271:L910–L917.

121. Cohen MD, Ciocca V, Panettieri RA Jr. TGF-β 1 modulates human airway smooth-muscle cell proliferation induced by mitogens. Am J Respir Cell Mol Biol 1997; 16:85–90.

122. Krymskaya VP, Hoffman R, Eszterhas A, Ciocca V, Panettieri RA Jr. TGF-β 1 modulates EGF-stimulated phosphatidylinositol 3-kinase activity in human airway smooth muscle cells. Am J Physiol 1997; 273:L1220–L1227.

123. Okona-Mensah KB, Shittu E, Page C, Costello J, Kilfeather SA. Inhibition of serum and transforming growth factor β (TGF-β1)-induced DNA synthesis in confluent airway smooth muscle by heparin. Br J Pharmacol 1998; 125:599–606.

124. Zuyderduyn S, Hiemstra PS, Rabe KF. TGF-β differentially regulates TH2 cytokine-induced eotaxin and eotaxin-3 release by human airway smooth muscle cells. J Allergy Clin Immunol 2004; 114:791–798.

125. Metzger WJ, Richerson HB, Worden K, Monick M, Hunninghake GW. Bronchoalveolar lavage of allergic asthmatic patients following allergen bronchoprovocation. Chest 1986; 89:477–483.

126. Kelly C, Ward C, Stenton CS, Bird G, Hendrick DJ, Walters EH. Number and activity of inflammatory cells in bronchoalveolar lavage fluid in asthma and their relation to airway responsiveness. Thorax 1988; 43:684–692.

127. Adams DH, Hathaway M, Shaw J, Burnett D, Elias E, Strain AJ. Transforming growth factor-β induces human T lymphocyte migration in vitro. J Immunol 1991; 147:609–612.

128. Cerwenka A, Bevec D, Majdic O, Knapp W, Holter W. TGF-β 1 is a potent inducer of human effector T cells. J Immunol 1994; 153:4367–4377.

129. Ahuja SS, Paliogianni F, Yamada H, Balow JE, Boumpas DT. Effect of transforming growth factor-β on early and late activation events in human T cells. J Immunol 1993; 150:3109–3118.

130. Cerwenka A, Kovar H, Majdic O, Holter W. Fas- and activation-induced apoptosis are reduced in human T cells preactivated in the presence of TGF-β 1. J Immunol 1996; 156:459–464.

131. Genestier L, Kasibhatla S, Brunner T, Green DR. Transforming growth factor β1 inhibits Fas ligand expression and subsequent activation-induced cell death in T cells via downregulation of c-Myc. J Exp Med 1999; 189:231–239.

132. Chen W, Jin W, Hardegen N et al. Conversion of peripheral CD4+CD25-naive T cells to CD4+CD25+ regulatory T cells by TGF-β induction of transcription factor Foxp3. J Exp Med 2003; 198:875–886.

133. Nakao A, Miike S, Hatano M et al. Blockade of transforming growth factor β/Smad signaling in T cells by overexpression of Smad7 enhances antigen-induced airway inflammation and airway reactivity. J Exp Med 2000; 192:151–158.

134. Scherf W, Burdach S, Hansen G. Reduced expression of transforming growth factor β 1 exacerbates pathology in an experimental asthma model. Eur J Immunol 2005; 35:198–206.

135. Hansen G, McIntire JJ, Yeung VP et al. Allergen-specific Th1 cells fail to counterbalance Th2 cell-induced airway hyperreactivity but cause severe airway inflammation. J Clin Invest 2000; 105:61–70.

136. Schramm C, Herz U, Podlech J et al. TGF-β regulates airway responses via T cells. J Immunol 2003; 170:1313–1319.

137. Jarman ER, Lamb JR. Reversal of established CD4+ type 2 T helper-mediated allergic airway inflammation and eosinophilia by therapeutic treatment with DNA vaccines limits progression towards chronic inflammation and remodelling. *Immunology* 2004; 112:631–642.

138. Metzger WJ, Zavala D, Richerson HB *et al*. Local allergen challenge and bronchoalveolar lavage of allergic asthmatic lungs. Description of the model and local airway inflammation. *Am Rev Respir Dis* 1987; 135:433–440.

139. Wahl SM, Hunt DA, Wakefield LM *et al*. Transforming growth factor type β induces monocyte chemotaxis and growth factor production. *Proc Natl Acad Sci USA* 1987; 84:5788–5792.

140. Postlethwaite AE, Seyer JM. Identification of a chemotactic epitope in human transforming growth factor-β 1 spanning amino acid residues 368–374. *J Cell Physiol* 1995; 164:587–592.

141. Beasley R, Roche WR, Roberts JA, Holgate ST. Cellular events in the bronchi in mild asthma and after bronchial provocation. *Am Rev Respir Dis* 1989; 139:806–817.

142. Bentley AM, Kay AB, Durham SR. Human late asthmatic reactions. *Clin Exp Allergy* 1997; 27(suppl 1):71–86.

143. Chu HW, Trudeau JB, Balzar S, Wenzel SE. Peripheral blood and airway tissue expression of transforming growth factor β by neutrophils in asthmatic subjects and normal control subjects. *J Allergy Clin Immunol* 2000; 106:1115–1123.

144. Carroll MP, Durham SR, Walsh G, Kay AB. Activation of neutrophils and monocytes after allergen- and histamine-induced bronchoconstriction. *J Allergy Clin Immunol* 1985; 75:290–296.

145. Papageorgiou N, Carroll M, Durham SR, Lee TH, Walsh GM, Kay AB. Complement receptor enhancement as evidence of neutrophil activation after exercise-induced asthma. *Lancet* 1983; 2:1220–1223.

146. Diaz P, Gonzalez MC, Galleguillos FR *et al*. Leukocytes and mediators in bronchoalveolar lavage during allergen-induced late-phase asthmatic reactions. *Am Rev Respir Dis* 1989; 139:1383–1389.

147. Balazovich KJ, Fernandez R, Hinkovska-Galcheva V, Suchard SJ, Boxer LA. Transforming growth factor-β1 stimulates degranulation and oxidant release by adherent human neutrophils. *J Leukoc Biol* 1996; 60:772–777.

148. Gruber BL, Marchese MJ, Kew RR. Transforming growth factor-β 1 mediates mast cell chemotaxis. *J Immunol* 1994; 152:5860–5867.

149. Berger P, Girodet PO, Begueret H *et al*. Tryptase-stimulated human airway smooth muscle cells induce cytokine synthesis and mast cell chemotaxis. *FASEB J* 2003; 17:2139–2141.

150. Brightling CE, Bradding P, Symon FA, Holgate ST, Wardlaw AJ, Pavord ID. Mast-cell infiltration of airway smooth muscle in asthma. *N Engl J Med* 2002; 346:1699–1705.

151. Birukova AA, Adyshev D, Gorshkov B, Birukov KG, Verin AD. ALK5 and Smad4 are involved in TGF-β1-induced pulmonary endothelial permeability. *FEBS Lett* 2005; 579:4031–4037.

152. Mead AL, Wong TT, Cordeiro MF, Anderson IK, Khaw PT. Evaluation of anti-TGF-β2 antibody as a new postoperative anti-scarring agent in glaucoma surgery. *Invest Ophthalmol Vis Sci* 2003; 44:3394–3401.

153. Yang YA, Dukhanina O, Tang B *et al*. Lifetime exposure to a soluble TGF-β antagonist protects mice against metastasis without adverse side effects. *J Clin Invest* 2002; 109:1607–1615.

154. Ruzek MC, Hawes M, Pratt B *et al*. Minimal effects on immune parameters following chronic anti-TGF-β monoclonal antibody administration to normal mice. *Immunopharmacol Immunotoxicol* 2003; 25:235–257.

155. Siriwardena D, Khaw PT, King AJ *et al*. Human antitransforming growth factor β(2) monoclonal antibody – a new modulator of wound healing in trabeculectomy: a randomized placebo controlled clinical study. *Ophthalmology* 2002; 109:427–431.

156. Preliminary Results from Phase I/II Trial of CAT-192 for Scleroderma. 2004; available at http://www.cambridgeantibody.com/html/news_and_resources/news_releases/2004/cambridge_antibody_technology_and_genzym.

157. Akagi Y, Isaka Y, Arai M *et al*. Inhibition of TGF-β 1 expression by antisense oligonucleotides suppressed extracellular matrix accumulation in experimental glomerulonephritis. *Kidney Int* 1996; 50:148–155.

158. Han DC, Hoffman BB, Hong SW, Guo J, Ziyadeh FN. Therapy with antisense TGF-β1 oligodeoxynucleotides reduces kidney weight and matrix mRNAs in diabetic mice. *Am J Physiol Renal Physiol* 2000; 278:F628–F634.

159. Takabatake Y, Isaka Y, Mizui M *et al*. Exploring RNA interference as a therapeutic strategy for renal disease. *Gene Ther* 2005; 12:965–973.

160. Fakhrai H, Dorigo O, Shawler DL *et al*. Eradication of established intracranial rat gliomas by transforming growth factor β antisense gene therapy. *Proc Natl Acad Sci USA* 1996; 93:2909–2914.

161. Liau LM, Fakhrai H, Black KL. Prolonged survival of rats with intracranial C6 gliomas by treatment with TGF-β antisense gene. *Neurol Res* 1998; 20:742–747.

162. Bogdahn U, Hau P, Brawanski A et al. Specific therapy for high-grade glioma by convection-enhanced delivery of the TGF-β2 specific antisense oligonucleotide AP 12009. J Clin Oncol 2004; 22:1514.

163. Schlingensiepen K-H, Bischof A, Egger T et al. The TGF-β1 antisense oligonucleotide AP 11014 for the treatment of non-small cell lung, colorectal and prostate cancer: Preclinical studies. J Clin Oncol 2004; 22:3132.

164. Yehualaeshet T, O'Connor R, Begleiter A, Murphy-Ullrich JE, Silverstein R, Khalil NA. CD36 synthetic peptide inhibits bleomycin-induced pulmonary inflammation and connective tissue synthesis in the rat. Am J Respir Cell Mol Biol 2000; 23:204–212.

165. Okuno M, Akita K, Moriwaki H et al. Prevention of rat hepatic fibrosis by the protease inhibitor, camostat mesilate, via reduced generation of active TGF-β. Gastroenterology 2001; 120:1784–1800.

166. Kondou H, Mushiake S, Etani Y, Miyoshi Y, Michigami T, Ozono KA. Blocking peptide for transforming growth factor-β1 activation prevents hepatic fibrosis in vivo. J Hepatol 2003; 39:742–748.

167. Nakamura T, Sakata R, Ueno T, Sata M, Ueno H. Inhibition of transforming growth factor β prevents progression of liver fibrosis and enhances hepatocyte regeneration in dimethylnitrosamine-treated rats. Hepatology 2000; 32:247–255.

168. Wang Q, Wang Y, Hyde DM et al. Reduction of bleomycin induced lung fibrosis by transforming growth factor β soluble receptor in hamsters. Thorax 1999; 54:805–812.

169. Ueno H, Sakamoto T, Nakamura T et al. A soluble transforming growth factor β receptor expressed in muscle prevents liver fibrogenesis and dysfunction in rats. Hum Gene Ther 2000; 11:33–42.

170. Giri SN, Hyde DM, Braun RK, Gaarde W, Harper JR, Pierschbacher MD. Antifibrotic effect of decorin in a bleomycin hamster model of lung fibrosis. Biochem Pharmacol 1997; 54:1205–1216.

171. Kolb M, Margetts PJ, Galt T et al. Transient transgene expression of decorin in the lung reduces the fibrotic response to bleomycin. Am J Respir Crit Care Med 2001; 163:770–777.

172. Tuxhorn JA, McAlhany SJ, Yang F, Dang TD, Rowley DR. Inhibition of transforming growth factor-β activity decreases angiogenesis in a human prostate cancer-reactive stroma xenograft model. Cancer Res 2002; 62:6021–6025.

173. Ezquerro IJ, Lasarte JJ, Dotor J et al. Synthetic peptide from transforming growth factor β type III receptor inhibits liver fibrogenesis in rats with carbon tetrachloride liver injury. Cytokine 2003; 22:12–20.

174. Border WA, Okuda S, Languino LR, Sporn MB, Ruoslahti E. Suppression of experimental glomerulonephritis by antiserum against transforming growth factor β 1. Nature 1990; 346:371–374.

175. Giri SN, Hyde DM, Hollinger MA. Effect of antibody to transforming growth factor β on bleomycin induced accumulation of lung collagen in mice. Thorax 1993; 48:959–966.

176. McMillan SJ, Xanthou G, Lloyd CM. Manipulation of allergen-induced airway remodeling by treatment with anti-TGF-β antibody: effect on the Smad signaling pathway. J Immunol 2005; 174:5774–5780.

177. Carrington LM, Albon J, Anderson I, Kamma C, Boulton M. Differential regulation of key stages in early corneal wound healing by TGF-β isoforms and their inhibitors. Invest Ophthalmol Vis Sci 2006; 47:1886–1894.

178. Reinhardt AK, Bottoms SE, Laurent GJ, McAnulty RJ. Contribution of TGF-isoforms to sub-epithelial airway remodelling. Am J Respir Crit Care Med 2004; 169:A265.

179. Howell JE, Reinhardt AK, Bottoms SE, Laurent GJ, McAnulty RJ. TGF-isoform specific effects on decorin deposition in a model of asthma. Proc Am Thorac Soc 2006; 3:A29.

180. Bonniaud P, Margetts PJ, Kolb M et al. Progressive transforming growth factor β1-induced lung fibrosis is blocked by an orally active ALK5 kinase inhibitor. Am J Respir Crit Care Med 2005; 171:889–898.

181. Mori Y, Ishida W, Bhattacharyya S, Li Y, Platanias LC, Varga J. Selective inhibition of activin receptor-like kinase 5 signaling blocks profibrotic transforming growth factor β responses in skin fibroblasts. Arthritis Rheum 2004; 50:4008–4021.

182. DaCosta BS, Major C, Laping NJ, Roberts AB. SB-505124 is a selective inhibitor of transforming growth factor-β type I receptors ALK4, ALK5, and ALK7. Mol Pharmacol 2004; 65:744–752.

183. Grygielko ET, Martin WM, Tweed CW et al. Inhibition of gene markers of fibrosis with a novel inhibitor of transforming growth factor-β type I receptor kinase in puromycin-induced nephritis. J Pharmacol Exp Ther 2005; 313:943–951.

184. de Gouville AC, Boullay V, Krysa G et al. Inhibition of TGF-β signaling by an ALK5 inhibitor protects rats from dimethylnitrosamine-induced liver fibrosis. Br J Pharmacol 2005; 145:166–177.

185. Gellibert F, de Gouville AC, Woolven J et al. Discovery of 4-{4-[3-(pyridin-2-yl)-1H-pyrazol-4-yl]pyridin-2-yl}-N-(tetrahydro-2H-pyran-4-yl)benzamide (GW788388): a potent, selective, and orally active transforming growth factor-β type I receptor inhibitor. J Med Chem 2006; 49:2210–2221.

186. Rosendahl A, Checchin D, Fehniger TE, Ten Dijke P, Heldin CH, Sideras P. Activation of the TGF-β/activin-Smad2 pathway during allergic airway inflammation. *Am J Respir Cell Mol Biol* 2001; 25:60–68.

187. Yeom SY, Jeoung D, Ha KS, Kim PH. Small interfering RNA (siRNA) targetted to Smad3 inhibits transforming growth factor-β signaling. *Biotechnol Lett* 2004; 26:699–703.

188. Zhang L, Graziano K, Pham T, Logsdon CD, Simeone DM. Adenovirus-mediated gene transfer of dominant-negative Smad4 blocks TGF-β signaling in pancreatic acinar cells. *Am J Physiol Gastrointest Liver Physiol* 2001; 280:G1247–G1253.

189. Nakao A, Sagara H, Setoguchi Y *et al*. Expression of Smad7 in bronchial epithelial cells is inversely correlated to basement membrane thickness and airway hyperresponsiveness in patients with asthma. *J Allergy Clin Immunol* 2002; 110:873–878.

190. Dong C, Zhu S, Wang T *et al*. Deficient Smad7 expression: a putative molecular defect in scleroderma. *Proc Natl Acad Sci USA* 2002; 99:3908–3913.

191. Nakao A, Fujii M, Matsumura R *et al*. Transient gene transfer and expression of Smad7 prevents bleomycin-induced lung fibrosis in mice. *J Clin Invest* 1999; 104:5–11.

192. Lan HY, Mu W, Tomita N *et al*. Inhibition of renal fibrosis by gene transfer of inducible Smad7 using ultrasound-microbubble system in rat UUO model. *J Am Soc Nephrol* 2003; 14:1535–1548.

193. Duan W, Chan JH, McKay K *et al*. Inhaled p38α mitogen-activated protein kinase antisense oligonucleotide attenuates asthma in mice. *Am J Respir Crit Care Med* 2005; 171:571–578.

194. Chialda L, Zhang M, Brune K, Pahl A. Inhibitors of mitogen-activated protein kinases differentially regulate costimulated T cell cytokine production and mouse airway eosinophilia. *Respir Res* 2005; 6:36.

195. Eynott PR, Xu L, Bennett BL *et al*. Effect of an inhibitor of Jun N-terminal protein kinase, SP600125, in single allergen challenge in sensitized rats. *Immunology* 2004; 112:446–453.

196. Underwood DC, Osborn RR, Kotzer CJ *et al*. SB 239063, a potent p38 MAP kinase inhibitor, reduces inflammatory cytokine production, airways eosinophil infiltration, and persistence. *J Pharmacol Exp Ther* 2000; 293:281–288.

197. Stambe C, Atkins RC, Tesch GH, Masaki T, Schreiner GF, Nikolic-Paterson DJ. The role of p38α mitogen-activated protein kinase activation in renal fibrosis. *J Am Soc Nephrol* 2004; 15:370–379.

198. Matsuoka H, Arai T, Mori M *et al*. A p38 MAPK inhibitor, FR-167653, ameliorates murine bleomycin-induced pulmonary fibrosis. *Am J Physiol Lung Cell Mol Physiol* 2002; 283:L103–L112.

199. Underwood DC, Osborn RR, Bochnowicz S *et al*. SB 239063, a p38 MAPK inhibitor, reduces neutrophilia, inflammatory cytokines, MMP-9, and fibrosis in lung. *Am J Physiol Lung Cell Mol Physiol* 2000; 279:L895–L902.

3

The role of transcription factors in asthma: can we modify them for therapeutic purposes?

M. Roth, J. L. Black

INTRODUCTION

The airways of patients with asthma narrow too easily and too much [1]. The provoking factors which are known to initiate this bronchoconstriction are diverse and include exercise, an array of allergens including pollens, dust mites, and inhalation of non-isotonic solutions. The reason for this exaggerated response, which is not observed in non-asthmatic individuals, is unknown, although it is widely held that chronic inflammation, allergy and infections – mostly viral – play an aetiological role. The asthmatic lung is characterized by the presence of an inflammatory cell infiltrate comprised of lymphocytes, mast cells, macrophages and eosinophils. Examination of bronchoalveolar lavage fluid has revealed increased levels of a number of pro-inflammatory and profibrotic cytokines such as interleukins (IL)-3, -4, and -5 and -6 and transforming growth factor (TGF)β. Much research has been focused on elucidating a genetic basis for asthma, but thus far evidence for a firm relationship between a specific gene or group of genes and the presence of asthma remains elusive. Nevertheless, a strong family history is a common finding in most asthmatic patients. The airways of some but not all asthma patients exhibit thickening of the basement membrane (lamina reticularis) which is due to increased deposition of extracellular matrix and fibrosis, an increased mass of bronchial smooth muscle, and an increased number of small blood vessels. In addition, there is metaplasia of the airway epithelium and an increase in the number of goblet cells [2–4]. These pathological features which are known collectively as remodelling could be explained on the basis of response of the lung to persistent inflammation. However, evidence is accumulating that factors other than inflammation such as mechanical stress or strain could lead to the development of these structural changes and thus a disconnect between inflammation and remodelling.

Animal models have been developed to study asthma for 20 years [5], but none of the current available models covers all pathological features documented in the human lung that are so characteristic of asthma. The animal models can be used to study the inflammatory aspect of asthma, however most of the histopathology seen in asthma is absent. Evidence from the study of animal models supports the T helper (Th)2 paradigm for allergic diseases with local and systemic increase and activation of Th2 lymphocytes that produce IL-4, -5, -9 and -13 that trigger in turn immunoglobulin (Ig)E production and

Michael Roth, PhD, Research Group Leader, Molecular Medicine, The Woolcock Institute for Medical Research, University of Sydney, Camperdown, NSW, Australia

Judith L. Black, MBBS, PhD, FRACP, Professor, Discipline of Pharmacology, Faculty of Medicine, Woolcock Institute of Medical Research, University of Sydney, NSW, Australia

eosinophil recruitment and activation. This hypothesis was supported by clinical studies showing that Th2-like cytokines were readily released from lymphocytes of patients with allergies or asthma [6–9]. However, other studies have produced inconsistent results, revealing enhanced levels of Th1-like cytokines [10–12].

The increased mass of smooth muscle may explain why the asthmatic airway constricts more forcefully to a stimulus, and the thickening of the airway wall may make airway narrowing less easy to reverse, but one could easily argue the opposite, i.e. a stiffened airway wall would hinder constriction. Airway smooth muscle cell (ASMC) contraction in asthma patients may thus be more forceful due to mere physical properties as a result of increased smooth muscle mass. In this context, we have demonstrated that human isolated bronchial smooth muscle cells obtained from patients with asthma proliferate faster under cell culture conditions than bronchial smooth muscle cells from non-asthma controls, including patients with COPD [13, 14]. This result indicates that proliferation control of bronchial smooth muscle cells is deregulated in asthma and, since it is maintained in isolated cells after several passages, this finding is likely to represent an aspect of asthma pathology that is independent of the inflammatory micro-environment in the asthmatic lung. However, the cause of the ongoing remodelling process in the asthmatic lung is largely unknown and cannot be explained merely by the Th2 paradigm.

Inhaled allergen can induce the airway epithelium to produce chemoattractants, pro-inflammatory ILs, and matrix-modifying proteins which influence the growth and activation state of airway structural cells, and which contribute to the influx of inflammatory cells and changes in structure of the asthmatic airway. In a recent study, gene expression in lung epithelial cells before and after allergen challenge was assessed using a gene micro-array system [15]. The study identified 141 upregulated and eight downregulated sequences. Besides known asthma associated pro-inflammatory factors (IL-3, -4 and -5 receptors, nuclear factor-kappa B (NF-κB), and lipocortin) the study indicated that a much wider array of genes is involved in the response to allergen, including many which had not been associated with asthma before [15].

The expression of multiple genes encoding for pro-inflammatory factors is orchestrated by transcription factors. Transcription factors are proteins that bind to promoter regions of genes and activate or silence their transcription into messenger RNA (mRNA). Several transcription factors have been implicated in the inflammatory process in asthma, including the glucocorticoid receptor (GR), NF-κB, activator protein-1 (AP-1), nuclear factor of activated T cells (NF-AT), cyclic AMP response element binding protein (CREB) and signal transduction-activated transcription factors (STAT) [16–18]. Recently, more transcription factors have been added to those that may play a role in asthma, the CCAAT/enhancer binding protein (C/EBP), peroxisome proliferator-activated receptor (PPAR) and the bZIP transcription factor, NF-E2-related factor-2 (Nrf2) [14, 19, 20–23] (Table 3.1). A summary of asthma-relevant transcription factors and their interaction has been provided by Popescu [23], and a special review of the interactions of the GR with NF-κB and AP-1 with regard to the transrepressive action of the GR has been provided by De Boesscher *et al.* [24].

The recent knowledge about transcription factors raises important questions which need to be addressed, *viz* could a pathological deregulation of one of these transcription factors explain the broad spectrum of asthma pathology and could any type of modulation of asthma-relevant transcription factors lead to better symptom control or even a cure for asthma. This overview will try to summarize knowledge of asthma-relevant transcription factors and their possible use for asthma therapy.

THE CCAAT/ENHANCER BINDING PROTEINS

The family of the C/EBPs consists of six known isoproteins (-α, -β, -γ, -δ, -ε, and -ζ) which are each subdivided into several isoforms. All C/EBPs are crucially involved in the balance

Table 3.1 Transcription factors with a role in asthma, together with their inhibitors and mechanisms of action

Transcription factor	Inhibitor	Function of inhibitor
AP-1	Cyclosporin A	Inhibits DNA binding
	Clarithromycin	Inhibits DNA binding
	Dehydroepiandrosterone	Inhibits DNA binding?
	MOL 294	Downregulates transcription
	PNRI-299	Species-specific inhibitory or activating effect ?
	SP100020	Inhibits activation
	Decoy oligonucleotides	Binds active transcription factors
C/EBP-α	Trichostatin A	Downregulation of transcription
	Valproic acid	Protein degradation or inhibition of synthesis
C/EBP-β	Ceramide	Inhibition of nuclear transport
C/EBP-α + -β	Curcumine	Interference with DNA binding
C/EBP (all)	Decoy oligonucleotides	Binds active transcription factors
GATA-3	None	
NF-κB	β$_2$-agonists	Inhibition of DNA formation/binding
	Flavonoids (silybin)	?
	Fosmycin	Activation
	Fumaric acid	Nuclear transport
	Glucocorticoids	Inhibition of DNA formation/binding, synthesis
	MOL 294	Downregulates transcription
	Kaurene diterpenoid	?
	Pyrrolydine thiocarbamate	?
	Sesquiterpene lactone	?
	SP10030	Inhibits activation
Nrf2/ARE	Ceramide	Inhibition of nuclear transport
PPAR-α/-γ	Rapamycin	?
STAT (all)	Glucocorticoids	?
SRF	None	

of cell proliferation–differentiation and may even be expressed in a cell type specific pattern in the lung [25–27]. The balance of C/EBP-isoforms is essential for smooth muscle cell and fibroblast phenotypes [28, 29] and may hold the clue to explain the often-discussed phenotype switch between asthma smooth muscle cells, myofibroblasts and fibroblasts as has been shown in other cell types [29].

C/EBPs have been implicated in asthma since several cytokines elevated in asthma are controlled by one or more C/EBP-isoproteins. They play a crucial role in eosinophil differentiation [30] and control the expression of eotaxin and IL-5 [19, 31]. IL-4 expression and simultaneous reduction of IL-2 and interferon (IFN) γ expression was mediated by C/EBP-β in a lymphocyte cell line which could shed some light on the Th1–Th2 cell paradigm for asthma as discussed above [32]. Interestingly IL-5 expression depends on the interaction, most probably dimer formation, of C/EBP-β with -δ and may be stimulated by human pathogenic viruses [19]. A hypothesis for the role of C/EBP-isoproteins in asthma has been presented elsewhere [33].

The hyperplasia of smooth muscle bundles in asthmatic airways might be explained by the observation of our group that ASMC obtained from patients with asthma proliferate at a rate of 2.5 times that of cells obtained from non-asthmatic patients, including those with COPD [13]. It seems that the signalling pathway that controls ASMC proliferation includes the formation of a complex consisting of the GR and C/EBP-α [34, 35], but since C/EBP-α is missing in ASMC of patients with asthma, glucocorticoids can not reverse this abnormality [14].

In non-pulmonary cells ceramide, a sphingolipid, inhibited the transport of activated C/EBP-β and Nrf2 into the nucleus [36]. Curcumine, an anti-oxidant, has been shown to interfere with C/EBP-α and -β binding to its DNA consensus sequence [37]. Trichostatin A inhibits C/EBP-α mRNA levels while valproic acid downregulated its protein expression in adipocytes [38]. Decoy oligonucleotide trapping transcription factors including C/EBPs have been used to control smooth muscle cell differentiation and are well tolerated *in vivo* as shown in animal models [39, 40] and in several pre-clinical therapeutic strategies as reviewed by Quarcoo and Hamelmann [41].

The possibility of modulation of C/EBPs as an intervention in asthma needs further investigation. A general blockade of all C/EBP-isoproteins, e.g. decoy oligonucleotides is not advisable since the various C/EBP-isoproteins exert distinct, often opposing, functions in cell biology. If the lack of C/EBP-α in smooth muscle cells of asthma patients could be proven to be cell type specific, then an overall inhibition of C/EBPs might even be counter-productive. The cell type specific expression and role of the various C/EBP-isoproteins and their isoforms will be a stimulus for the development of specific drugs or effector (cell type specific) delivery, and may also hold the key to a highly specific asthma drug.

NUCLEAR FACTOR-KAPPA B

Dysregulation of members of the NF-κB transcription factor family is associated with many diseases including AIDS, atherosclerosis, asthma, arthritis, cancer, diabetes, inflammatory bowel disease, muscular dystrophy, stroke, and viral infections [42, 43]. NF-κB is a ubiquitous transcription factor regulating the expression of multiple inflammatory and immune genes, and it plays a critical role in host defence and in chronic inflammatory diseases. Therefore, appropriate regulation and control of NF-κB activity by gene modification or drugs was suggested as a potential approach for some of the above mentioned diseases [24, 42]. NF-κB is a heterodimer, residing in the cytoplasm in an inactive form complexed to its inhibitor, IκB. Viruses, oxidants, inflammatory cytokines and immune stimuli activate NF-κB [24, 43, 44]. Once activated, it binds to recognition elements in the promoter regions of genes encoding for pro-inflammatory cytokines, chemokines, inflammatory enzymes and adhesion molecules.

In airway epithelial cells of patients with asthma, there is increasing evidence that NF-κB plays a pivotal role in the expression of inflammatory genes and NF-κB may be a major target for glucocorticoids to exert their anti-inflammatory effect [45]. In an animal model of asthma, persistent NF-κB activation in bronchi was driven by granulocytes *via* IL-1β and TNFα, which both induce the degradation of IκB-β, thereby perpetuating the immune response in asthmatic airways [46]. NF-κB activation in epithelial cells was demonstrated by immunohistochemistry in patients with asthma but was absent in control subjects, and active NF-κB was confirmed by electrophoretic DNA mobility shift assay [47, 48]. However, some studies suggest that NF-κB is essential for the inflammatory reaction in asthma but does not contribute to the structural changes of the lung in long-standing asthma or participate in steroid unresponsive asthma [49].

Using transgenic mice, suppression of NF-κB over 15 months did not result in a significantly lower immune response to allergens [50]. In a different transgenic mouse model, airway epithelium specific suppression of NF-κB resulted in significant reduced airway inflammation compared to controls, and reduced levels of chemokines, T cell cytokines, mucus cell metaplasia, and circulating IgE, but the lack of NF-κB did not alter airway hyper-responsiveness [51]. A similar result with cytokine release and IgE production was obtained in another animal model after the application of antisense oligonucleotides to mice [52]. In contrast, intratracheal NF-κB decoy oligodeoxynucleotides administered to OVA-sensitized mice demonstrated an efficient nuclear transfection of airway immune cells, but not of structural lung cells. NF-κB decoy treatment was followed by strong attenuation of allergic lung inflammation, airway hyperresponsiveness, and local production of mucus, IL-5, -13, and eotaxin. Surprisingly IL-4 and OVA-specific IgE and IgG$_1$ production were not reduced [53].

In addition to glucocorticoids, which inhibit NF-κB activity by binding to the activated GR (for review see [24, 54, 55]) other chemicals and drugs inhibit NF-κB. Together with a long-acting β$_2$-agonist, glucocorticoids seem to inhibit NF-κB more efficiently [56]. Pranlukast was also reported to inhibit NF-κB activity and thereby downregulate the release of pro-inflammatory mediators [57, 58]. Antibiotics may also be able to downregulate NF-κB activity as demonstrated by fosfomycin [59]. Pyrrolydine dithiocarbamate inhibits NF-κB activation by an unclear mechanism in human ASMC [60]. An interesting approach to inhibiting NF-κB activity was used with an 11 amino acid long artificial peptide that was derived from an IκB protein and used in eosinophils to induce apoptosis [61]. A large number of NF-κB modulators belong to the isoprenoids, more specifically to the kaurene diterpenoid and sesquiterpene lactone class and flavonoids such as silybin, but their mode of action has to be further investigated before they can be used to modify NF-κB activity [62].

ACTIVATOR PROTEIN-1

An imbalance of oxidants/anti-oxidants has been suggested to contribute to the pathology of asthma [63, 64], and to activate redox-sensitive transcription factors such as AP-1. AP-1 induction, at least in the human lung epithelial cell line A549, has, as a prerequisite, the activation of the pro-inflammatory neuropeptide substance P [65]. AP-1 together with histone acetyltransferase, CBP/p300 and the transcription factors C/EBP, NF-AT controls the expression of the asthma-associated cytokine IL-5 [66, 67]. In a cell culture model Oudin and Pugin [68] claimed that overstretching of the airway can induce AP-1 expression and activation in epithelial cells. Interestingly, rhinovirus, which can trigger asthma attacks or increase the severity of the disease [69, 70] has been shown to stimulate AP-1 and subsequently IL-8 and granulocyte-macrophage colony-stimulating factor (GM-CSF) *via* one of its proteases [44].

The action of AP-1 can be blocked by two mechanisms: (i) suppression of its activation and (ii) inhibition of AP-1 binding to its DNA consensus sequence in a gene promoter. Both concepts have been demonstrated in animal and cell culture models but not yet in patients. The activation of AP-1 by a small-molecule inhibitor, PNRI-299, directly targeting the oxidoreductase, redox effector factor-1, was reported in human lung epithelial A549 cells with an IC$_{50}$ of 20 μM [63]. PNRI-299 also inhibited AP-1 in a mouse asthma model significantly reducing eosinophil infiltration into the airways, mucus hypersecretion, oedema, and IL-4 levels [63]. MOL 294 is another AP-1/NF-κB inhibitor, controlling both factors at the transcriptional level, resulting in reduced airway inflammation and airway hyperreactivity in a mouse model of asthma [71]. Similarly, SP100030 at a concentration of 20 mg/kg/day (3 days, intraperitoneal prior to allergen challenge) inhibits allergen-induced AP-1 and NF-κB activation in sensitized Brown-Norway rats [72]. In this animal model, AP-1/NF-κB inhibition seemed to be CD8(+) T cell specific and resulted in downregulation of mRNA of both Th1 and Th2 cytokines *in vivo*, but did not inhibit allergen-induced airway eosinophilia or bronchial hyperresponsiveness [72].

Several well-known drugs have recently been reported to inhibit the binding of AP-1 to its DNA binding sequences, but the underlying mechanism remains unclear. Cyclosporin A suppressed the DNA-binding activity of AP-1 to the NF-AT/AP-1 site in the IL-5 gene promoter [67]. In human epithelial cells the macrolide clarithromycin has been reported to repress IL-8 gene transcription by preventing binding of AP-1 to its DNA consensus sequence [73]. The adrenal steroid dehydroepiandrosterone and its analogue 16 α-bromoepiandrosterone reduced growth of ASMC by decreasing DNA binding of AP-1 which led the author to suggest that non-glucocorticoid steroids may be a new tool in asthma therapy [74]. Decoy oligonucleotides have also been used to trap activated AP-1 in the cytosol thereby inhibiting its transport into the nucleus and the binding to its DNA consensus sequence [75].

PEROXISOME PROLIFERATOR-ACTIVATED RECEPTOR

PPAR-isoproteins, PPAR-α, -δ, -γ, -ζ, interact with the GR and with C/EBPs and may have a similar critical role in the pathology of asthma as the GR and CEBPs [26, 76]. PPAR-γ is mainly expressed in airway epithelium following antigen sensitization [77]. PPARs and C/EBPs play a central but yet to be resolved function in the balance of cell proliferation–differentiation, as has been demonstrated in adipocytes and suggested for other cell types. With regard to inflammation, C/EBP-α and PPAR-γ stimulate each other's expression in a positive feedback system, which interestingly can be interrupted by rapamycin [26, 78]. Cytokine expression in human bronchial smooth muscle cells is inhibited by PPAR-γ, but it is as yet unclear which role such a complex formed by C/EBP-α and PPAR-γ plays in the control mechanism of cytokines [78].

PPAR-γ agonists, glucocorticoids, and β_2-agonists synergistically suppress the expression of most asthma-associated cytokines at the transcriptional level and constitute a new therapeutic approach [76]. Furthermore, the benefit with regard to the development of the new anti-asthma drugs on the basis of PPARs is the fact that there are specific PPAR-isoform inhibitors and activators available [22]. However their safety in clinical use has yet to be demonstrated. The PPAR-γ agonists 15-deoxy-δ (12, 3)-PGJ(2) (15d-PGJ(2)) and troglitazone inhibited TNFα-induced production of eotaxin and monocyte chemotactic protein-1 but not of IL-8. Co-immunoprecipitation revealed that 15d-PGJ [79] induced a protein–protein interaction between PPAR-γ and the GR [76]. In an animal model of asthma ciglitazone and GW9662, two other PPAR-γ agonists, were administered by nebulization together with antigen challenge and decreased airway hyperresponsiveness, basement membrane thickness, mucus production, collagen deposition, and TGFβ synthesis significantly [77]. Importantly for asthma therapy, PPAR-γ prevents induction of Th2-dependent eosinophilic airway inflammation and might contribute to immune homeostasis in the lung [80].

PPAR-α is the second anti-inflammatory transcription factor in this family and has been shown to mediate the anti-inflammatory effect of statins on LPS-stimulated macrophages and neutrophils. PPAR-α may achieve this effect *via* the inhibition of NF-κB activity [81].

In contrast to PPAR-γ, and -α, PPAR-δ functions as a pro-inflammatory factor and binds to the same targets as PPAR-γ, and its enhanced expression would be of no benefit for asthma [21]. However, there are opposing results for the action of PPARs on inflammation. Under certain conditions the PPAR-γ agonist troglitazone counteracts the inhibitory effect of rapamycin on the PPAR-γ–C/EBP-α interaction, raising the possibility of problems when certain drugs may be combined for therapy [78]. PPAR-γ in particular seems to be a possible new anti-asthmatic factor, but has to be approached with caution because of its interaction with other transcription factors.

THE SIGNAL TRANSDUCER AND ACTIVATOR OF TRANSCRIPTION

The possible role of the JAK-STAT system was reviewed by Pernis and Rothman [82], and then the suggested correlation with asthma could be confirmed. TNFα and IL-4, two asthma-relevant cytokines, stimulate expression of the eotaxin gene by activating NF-κB and STAT6 [83]. TGFβ and IL-13 are also potent activators of STAT6 [84]. STAT6 signalling by IL-4 is essential for enhanced IgE production in asthma. A polymorphism in the STAT6 gene may be the first that could explain the long acknowledged genetic predisposition of high IgE levels in asthma patients and their siblings [85]. In an animal knockout model of asthma

STAT6$^{-/-}$ mice revealed significantly reduced airway responsiveness, low eosinophil infiltration and a shift from Th2 to Th1 cytokines [86].

The action of STAT6 is inhibited by glucocorticoids but the underlying mechanism is unclear [87, 88] and no other specific inhibitors for STAT6 have so far been reported.

Apart from STAT6, the other members of the STAT family and their link to asthma and inflammation are not well-studied. STAT3 seems to participate in IL-6 receptor gp130 mediated signalling [89], but also in the production of IL-10 which leads to inhibition of IgE synthesis in dendritic cells [90]. In a population study, a link was found between STAT3 polymorphisms and FEV$_1$ and lung function in asthma patients [91]. A polymorphism suggested a link between STAT4 and asthma [92, 93] and had been assessed in a cohort of 502 asthma patients and 164 controls, indicating its relevance for IgE control in response to house dust mite [92]. STAT5 was suggested to control proliferation of lymphocytes in two asthma animal models [94, 95]

GATA-3

GATA-3 was identified as a cell lineage specific factor selectively expressed and activated in the Th2 lineage as a consequence of STAT6 activation [96, 97]. GATA-3 is upregulated in asthmatic lung where it was associated with increased IL-5 expression [98]. Its expression can be induced by allergens such as ragweed pollen [99], and it activates the expression of IL-4, -5, and -13, all Th2 cytokines, by an IL-4 independent pathway [100–102]. However, its role in inflammation seems to be cell type specific since it is not upregulated by stimulation in lung structural cells [103].

In a mouse asthma model downregulation of GATA-3 by antisense oligonucleotides resulted in a blockade of GATA-3 expression and abrogated signs of lung inflammation such as eosinophil infiltration and Th2 cytokine production [104]. There are no known synthetic inhibitors of GATA-3. GATA-3 is assumed to be a major differentiation factor for Th1 and Th2 cells although its contribution to allergen-induced airway remodelling could not be supported in another mouse model [105]. It also became apparent that GATA-3 alone seems to be less effective in the regulation of asthma-related cytokines IL-4, -5 and -13, which needed its interaction with additional transcription factors Gfi-1 and STAT5 [106]. Furthermore, a study using high-altitude asthma therapy found that the expression of GATA-3 did not change while the severity of asthma and cytokine release was significantly reduced [107].

SERUM RESPONSE FACTOR

Serum response factor (SRF) seems to control smooth muscle cell differentiation, apoptosis, and proliferation and has been reviewed by Camoretti-Mercado *et al.* [108]. However, to exert its effects on smooth muscle cell specific proteins such as SM22, tetelokin and smooth muscle α-actin SRF requires interaction with other transcription factors, e.g. Elk-1 [109] and possibly Smads [110]. A summary of the potential interactions is shown in Figure 3.1.

SMADS

Smads are assumed to be one of the major cellular signal transducers of TGFβ and are therefore of interest in asthma. As mentioned above, it had been suggested that Smad7 interacts with SRF to control smooth muscle cell differentiation [110]. Smad7 inhibits the signalling cascade triggered by TGFβ *via* Smad2/3 and Smad4 linked to cell proliferation and thereby mediates some effects of glucocorticoids on inflammatory cytokine expression, IL-4, -13 and eotaxin [111]. Smad2 has a yet to be defined role in TGFβ mediated tissue remodelling [112, 113].

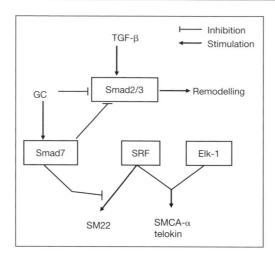

Figure 3.1 Multiple transcription factor interactions may occur in asthma.

NUCLEAR FACTOR E2 P45-RELATED FACTOR 2/ANTI-OXIDANT RESPONSE ELEMENT

Nrf2/anti-oxidant response element (ARE) is a transcription factor involved in the oxidative stress response which has also been suggested as a target for asthma therapy [114, 115]. Nrf2/ARE is assumed to induce anti-oxidant phase II enzyme expression which protects against the pro-inflammatory effects of particulate air pollutants in allergic inflammation of the lung including asthma [116, 117]. In response to oxidative stress Nrf2 can escape its proteosomal degradation and accumulate in the nucleus and therefore it was suggested that stimulation of Nrf2 may be beneficial in inflammatory diseases such as asthma [118]. Interestingly disruption of the Nrf2 gene in an animal model caused an increase in Th2 cells, IL-4 and -13 synthesis with an even stronger effect in asthmatic animals [119].

TRANSCRIPTION FACTORS WITH NON-CONFIRMED LINKS TO ASTHMA

EARLY GROWTH RESPONSE 1

Fast activation of early growth response 1 (Egr-1) by pro-inflammatory mediators such as platelet-derived growth factor (PDGF) and angiotensin II has been reported [120, 121]. While previously Egr-1 was assumed to be a T cell specific transcription factor, its expression was induced by angiotensin II in human ASMC which suggested a role in asthma [120]. Further studies also demonstrated Egr-1 expression in airway epithelial cells and its function to mediate inflammatory gene activity [121]. However, in the latter study the role of Egr-1 in asthma was not confirmed.

ETS-1, -2, -3

Ets-1 is a T cell and mast cell specific transcription factor and it had been suggested that it is linked to asthma and other chronic inflammatory diseases [122]. Ets-1 raised some interest as it regulates the autocrine loop of IL-3 and GM-CSF [122] and also TNFα-induced synthesis of matrix metalloproteinase-9 and tenascin which could contribute to remodelling in asthma [123]. Ets-2 and -3 are epithelium specific transcription factors but their possible role in asthma was not confirmed by polymorphism analysis in 311 asthma patients and 117 controls of Caucasian origin [124].

INTERFERON REGULATORY FACTOR

Interferon regulatory factors (IRFs) have a potential role in the regulation of IgE and IL-4 synthesis and therefore became of interest for asthma research. IRF-1 deficiency was linked with elevated Th2 cytokines, but a polymorphism analysis did not support the link of IRF-1 and asthma or atopy [125]. IFR-2, however, may have the potential to participate in the maternal inheritance of the IgE high affinity receptor [126].

SUMMARY

Several transcription factors have been identified as important regulators of the immune response, inflammation and airway remodelling and a summary of their interactions is provided in Figure 3.2. The inhibition or stimulation of a specific transcription factor in order to cure asthma or control its symptoms, while avoiding the side-effects of standard drugs such as inhaled glucocorticoids and β₂-agonists has not yet been realised. Although some of the transcription factors seem to be valid targets (NF-κB, Nrf2, or STAT6) or tools (PPAR-γ, -α and C/EBP-α) for new therapeutic approaches it is too early to draw conclusions. At this point, since all the described transcription factors play a central role in tissue and organ

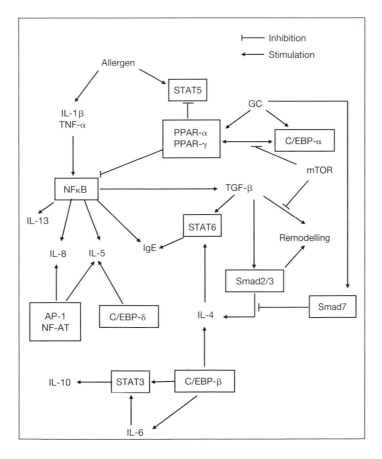

Figure 3.2 Transcription factors are important regulators of the immune response, inflammation and airway remodelling.

homeostasis, a long-term general suppression or overexpression, as would be needed for asthma therapy, would be most likely to cause severe side-effects in other organs.

Cell type specific application of decoy or antisense oligonucleotides for NF-κB, Nrf2 or STAT6, or specific agonists for PPAR-γ and -α may help to control the inflammatory response in lung epithelial cells and infiltrated immune cells, but an additional effect on other resident cells of the lung with unwanted side-effects cannot be excluded and a beneficial effect over known anti-asthma drugs has first to be proven. In order to progress with such novel therapeutic strategies, the only option seems to be to link transcription factor inhibitors/activators to a cell type specific delivery system, similar to those used in tumour therapy. However, such systems are mostly at an early stage of development and need further development.

REFERENCES

1. WHO/NHLBI Workshop Report 1995. Global strategy for asthma management and prevention. National Institute of Health, National Heart, Lung and Blood Institute, Bethesda, MD. Publication No. 95-3659.
2. Black J, Marthan R, Armour C, Johnson P. Is airway hyperresponsiveness a smooth muscle abnormality? *Prog Clin Biol Res* 1988; 263:267–280.
3. Fish JE, Peters SP. Asthma severity: histopathologic correlations. *Drugs Today (Barc)*. 1999; 35:585–594.
4. Sidebotham HJ, Roche WR. Asthma deaths; persistent and preventable mortality. *Histopathology* 2003; 43:105–117.
5. Mosmann TR, Cherwinski H, Bond MW, Giedlin MA, Coffman RL. Two types of murine helper T cell clone. I. Definition according to profiles of lymphokine activities and secreted proteins. *J Immunol* 1986; 136:2348–2357.
6. Hamid Q, Azzawi M, Ying S et al. Expression of mRNA for interleukin-5 in mucosal bronchial biopsies from asthma. *J Clin Invest* 1991; 87:1541–1546.
7. Robinson DS, Hamid Q, Ying S et al. Predominant TH2-like bronchoalveolar T-lymphocyte population in atopic asthma. *N Engl J Med* 1992; 326:298–304.
8. Ying S, Durham SR, Corrigan CJ, Hamid Q, Kay AB. Phenotype of cells expressing mRNA for TH2-type (interleukin 4 and interleukin 5) and TH1-type (interleukin 2 and interferon gamma) cytokines in bronchoalveolar lavage and bronchial biopsies from atopic asthmatic and normal control subjects. *Am J Respir Cell Mol Biol* 1995; 12:477–487.
9. Umetsu DT and DeKruyff RH. TH1 and TH2 CD4+ cells in human allergic diseases. *J Allergy Clin Immunol* 1997; 100:1–6.
10. Hakonarson H, Maskeri N, Carter C, Grunstein MM. Regulation of TH1- and TH2-type cytokine expression and action in atopic asthmatic sensitized airway smooth muscle. *J Clin Invest* 1999; 103:1077–1087.
11. Laaksonen K, Waris M, Makela MJ, Terho EO, Savolainen J. In vitro kinetics of allergen- and microbe-induced IL-4 and IFN-gamma mRNA expression in PBMC of pollen-allergic patients. *Allergy* 2003; 58:62–66.
12. Prescott SL. New concepts of cytokines in asthma: is the Th2/Th1 paradigm out the window? *Allergy* 2003; 58:62–66.
13. Johnson PR, Roth M, Tamm M et al. Airway smooth muscle cell proliferation is increased in asthma. *Am J Respir Crit Care Med* 2001; 164:474–477.
14. Roth M, Johnson PR, Borger P et al. Dysfunctional interaction of C/EBPalpha and the glucocorticoid receptor in asthmatic bronchial smooth-muscle cells. *N Engl J Med* 2004; 351:560–574.
15. Lilly CM, Tateno H, Oguma T, Israel E, Sonna LA. Effects of allergen challenge on airway epithelial cell gene expression. *Am J Respir Crit Care Med* 2005; 171:579–586.
16. Barnes PJ, Adcock IM. Transcription factors and asthma. *Eur Respir J* 1998; 12:221–234.
17. Rahman I, MacNee W. Role of transcription factors in inflammatory lung diseases. *Thorax* 1998; 53:601–612.
18. Barnes PJ. Nuclear factor-kappa B. *Int J Biochem Cell Biol* 1997; 29:867–870.
19. Li-Weber M, Giaisi M, Krammer PH. Roles of CCAAT/enhancer-binding protein in transcriptional regulation of the human IL-5 gene. *Eur J Immunol* 2001; 31:3694–3703.
20. Benayoun L, Letuve S, Druilhe A et al. Regulation of peroxisome proliferator-activated receptor gamma expression in human asthmatic airways: relationship with proliferation, apoptosis, and airway remodeling. *Am J Respir Crit Care Med* 2001; 164(pt 1):1487–1494.

21. Woerly G, Honda K, Loyens M *et al.* Peroxisome proliferator-activated receptors alpha and gamma down-regulate allergic inflammation and eosinophil activation. *J Exp Med* 2003; 198:411–421.

22. Trifilieff A, Bench A, Hanley M, Bayley D, Campbell E, Whittaker P. PPAR-alpha and -gamma but not -delta agonists inhibit airway inflammation in a murine model of asthma: in vitro evidence for an NF-kappaB-independent effect. *Br J Pharmacol* 2003; 139:163–171.

23. Popescu F-D. New asthma drugs acting on gene expression. *J Cell Mol Med* 2003; 7:475–486.

24. De Boesscher K, Vanden Berghe W, Haegeman G. The interplay between the glucocorticoid receptor and Nuclear factor-KB or activator protein-1: molecular mechanisms for gene repression. *Endocr Rev* 2003; 24:488–522.

25. Cassel TN, Nord M. C/EBP transcription factors in the lung epithelium. *Am J Physiol Lung Cell Mol Physiol* 2003; 285:L773–L781.

26. Barlier-Mur AM, Chailley-Heu B, Pinteur C, Henrion-Caude A, Delacourt C, Bourbon JR. Maturational factors modulate transcription factors CCAAT/enhancer-binding proteins alpha, beta, delta, and peroxisome proliferator-activated receptor-gamma in fetal rat lung epithelial cells. *Am J Respir Cell Mol Biol* 2003; 29:620–626.

27. Rosenberg E, Li F, Reisher SR *et al.* Members of the C/EBP transcription factor family stimulate expression of the human and rat surfactant protein A (SP-A) genes. *Biochim Biophys Acta* 2002; 1575:82–90.

28. Hu B, Wu Z, Jin H, Hashimoto N, Liu T, Phan SH. CCAAT/enhancer-binding protein beta isoforms and the regulation of alpha-smooth muscle actin gene expression by IL-1 beta. *J Immunol* 2004; 173:4661–4668.

29. Takeji M, Kawada N, Moriyama T *et al.* CCAAT/enhancer-binding protein delta contributes to myofibroblast transdifferentiation and renal disease progression. *J Am Soc Nephrol* 2004; 15:2383–2390.

30. Hamaguchi-Tsuru E, Nobumoto A, Hirose N *et al.* Development and functional analysis of eosinophils from murine embryonic stem cells. *Br J Haematol* 2004; 124:819–827.

31. Hein H, Schluter C, Kulke R, Christophers E, Schroder JM, Bartels J. Genomic organization, sequence, and transcriptional regulation of the human eotaxin gen. *Biochem Biophys Res Commun* 1997; 237:537–542.

32. Berberich-Siebelt F, Klein-Hessling S, Hepping N *et al.* C/EBPbeta enhances IL-4 but impairs IL-2 and IFN-gamma induction in T cells. *Eur J Immunol* 2000; 30:2576–2585.

33. Borger P, Black JL, Roth M. Asthma and the CCAAT-enhancer binding proteins: a holistic view on airway inflammation and remodeling. *J Allergy Clin Immunol* 2002; 110:841–846.

34. Ruediger JJ, Roth M, Bihl MP *et al.* Glucocorticoids act through a C/EBP-α-glucocorticoid receptor complex. *FASEB J* 2002; 16:177–184.

35. Roth M, Johnson PRA, King G *et al.* Synergism between glucocorticoids and β₂-agonists on bronchial airway smooth muscle cells through synchronised cellular signalling. *Lancet* 2002, 360:1293–1299.

36. Park IN, Cho IJ, Kim SG. Ceramide negatively regulates glutathione S-transferase gene transactivation via repression of hepatic nuclear factor-1 that is degraded by the ubiquitin proteasome system. *Mol Pharmacol* 2004; 65:1475–1484.

37. Balasubramanian S, Eckert RL. Green tea polyphenol and curcumin inversely regulate human involucrin promoter activity via opposing effects on CCAAT/enhancer-binding protein function. *J Biol Chem* 2004; 279:24007–24014.

38. Lagace DC, Nachtigal MW. Inhibition of histone deacetylase activity by valproic acid blocks adipogenesis. *J Biol Chem* 2004; 279:18851–18860.

39. Kelkenberg U, Wagner AH, Sarhaddar J, Hecker M, von der Leyen HE. CCAAT/enhancer-binding protein decoy oligodeoxynucleotide inhibition of macrophage-rich vascular lesion formation in hypercholesterolemic rabbits. *Arterioscler Thromb Vasc Biol* 2002; 22:949–954.

40. Wagner AH, Krzesz R, Gao D, Schroeder C, Cattaruzza M, Hecker M. Decoy oligodeoxynucleotide characterization of transcription factors controlling endothelin-B receptor expression in vascular smooth muscle cells. *Mol Pharmacol* 2000; 58:1333–1340.

41. Quarcoo D, Hamelmann E. Transcription factors: new targets for antiallergic therapy. *Pathobiology* 2002–2003; 70:293–296.

42. Kumar A, Takada Y, Boriek AM, Aggarwal BB. Nuclear factor-kappaB: its role in health and disease. *J Mol Med* 2004; 82:434–448.

43. Yamamoto Y, Gaynor RB. IkappaB kinases: key regulators of the NF-kappaB pathway. *Trends Biochem Sci* 2004; 29:72–79.

44. Funkhouser AW, Kang JA, Tan A *et al.* Rhinovirus 16 3C protease induces interleukin-8 and granulocyte-macrophage colony-stimulating factor expression in human bronchial epithelial cells. *Pediatr Res* 2004; 55:13–18.

94. Li G, Liu Z, Ran P, Qiu J, Zhong N. Activation of signal transducer and activator of transcription 5 (STAT5) in splenocyte proliferation of asthma mice induced by ovalbumin. *Cell Mol Immunol* 2004; 1:471–474.

95. Eriksson U, Egermann U, Bihl MP *et al.* Human bronchial epithelium controls TH2 responses by TH1-induced, nitric oxide-mediated STAT5 dephosphorylation: implications for the pathogenesis of asthma. *J Immunol* 2005; 175:2715–2720.

96. Finotto S, Glimcher L. T cell directives for transcriptional regulation in asthma. *Springer Semin Immunopathol* 2004; 25:281–294.

97. Taha R, Hamid Q, Cameron L, Olivenstein R. T helper type 2 cytokine receptors and associated transcription factors GATA-3, c-MAF, and signal transducer and activator of transcription factor-6 in induced sputum of atopic asthmatic patients. *Chest* 2003; 123:2074–2082.

98. Nakamura Y, Ghaffar O, Olivenstein R *et al.* Gene expression of the GATA-3 transcription factor is increased in atopic asthma. *J Allergy Clin Immunol* 1999; 103(pt 1):215–222.

99. Justice JP, Borchers MT, Lee JJ, Rowan WH, Shibata Y, Van Scott MR. Ragweed-induced expression of GATA-3, IL-4, and IL-5 by eosinophils in the lungs of allergic C57BL/6J mice. *Am J Physiol Lung Cell Mol Physiol* 2002; 282:L302–L309.

100. Kishikawa H, Sun J, Choi A, Miaw SC, Ho IC. The cell type-specific expression of the murine IL-13 gene is regulated by GATA-3. *J Immunol* 2001; 167:4414–4420.

101. Zhang DH, Cohn L, Ray P, Bottomly K, Ray A. Transcription factor GATA-3 is differentially expressed in murine Th1 and Th2 cells and controls Th2-specific expression of the interleukin-5 gene. *J Biol Chem* 1997; 272:21597–21603.

102. Zhang DH, Yang L, Cohn L *et al.* Inhibition of allergic inflammation in a murine model of asthma by expression of a dominant-negative mutant of GATA-3. *Immunity* 1999; 11:473–482.

103. Caramori G, Lim S, Ito K *et al.* Expression of GATA family of transcription factors in T-cells, monocytes and bronchial biopsies. *Eur Respir J* 2001; 18:466–473.

104. Finotto S, De Sanctis GT, Lehr HA *et al.* Treatment of allergic airway inflammation and hyperresponsiveness by antisense-induced local blockade of GATA-3 expression. *J Exp Med* 2001; 193:1247–1260.

105. Kiwamoto T, Ishii Y, Morishima Y *et al.* Transcription factors T-bet and GATA-3 regulate development of airway remodeling. *Am J Respir Crit Care Med* 2006; 174:142–151.

106. Zhu J, Yamane H, Cote-Sierra J, Guo L, Paul WE. GATA-3 promotes Th2 responses through three different mechanisms: induction of Th2 cytokine production, selective growth of Th2 cells and inhibition of Th1 cell-specific factors. *Cell Res* 2006; 16:3–10.

107. Karagiannidis C, Hense G, Rueckert B *et al.* High-altitude climate therapy reduces local airway inflammation and modulates lymphocyte activation. *Scand J Immunol* 2006; 63:304–310.

108. Camoretti-Mercado B, Dulin NO, Solway J. Serum response factor function and dysfunction in smooth muscle. *Respir Physiol Neurobiol* 2003; 137:223–235.

109. Zhou J, Hu G, Herring BP. Smooth muscle-specific genes are differentially sensitive to inhibition by Elk-1. *Mol Cell Biol* 2005; 25:9874–9885.

110. Camoretti-Mercado B, Fernandes DJ, Dewundara S *et al.* Inhibition of TGFbeta-enhanced SRF-dependent transcription by SMAD7. *J Biol Chem* 2006; 281:20383–20392.

111. McMillan SJ, Xanthou G, Lloyd CM. Therapeutic administration of Budesonide ameliorates allergen-induced airway remodelling. *Clin Exp Allergy* 2005; 35:388–396.

112. Johnson PR, Burgess JK, Ge Q *et al.* Connective tissue growth factor induces extracellular matrix in asthmatic airway smooth muscle. *Am J Respir Crit Care Med* 2006; 173:32–41.

113. Karagiannidis C, Hense G, Martin C *et al.* Activin A is an acute allergen-responsive cytokine and provides a link to TGF-beta-mediated airway remodeling in asthma. *J Allergy Clin Immunol* 2006; 117:111–118.

114. Cho HY, Jedlicka AE, Reddy SP *et al.* Role of NRF2 in protection against hyperoxic lung injury in mice. *Am J Respir Cell Mol Biol* 2002; 26:175–182.

115. Cho HY, Reddy SP, Debiase A, Yamamoto M, Kleeberger SR. Gene expression profiling of NRF2-mediated protection against oxidative injury. *Free Radic Biol Med* 2005; 38:325–343.

116. Chen XL, Kunsch C. Induction of cytoprotective genes through Nrf2/antioxidant response element pathway: a new therapeutic approach for the treatment of inflammatory diseases. *Curr Pharm Des* 2004; 10:879–891.

117. Li N, Alam J, Venkatesan MI *et al.* Nrf2 is a key transcription factor that regulates antioxidant defense in macrophages and epithelial cells: protecting against the proinflammatory and oxidizing effects of diesel exhaust chemicals. *J Immunol* 2004; 173:3467–3481.

118. Li N, Nel AE. Role of the Nrf2-mediated signaling pathway as a negative regulator of inflammation: implications for the impact of particulate pollutants on asthma. *Antioxid Redox Signal* 2006; 8:88–98.

119. Rangasamy T, Guo J, Mitzner WA *et al.* Disruption of Nrf2 enhances susceptibility to severe airway inflammation and asthma in mice. *J Exp Med* 2005; 202:47–59.

120. McKay S, de Jongste JC, Saxena PR, Sharma HS. Angiotensin II induces hypertrophy of human airway smooth muscle cells: expression of transcription factors and transforming growth factor-beta1. *Am J Respir Cell Mol Biol* 1998; 18:823–833.

121. Hjoberg J, Le L, Imrich A *et al.* Induction of early growth-response factor 1 by platelet-derived growth factor in human airway smooth muscle. *Am J Physiol Lung Cell Mol Physiol* 2004; 286:L817–L825.

122. McKinlay LH, Tymms MJ, Thomas RS *et al.* The role of Ets-1 in mast cell granulocyte–macrophage colony-stimulating factor expression and activation. *J Immunol* 1998; 161:4098–4105.

123. Nakamura Y, Esnault S, Maeda T, Kelly EA, Malter JS, Jarjour NN. Ets-1 regulates TNF-alpha-induced matrix metalloproteinase-9 and tenascin expression in primary bronchial fibroblasts. *J Immunol* 2004; 172:1945–1952.

124. Baron RM, Palmer LJ, Tantisira K *et al.* Epithelium. *Am J Respir Crit Care Med* 2002; 166:927–932.

125. Noguchi E, Shibasaki M, Arinami T *et al.* Mutation screening of interferon regulatory factor 1 gene (IRF-1) as a candidate gene for atopy/asthma. *Clin Exp Allergy* 2000; 30:1562–1567.

126. Traherne JA, Hill MR, Hysi P *et al.* LD mapping of maternally and non-maternally derived alleles and atopy in FcepsilonRI-beta. *Hum Mol Genet* 2003; 12:2577–2585.

4

Is IKKβ a feasible therapeutic target for allergic asthma?

Y. Amrani

INTRODUCTION

The maintenance of airway inflammation is a hallmark of allergic asthma, and anti-inflammatory drugs, such as steroids, remain the sole effective treatment to treat the disease. Steroid treatment also has downsides: failure to treat a subset of asthmatic patients (called cortico-resistant) as well as serious side-effects in severe patients requiring long-term treatment with high oral doses. Alternative therapeutic strategies are therefore needed to more safely suppress the ongoing airway inflammation in asthma. Acting on defined signalling molecules that are critical for the orchestration and/or perpetuation of the inflammatory process may represent a promising therapeutic approach. The ubiquitously expressed transcription factor nuclear factor-κB (NF-κB) plays a foremost role in the expression of a number of cellular genes involved in immune, inflammatory pro- and anti-apoptotic responses. This observation prompted many investigators to suggest that interfering with the NF-κB activating cascade could have therapeutic implications for treating different chronic inflammatory diseases including rheumatoid arthritis and inflammatory bowel disease. In recent years, studies in both human and animals demonstrated that activation and/or expression of NF-κB are dramatically increased in structural lung tissues as well as in infiltrated inflammatory cells in asthma. The importance of NF-κB in the pathogenesis of asthma was further confirmed in animal models of asthma where a variety of NF-κB inhibitors significantly suppressed allergen-induced airway inflammation and airway hyperresponsiveness, the two cardinal features of asthma. This review will not describe the molecular mechanisms that regulate NF-κB pathways but will focus on the current evidence in the literature that supports the therapeutic potential of NF-κB inhibitors in allergic asthma, with emphasis on the obligatory molecules for NF-κB activation: the upstream activating kinase IKKβ (or IKK2).

IKKβ IS A NECESSARY STEP IN THE REGULATION OF INFLAMMATORY SIGNALS

DIFFERENTIAL ROLE OF IKKβ AND IKKα IN MEDIATING NF-κB-DEPENDENT INFLAMMATORY RESPONSES

NF-κB, which belongs to the Rel protein family comprising RelA (p65), RelB, c-Rel, NF-κB1 (p50) and NF-κB2 (p52), regulates the expression of a plethora of genes involved in inflammation [1, 2]. In most cells, Rel/NF-κB is present in the cytoplasm as an inactive form

Yassine Amrani, PhD, Research Assistant and Professor of Medicine, Pulmonary, Allergy and Critical Care Division, University of Pennsylvania, Philadelphia, Pennsylvania, USA

through the association with inhibitory proteins called inhibitors of NF-κB (IκBs), the function of which is to mask the NF-κB nuclear localization signal. Various stimuli through the activation of IκB upstream kinase (IKK) induce rapid phosphorylation, ubiquitination, and degradation of IκBs, resulting in nuclear translocation of NF-κB proteins and transcription activation. The IκB kinase (IKK) complex, an obligatory NF-κB activating step, is composed of a regulatory subunit IKKγ and two different catalytic subunits called IKKα (or IKK1) and IKKβ (or IKK2) that have similar structures (52% homology). IKKα and IKKβ are themselves phosphorylated and activated by different kinases called NF-κB-inducing kinase (NIK) and transforming growth factor (TGF)β-activated kinase 1 (TAK1), respectively [1–4]. The role of each IKK in the regulation of NF-κB-dependent inflammatory genes is still a matter of extensive research. The classical or canonical NF-κB activating pathway involves both IKKβ and IKKγ (NEMO) of the IKK complex and is typically activated by pro-inflammatory stimuli such as tumour necrosis factor (TNF)α and interleukin (IL)-1β. In contrast, IKKα, the downstream target of NIK, participates in the alternative NF-κB activation *via* the p100 processing (to mature p52) which is triggered mainly by CD40, B cell receptor for BAFF (BAFFR), and lymphotoxin β receptor [5–8]. Genetic studies showed the importance of IKKα in lymphoid organ development and B cell maturation [9]. In contrast to the acknowledged role of IKKβ in NF-κB-dependent inflammatory genes, there are still gaps to be filled about the implication of IKKα in this canonical pathway. Recent convincing studies showed that IKKα, through its ability to change chromatin structure, participates in the transcriptional regulation of TNFα-inducible genes [10–13]. More surprising is the latest interesting report describing a protective role of IKKα in suppressing inflammation. It was found that mice expressing the mutated form of IKKα have an augmented susceptibility to bacterial infection when compared to wild type mice [14]. Another debate resides in the nature of the upstream kinases that activate IKK activation, such as NIK [15]. Knockout studies, however, demonstrated the failure of NIK-deficient cells to respond to canonical activators but its implication in the alternative NF-κB-activating pathway [16]. These studies indicate that in addition to being critical for the alternative NF-κB pathway, IKKα may also modulate the canonical activation of NF-κB target genes induced by inflammatory cytokines. Figure 4.1 shows a schematic description of the role of IKKs in the NF-κB-activating pathways and their physiological roles.

INTRICACIES SURROUNDING THE UPSTREAM PROTEINS THAT REGULATE IKKβ FUNCTION

Despite intense research in the field, the precise molecular mechanisms that regulate IKKβ function have not been completely characterized. Numerous reports discovered that a surprisingly increased number of different proteins can in fact control NF-κB pathways in part *via* direct physical interaction with IKKβ. Earlier reports demonstrated that NF-κB activation by TNFα can occur through pathways that are independent of the traditional TRADD/TRAF-2 pathway, including members of IL-1β signalling complex such as IRAK (interleukin receptor-associated kinase)-TRAF-6 proteins, which mediates IL-1β-induced IKKβ activation [4]. The latest studies confirmed that TRAF-6 is essential for NF-κB activation, in part, through its capacity to physically assemble with IKKβ [17–19]. The other kinase TAK1, also associated with both IL-1β- and TGFβ-signalling pathways, also mediates IKKβ-dependent activation of NF-κB in response to different stimuli including TNFα [20]. TAK1-deficient embryonic fibroblasts failed to activate NF-κB pathways in response to TNFR1, IL-1R, TLR3 and TLR4 stimulation strongly suggesting a more ubiquitous role for TAK1 in the canonical activation of NF-κB [21]. Ea *et al.* [22] found that TIFA (TRAF-interacting protein with a forkhead-associated domain) is a novel intermediate protein that stimulates TAK1 and IKKβ activation indirectly *via* the activation of TRAF-6 ligase. Soond *et al.* [23] found a novel scaffolding protein, called TNFR1-Ubiquitous Scaffolding and Signalling Protein (TRUSS), that mediates TNFα-induced NF-κB activation in 3T3 cells *via* the interaction

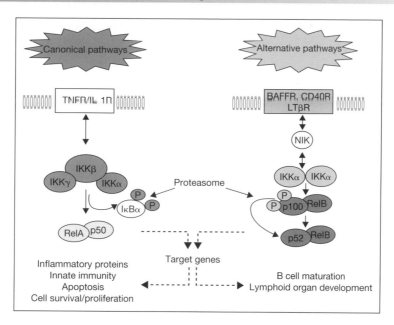

Figure 4.1 NF-κB activating pathways: two signalling pathways regulate NF-κB activation. The classical or canonical activation of NF-κB (p65/p50 heterodimer) results from the activation of IKKβ which phosphorylates and inactivates the cytosolic IκBα. IκBα is then degraded by the proteasome to free NF-κB that can translocate to the nucleus to activate a set of target genes essential for various cellular responses including inflammation (cytokines, adhesion molecules), apoptosis, cell survival and cell proliferation. The alternative pathway involves NIK-dependent activation of IKKα homodimers which then stimulates the processing of p100 by the proteasome leading to the mature subunit p52. RelB/p52 heterodimers migrate to the nucleus to activate genes that are important for B cell maturation and lymphoid organ development.

with NF-κB-regulatory proteins, TRADD, TRAF2 and surprisingly with all three IKK sub-units. Another report uncovered a novel function for PAX-4 (p21 activated kinase), a protein that has important roles in embryonic development, cell adhesion and cytoskeleton organi-zation. It was shown that PAX-4 mediates TNFα-induced pro-survival signals, in part *via* its ability to activate NF-κB in a TRADD-dependent manner [24]. Whether PAX-4 directly binds to IKKβ to activate NF-κB remains to be investigated. Additional recently described IKKβ regulatory proteins include the kinase NAP (NAK-associated protein 1) [25] and NIBP (NIK and IKKβ-binding protein) [26] that were reported to act as signalling amplifiers of NF-κB-dependent cellular responses including neuronal differentiation, and cell survival. These observations suggest that the role of IKKβ in NF-κB function is complex and requires the intimate involvement of a multitude of regulatory proteins that have just recently been uncovered (Figure 4.2).

IKKβ–NF-κB SIGNALLING PATHWAYS: A VITAL AXIS IN THE PATHOGENESIS OF ALLERGIC ASTHMA

TECHNIQUES USED TO ASSESS NF-κB FUNCTION IN THE LUNGS

NF-κB is considered a central regulator of inflammation and immune processes, indubitably *via* its transcriptional regulation of several inflammatory genes encoding for adhesion mol-ecules, cytokines and chemokines [27, 28]. A growing number of 'lung' investigators have

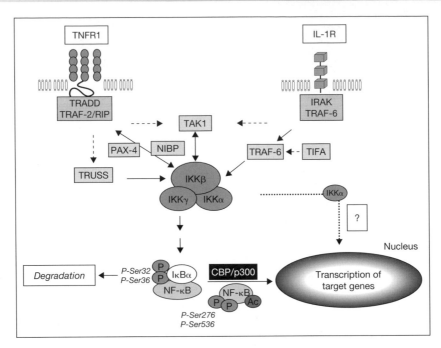

Figure 4.2 Complexity of the upstream signalling mechanisms that regulate IKK function in cytokine-induced inflammatory gene expression: in cytokine-stimulated cells, IKKβ activation leads to the phosphorylation and degradation of IκBα allowing the unbound NF-κB to translocate to the nucleus where it can regulate gene transcription. In the nucleus, a set of phosphorylation (P), acetylation (Ac) as well as recruitment of different co-activators (CBP/p300) enhance NF-κB transcriptional activity. IKKα was also described to be part of the classical activation of NF-κB *via* its chromatin-modifying function (?). Recent evidence shows that IKKβ function is regulated by a variety of upstream regulatory proteins that can affect NF-κB activation *via* direct protein–protein interaction with IKKβ. Upon stimulation by TNFα, the recently uncovered proteins TRUSS (TNFR1-Ubiquitous Scaffolding and Signalling Protein), PAX-4 (p21 activated kinase), NIBP (NIK and IKKβ-binding protein) were shown to directly or indirectly assemble with IKKβ. TAK1, a member of both TGFβ and IL-1 receptor signalling pathways, has been shown to be involved in mediating TNFα-induced NF-κB activation. TAK1 usually serves as an adapter bridge between TRAF-6 and IKK complex in the IL-1R signalling. Another report showed, however, that TRAF-6 could also activate NF-κB pathways through its direct physical interaction with IKKβ. The implication of TRAF-6 in IKKβ function seems to be very complex since another protein called TIFA (TRAF-interacting protein with a forkhead-associated domain) was recently described to be essential in TAK1 and IKKβ activation *via* TRAF-6 oligomerization and ubiquitination. Together, these studies shows the complexity of protein–protein interactions between IKKβ and upstream signalling molecules in the regulation of NF-κB activation and function.

examined whether abnormal NF-κB activity may exist in asthmatics vs. normal subjects and whether or not these changes correlate with the disease state and/or progression. The majority of studies have used different experimental strategies to examine the presence of functionally active NF-κB in the asthmatic airways: (i) *immunohistochemistry* techniques applied to bronchial biopsies to determine the tissue distribution of activated NF-κB in the airways, (ii) *gel shift* assays using nuclear fractions from cells or biopsies to assess NF-κB/DNA binding activity and, (iii) *immunoblot* analysis to determine any quantitative changes in NF-κB protein (p65 or p50 subunit) content. Another elegant approach is the use of NF-κB receptor mice that stably expresses a transgene containing two copies of the κB motifs from the κ light chain enhancer in front of a minimal fos promoter driving the luciferase gene [29]. These mice can be used to monitor NF-κB activation in different tissues and experimental conditions. A recent study used these reporter mice to show an increased NF-κB activity in sensitized lungs after allergen treatment [30].

ABERRANT NF-κB ACTIVATION IN HUMAN AND EXPERIMENTAL ASTHMA

INCREASED NF-κB ACTIVATION IN ASTHMATIC PATIENTS

Different studies have convincingly demonstrated the presence of activated NF-κB in 'asthmatic' lungs especially in the epithelium as well as in numerous inflammatory cells present within the submucosa including T cells, mast cells, macrophages and eosinophils [31–33]. Interestingly, some of these studies have been performed in patients who did not receive any inhaled or oral corticosteroids, suggesting that mechanisms that lead to persistent NF-κB activation are still present in stable subjects with mild asthma. *In vitro* studies using isolated asthmatic epithelial cells or peripheral blood mononuclear cells (PBMCs) confirmed that allergen exposure is a key event in stimulation of NF-κB activation [34–35]. Further studies reported that abnormal NF-κB activation could also be detected in other tissues such as the endothelium [31], or peripheral blood mononuclear cells [36]. More importantly, Gagliardo *et al.* [36], who performed their study in asthmatic patients at different stages of the disease (mild, moderate and severe), provided the first evidence of a strong correlation between the status of NF-κB activation and the severity of disease. Indeed, it was found that peripheral blood monocytes of severe asthmatics exhibited a greater NF-κB activity that was associated with an enhanced expression of key regulatory NF-κB molecules, p65 subunit and IKKβ as well as phosphorylation of IκBα [36]. Another important finding from these studies is the lack of effect of steroid treatment on the abnormal NF-κB activation in the airways. NF-κB binding activity was still present in alveolar macrophages or epithelium of asthmatics treated with inhaled fluticasone (500 μg twice daily, 4 weeks) or with prednisolone (1 mg/kg, 10 days) [33, 36]. Similarly, Hancox *et al.* [37] using gel shift assays found that a 6-week treatment with inhaled budesonide (400 μg twice daily) partially suppressed NF-κB activity in asthmatic lung biopsies [37]. In severe asthmatics, Vignola *et al.* [38] found an increased epithelial NF-κB activation despite the use of high doses of corticosteroids (1000 μg inhaled fluticasone and 10–80 mg daily oral prednisone) [38]. These studies show an aberrant steroid-insensitive NF-κB function in asthmatic airways, with functional and quantitative changes that seem to correlate with the severity of disease (Table 4.1).

INCREASED NF-κB ACTIVATION IN THE LUNGS OF DIFFERENT ANIMAL MODELS OF ASTHMA

The study of NF-κB in animal models of allergic asthma has led to the description of clinically relevant facts about NF-κB activity in asthmatic lungs, including the kinetics of activation, the potential stimuli, as well as the mechanisms that may explain its activation in asthmatics with stable conditions. Similar to the assumptions made with studies from asthmatic patients, several animal reports clearly supported the notion that allergen challenge is playing an essential role in the initiation of NF-κB activation in asthmatic airways [30, 39–44]. Poynter *et al.* [30] found that a single allergen challenge is able to induce a rapid NF-κB activation as well as NF-κB-inducible genes (MIP-2 and eotaxin) in ovalbumin-sensitized mice. The authors found that antigen exposure induced a rapid nuclear translocation of NF-κB p65 subunit that correlates with increased IKK activation in sensitized lungs; interestingly, both responses were detected within 15 min, and were sustained for up to 24 h following antigen exposure. Similarly, NF-κB activity dramatically increased in the bronchi of heaves-affected horses following allergen challenge, a response that was surprisingly maintained for up to 21 days despite the absence of allergen [42]. Another study from the same group also found that increased NF-κB activity also persists *in vitro* in cultured bronchial brushing samples derived from allergen-exposed horses for up to 24–48 h following

Table 4.1 NF-κB activation in asthmatic airways: sensitivity to steroids

Number of patients/ disease state	Steroid treatment	NF-κB status/ steroid sensitive	Positive tissue/cells	References
9/Stable	None	Nuclear staining	Epithelial cells Bronchial biopsies	Hart *et al.* [32]
10/Mild	Budesonide (400 μg twice, 8 weeks)	Increased p65/ sensitive Increased P-p65/ insensitive	Epithelium, T and B cells Eosinophils, macrophages	Wilson *et al.* [31]
7/Moderate	Budesonide (400 μg twice, 6 weeks)	Nuclear activation/ partial Sensitivity (34%)	Bronchial mucosa Samples	Hancox *et al.* [37]
6/Mild	None	Increased P-IκB	PBMC	Gagliardo *et al.* [36]
8/Moderate	Prednisolone (1 mg/kg, 10 days)	Increased P-IκB/ insensitive Increased p65/ insensitive Increased IKKβ/ insensitive	PBMC	Gagliardo *et al.* [36]
14/Severe	Prednisolone (1 mg/kg, daily) Beclomethasone, (3 mg, daily)	Increased P-IκB/ Increased p65/ insensitive Increased IKKβ/ insensitive	PBMC	Gagliardo *et al.* [36]
15/Stable	Fluticasone (500 μg twice, 4 weeks)	p65 staining/ insensitive Nuclear activation/ insensitive	Epithelium Alveolar macrophages	Hart *et al.* [33]

allergen challenge [43]. In addition, Lee *et al.* [40] reported that the increased NF-κB activity in the lung of sensitized mice could be maintained for up to 72 h after allergen inhalation. These studies demonstrated that NF-κB activation in allergen-exposed lungs is rapid and abnormally maintained for long time periods after allergen challenge. These observations are somewhat in agreement with studies performed in asthmatics who showed a similar maintenance of NF-κB activation in the airways of patients with stable conditions [31–33]. *In vitro* studies demonstrated that excessive production of pro-inflammatory stimuli such as TNFα or IL-1β as well as impaired synthesis of the NF-κB inhibitor, IκBα, could explain the sustained NF-κB activation observed in cells derived from asthmatic lungs [43]. Cysteinyl leukotrienes (cysLT) also seem to be important in mediating allergen-induced NF-κB activation as pre-treatment with the cysLT antagonist pranlukast completely abrogated this response in mononuclear cells [45]. Additional studies are clearly needed to define the factors and the molecular mechanisms that maintain NF-κB activation in the challenged animals.

THERAPEUTIC BENEFIT OF TARGETING NF-κB PATHWAYS IN ALLERGIC ASTHMA

In addition to describing NF-κB activation in asthmatic airway tissues, parallel studies have used different blocking approaches to evaluate the therapeutic potential of NF-κB inhibition in allergic asthma. As described below, several strategies have been used successfully to support the key contribution of NF-κB pathways in mediating allergen-induced airway inflammatory responses. Studies have used (i) knockout mice deficient in NF-κB/Rel genes, (ii) transgenic mice selectively overexpressing NF-κB regulatory proteins in the lung epithelial cells, and (iii) a variety of inhibitors; some acting directly on NF-κB proteins by blocking its nuclear translocation or increasing IκBα function, others by indirectly interfering with upstream regulatory kinases (IKKs), required for NF-κB activation.

EVIDENCE FROM THE USE OF TRANSGENIC MICE OR MICE DEFICIENT IN NF-κB/rel GENES

Studies using knockout mice showed that allergen-challenged mice deficient in the p50 subunit of NF-κB, classically composed of p65(relA)/p50 heterodimers, were incapable of mounting an eosinophilic airway inflammation, possibly because of their lack of production of T helper 2 (Th2) cytokines, IL-5 and eotaxin, when compared to the wild type controls [46]. A second study from the same group using the same p50-deficient mice demonstrated that, in fact, NF-κB was critical in mediating allergen-induced Th2 type cytokine (IL-4, IL-5, and IL-13) production by promoting lymphocyte Th2 differentiation via the upregulation of the transcription factor GATA3 [47]. Donovan et al. [44] confirmed the 'pro-asthmatic' role of NF-κB in T cells by showing that mice deficient in c-Rel protein, the Rel family member that is important for T cell activation and proliferation, failed to develop important features of asthma including airway inflammation and airway hyperresponsiveness.

The use of transgenic mice overexpressing the IκBα inhibitor in epithelial cells (under the transcriptional control of CC10 promoter) allowed others to show that blocking NF-κB activity specifically in the airway epithelium was sufficient to prevent the development of airway inflammation induced by either allergen [48] or lipopolysaccharide (LPS) [49]. Interestingly, the authors also made the observation that allergen-associated airway hyperresponsiveness, a cardinal feature of asthma, was unaffected despite complete NF-κB activation in the epithelium [48]. Among the first to implicate IKKs in the pathogenesis of asthma, Sadikot et al. [50] showed that overexpressing either IKKα and IKKβ kinases selectively in the epithelium (using intra-tracheal administration of replication-deficient expressing adenoviral vectors) led to increased NF-κB activation with subsequent inflammatory cytokine production and neutrophilic airway inflammation. These different observations suggest that abnormal activation of IKK leading to increased NF-κB-dependent signals could play a determinant function in the initiation and/or maintenance of airway inflammation in asthma.

EVIDENCE FROM THE IN VIVO USE OF NF-κB INHIBITORS

The putative role of NF-κB in inflammatory diseases also has been confirmed using a variety of soluble inhibitors. For example, the intranasal administration of MOL 294, a selective nonapeptide combined inhibitor of both NF-κB and AP-1, was found to reduce many pathological features associated with asthma, including airway eosinophilia, mucus hypersecretion and cytokine secretion in the bronchoalveolar lavage (BAL) in a mouse model of asthma [51]. Another AP-1/NF-κB inhibitor, named SP100030, when administered intraperitoneally also exhibited similar protective results by decreasing allergen-induced inflammatory cytokine production (IL-2, IL-5 and IL-10) and T cell infiltration in the airway submucosa of sensitized rats [52]. Administration of more specific NF-κB inhibitors, such as specific decoy oligodeoxynucleotides to prevent nuclear binding [53] or NF-κB inhibitory protein (ABIN-1), delivered specifically in the epithelium using recombinant adenoviral vectors [54] was associated with a drastic reduction of airway inflammatory reactions. Another promising NF-κB blocking approach is use of the cell-permeable peptides carrying

Table 4.2   Successful NF-κB inhibitory strategies in animal models of allergic asthma

Compound	Pharmacological profile	Treatment and duration	References
MOL294	Dual NF-κB/AP-1 inhibitor	0.075 mg/kg, intranasal on days 25, 26, 27 prior each Ag challenge	Henderson *et al.* [51]
SP100030	Dual NF-κB/AP-1 inhibitor	20 mg/kg, intraperitoneal on days 15–17 prior each Ag challenge	Huang *et al.* [52]
Selenite	Environmental metal and anti-oxidant	2.5 mg/kg, intraperitoneal 1 day prior Ag challenge	Jeong *et al.* [39]
ABIN-1 expressing adenovirus	NF-κB inhibitory protein	2×10^9 pfu adenovirus intratracheal 2 days prior last Ag challenge	El Bakkouri *et al.* [54]
NF-κB decoy oligodeoxynucleotides	Impair NF-κB/ DNA interaction	15 nmol, intratracheal on days 28, 30 prior each Ag challenge	Desmet *et al.* [53]
L-2-oxothiazolidine-4-carboxylic acid (OTC)	Prodrug of cysteine	40, 80, 160 mg/kg, intraperitoneal on days 21–24 prior each Ag challenge	Lee *et al.* [40]
Activated protein C	Blood coagulation regulator	120 μg/ml, aerosolized on days 22–26 prior Ag challenge	Yuda *et al.* [41]

the nuclear localization sequence (NLS) that prevent NF-κB nuclear translocation [55]. These peptides were found to be effective in preventing LPS-induced lung production of inflammatory cytokines. Other recent studies found that the decreased immunologic and inflammatory responses exerted by other compounds such as a prodrug of cysteine, L-2-oxothiazolidine-4-carboxylic acid [40], selenite [39] or activated protein C [41] in murine animal models of allergic asthma could be ascribed to their suppressive action on NF-κB pathways. Table 4.2 summarizes the different inhibitory strategies used in the animal models of asthma. These studies again strongly support the notion that NF-κB-inducible inflammatory pathways are critically important for the pathogenesis of chronic lung diseases.

THERAPEUTIC ACTION OF IKKβ INHIBITORS IN ALLERGIC ASTHMA

In the single year of 2005, there has been a veritable explosion of convincing reports describing the therapeutic value of inhibitory strategies directed specifically against IKKβ in both *in vivo* and *in vitro* models of inflammation. The recently developed IKKβ inhibitor TPCA-1 (2-[(aminocarbonyl)amino]-5-[fluorophenyl]-3-thiophenecarboxamide) exhibits promising results by reducing in a dose-dependent manner collagen-induced arthritis *in vivo* in DBA/1 mice (doses 3–20 mg/kg) as well as LPS-induced inflammatory cytokine release in human monocytes ($IC_{50} = 17$ nM) [56]. The same inhibitor also manifested protective effects in a rat model of allergic asthma where TPCA-1 suppressed ovalbumin-induced cytokine production, airway eosinophilia, and late asthmatic reactions [57]. Similarly, another newly synthesized IKKβ inhibitor called COMPOUND A ($IC_{50} = 40$–240 nM) inhibited the development of airway inflammation, airway hyperresponsiveness induced by cockroach allergen exposure [58]. The validation of IKKβ as a potential therapeutic target was also confirmed using adenoviral transfer of dominant negative IKKβ in epithelial A549 cells, which exhibited reduced expression of inflammatory genes such as ICAM-1, IL-8,

GM-CSF and COX-2 [59]. Surprisingly, the authors failed to demonstrate any inhibitory effect of IKKα dominant negative. The implication of IKKβ in asthmatic reactions was also supported in transgenic mice lacking active IKKβ in the airway epithelium [60]. This study convincingly demonstrates a diminished inflammatory response, as well as peribronchial fibrosis and mucus production in allergen-challenged IKKβ-deficient mice compared to their wild-type counterparts.

SUMMARY

Growing evidence shows that asthmatic patients exhibit an exaggerated NF-κB activity and/or expression of NF-κB regulatory proteins (p65) in airway structural tissues as well as infiltrated inflammatory cells. In some patients, NF-κB activation appears to correlate with the severity of the disease and to be refractory to the anti-inflammatory action of steroids. It is likely that aberrant steroid-insensitive NF-κB activation will be playing a central role in the orchestration and/or progression of asthma. Thus, there is no doubt that the IKKβ–NF-κB axis will provide an excellent target for the development of therapeutic drugs that would be effective for the treatment of asthma (Figure 4.3). In addition to the gene-therapy based approaches (adenovirus), the recent development of potent inhibitors of IKKβ led to

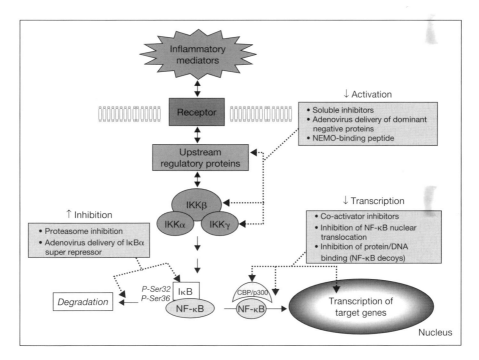

Figure 4.3 Potential therapeutic strategies for suppressing inflammation-linked NF-κB activation: based on the recent studies, different molecular strategies could be developed to interfere with NF-κB function. First, effective inhibitors could be used to block IκBα phosphorylation by acting on upstream kinases IKKβ and IKKγ using soluble molecules or NEMO-binding peptides, respectively. The inhibitors could also be designed to target one of the recently discovered IKKβ regulatory proteins (see Figure 4.1) that serve as bridges between the receptors and the IKKβ. A second pathway could be to prevent NF-κB translocation by maintaining high IκBα levels, either through proteasome inhibition or *via* adenovirus delivery of a IκBα super-repressor. Finally, inhibitors could also target NF-κB-dependent gene transcription by inhibiting NF-κB nuclear translocation, NF-κB/DNA interaction and activation of co-activators, indirectly preventing the recruitment of additional transcription factors that are required for full transcriptional activity.

5

Protease-activated receptors: targets for therapeutic intervention in asthma

J. M. Tunon de Lara, P. Berger

INTRODUCTION

Protease proteinase-activated receptors (PARs) are members of a family of hepta-helical receptors and were first identified as a mechanism for the interaction between blood clotting and platelet activation. These receptors were initially investigated for their role in injury and wound healing but, more recently, their role in chronic inflammation has become a focus of attention. Cell surface PARs appear to have evolved to detect extracellular enzymatically active serine proteases including thrombin, trypsin and tryptase. They are expressed extensively in various tissues and cells throughout the mammalian body with a predominant location on endothelia and epithelia. Activated upon the proteolytic activity of enzymes, PARs are different from other protease receptors and may be considered as sensors of proteolytic activity rather than receptors in the traditional sense [1].

In the respiratory system, PAR-1 and PAR-2 are expressed in both epithelial and smooth muscle cells and may detect exogenous or endogenous protease activity. For example, dust mite allergens such as Der p 1, Der p 3 or Der p 9 could be exogenous agonists for PAR-2 expressed at the surface of bronchial epithelium. Mast cells that infiltrate bronchial mucosa in asthma are a major source of tryptase, a serine protease which can activate PARs expressed at the surface of smooth muscle cells. In this respect, recent investigations have provided strong evidence that PARs could play an important role in the pathophysiology of asthma [2] and may thus be considered as a new therapeutic target.

PAR FAMILY: STRUCTURE, DISTRIBUTION, LIGANDS AND SIGNALLING

Among seven transmembrane G protein-coupled receptors, PARs have been shown to have a unique mechanism of activation. PAR is activated through its proteolysis by serine proteases, a family of enzymes that require serine within the active site [3]. Serine proteases cleave the amino acids at a specific site of the extra cellular NH2-terminus of the molecule leading to the exposure of a new NH2-terminus that acts as a tethered ligand, which binds and activates the cleaved receptor molecule (Figure 5.1). The amino-acid sequence of each cleavage site is specific for each particular PAR.

Four PARs have been identified and cloned so far. These receptors are widely expressed by epithelial and endothelial cells, fibroblasts, smooth muscle cells, leucocytes and a variety

J. Manuel Tunon de Lara, MD, PhD, Professor of Respiratory Medicine, Laboratory of Cell Physiology (INSERM 356), University of Bordeaux 2, Department of Respiratory Medicine, Bordeaux Teaching Hospital, Bordeaux, France

Patrick Berger, MD, PhD, Laboratory of Cell Physiology (INSERM 356), University of Bordeaux 2, Department of Respiratory Medicine, Bordeaux Teaching Hospital, Bordeaux, France

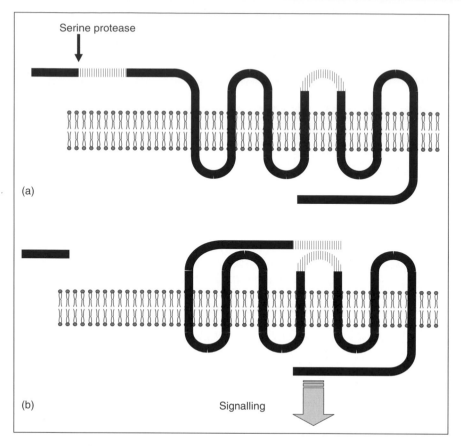

Serine protease

(a)

(b)   Signalling

Figure 5.1 Mechanism of activation of PAR. The tethered ligand sequence (hatched box) is exposed following serine protease cleavage (a) and then binds to a specific site on the second extracellular loop to initiate cell signalling (b).

of cells present in airways and playing a role in allergic inflammation. The properties and distribution of PAR-1–4 are presented in Table 5.1.

The proteolytic activation of PAR is irreversible and, once cleaved, the receptors are degraded in lysosomes. Activated PARs interact with both types of hetero trimeric G proteins in the plasma membrane, i.e. G_q and G_i. G_q-signalling cascade activates phospholipase C leading to an increase in intracellular Ca^{++} level [4]. G_i-signalling cascade generates transcriptional responses through extracellular signal-regulated kinase, mitogen-activated protein (MAP) kinase and nuclear factor-κB (NF-κB)[5]. Coupling to specific G proteins varies between different PARs. The best documented pathway includes activation of phospholipase Cβ *via* $G_{q/11}$ protein, which produces inositol triphosphate followed by Ca^{2+} mobilization and di-acylglycerol followed by activation of protein kinase C. Nevertheless, other signalling pathways have also been described, particularly for PAR-1 and -2. PAR-1 interacts with multiple α-subunits of G proteins such as $G_{12/13}\alpha$ and $G_i\alpha$. $G_{12/13}\alpha$ coupled to PAR-1 interacts with Rho guanine-nucleotide exchange factors leading to Rho-mediated control of cell shape and migration [6]. PAR-1 also triggers activation of the MAP kinase cascades and is capable of transactivating epidermal growth factor receptors [7]. In different tissues including airways, PAR-2 activation causes arachidonic acid release and prostanoid formation and stimulates the MAP kinase cascades [8, 9].

Table 5.1 Properties and distribution of PARs

Subtype	PAR-1	PAR-2	PAR-3	PAR-4
Chromosome	5q13	5q13	5q13	19p12
Enzymatic activators	Thrombin Trypsin Mast cell tryptase	Trypsin Mast cell tryptase Neutrophil elastase	Thrombin	Thrombin Trypsin
Cleavage site	Arg 41–Ser 42	Arg 34–Ser35	Lys 38–Thr39	Arg 47–Gly48
Tethered ligand sequences	SFLLRN	SLIGKV	TFRGAP	GYPGQV
Actvivity of synthetic peptides	Yes	Yes	No	Yes
Airway epithelium	+	+	+	+
Mast cell	+	+		
Eosinophil	+	+	+	
Neutrophil		+		
Alveolar macrophage	+	+		
Monocyte and dendritic cell	+	+	+	
T & B lymphocyte	+	+		
Airway smooth muscle	+	+	+ (cultured cells)	
Endothelial cell	+	+		
Vascular smooth muscle	+	+		
Fibroblast	+	+		
Neuron	+	+		

PAR IN ASTHMA

Mast cell infiltration is an important component of inflammation in asthma, a disease characterized by bronchial hyperresponsiveness (BHR) and infiltration of airway mucosa by several cell types including eosinophils and activated mast cells [10]. It has been clearly demonstrated that inflammatory infiltration also concerns the smooth muscle layer and that the number of mast cells infiltrating the bronchial smooth muscle is higher in asthmatic patients than in normal subjects and closely related with BHR [11]. The mechanism of mast cell infiltration involves the secretion of chemotactic factors such as transforming growth factor $\beta1$, stem cell factor, CX_3CL1 and CXCL10 by human airway smooth muscle cells (HASMC) [12–14]. Mast cell-derived products play a major role in this chemotactic activity of HASMC (Figure 5.2).

The neutral serine protease tryptase triggers a calcium response in airway and promotes proliferation [15, 16]. Tryptase also induces BHR both *in vitro* in dog [17] or in human [18] and *in vivo* in sheep [19]. Most of these effects are likely mediated by PAR-2 since the peptide agonist SLIGKV corresponding to the tethered ligand in human PAR-2 mimics the effects of tryptase on HASMC, i.e. calcium rise [4], proliferation [15], and cytokine synthesis [12].

PAR EXPRESSION IN ASTHMATIC TISSUE

PAR-1–4 are expressed on epithelium and smooth muscle in human endobronchial biopsy specimens from asthmatic patients and normal subjects. PAR-1 and -3 expression is predominately localized to defined foci within the apical regions of columnar epithelial cells, whereas PAR-2 and -4 staining is generally more widespread and diffuse. The intensity of PAR-1, -3, and -4 expression is not altered in asthma by contrast with the intensity of PAR-2 staining in epithelium that is significantly upregulated in biopsy specimens taken from asthmatics [20].

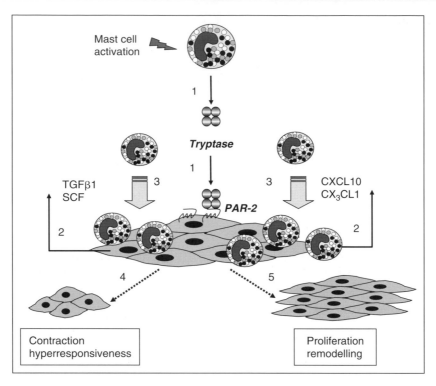

Figure 5.2   Pathophysiology of mast cell myositis in atopic asthma. Upon mast cell activation, tryptase activates PAR-2 expressed at the surface of human airway smooth muscle cells (1). As a consequence, smooth muscle cells synthesize chemotactic factors for mast cells (2) leading to an infiltration of the smooth muscle layer (3) so-called 'mast cell myositis'. Mast cell-derived products participate to the alteration of the contractile response (4) and contribute to the airway remodelling by facilitating smooth muscle cell proliferation (5). SCF = Stem cell factor; TGFβ1 = transforming growth factor β1.

The intensity and distribution of staining for all four PARs in the airway smooth muscle is similar in biopsy specimens from normal and asthmatic subjects [20]. PAR-2 is also localized in primary cultures of HASMC using both RT-PCR and an antiserum to PAR-2 [21]. In addition, studies performed with trypsin and tryptase show Ca^{++} mobilization in HASMC confirming the expression of functional PAR-2 [4]. Schmidlin *et al.* [22] have also demonstrated that PAR-2 is present and is functional in human bronchial smooth muscle cells in culture.

THE ROLE OF PARS IN AIRWAYS

Expression of PAR-1 and -2 has been detected in a variety of inflammatory cells, including T cells, eosinophils, monocytes, and mast cells. PAR-2 agonist peptides inhibit the synthesis of interferon-γ and suppress the expression of the adhesion molecule CD44 from activated T cells [23]. By contrast, activation of PAR-2 on eosinophils induces superoxide anion production and cellular degranulation [24]. Activation of PAR-1 can also stimulate recruitment and cellular proliferation in monocytes [25]. The effects of PAR activation on mast cell function are not clear. Experimental results obtained in rats suggest that PAR activation promotes oedema through mast cell activation and degranulation [26]. In contrast, other studies showed little histological evidence of mast cell degranulation with PAR-1 or -2 agonist peptides [27]. These discrepancies may be explained by the fact that PAR activation may depend on mast cell phenotype and may stimulate controlled secretion of selective mediators. Taken together, these observations indicate that PAR activation may alternately stimulate or suppress inflammatory cell activity, depending on the inflammatory cell type and its state of activation.

There is strong evidence that PARs modulate airway smooth muscle tone, but this effect appears to differ significantly between species and the type of airway tissue examined. Activation of PAR 1 evokes contraction mainly through a direct activation of PAR-1 localized on the airway smooth muscle [28].

The effects of PAR-2 activation in airways also illustrate the 'double edge sword' nature of PARs with respect to airway tone and inflammation. On the one hand, activation of PAR-2 on epithelial cells has been shown to induce the release of PGE_2, which correlates with a reduction in airway smooth muscle contraction. In this respect, it has been argued that one of the major functions of epithelium-expressed PAR-2 is bronchoprotection [29]. In fact, PAR-2 activation causes bronchodilation *in vivo* and epithelium-dependent bronchial relaxation *in vitro*, without direct contraction [30]. This effect appears mediated by activation of epithelial PAR-2 and resembles that of the endothelium-dependent relaxation of blood vessels [31].

On the other hand, PAR-2 stimulation might also result in pro-inflammatory responses and bronchial hyperresponsiveness as suggested by the observations made in mice over-expressing PAR-2 [32]. Activation of PAR-2 on epithelial cells is also associated with interleukin (IL)-6 and IL-8 release [33], matrix metalloproteinase-9 release [34] and platelet-derived growth factor release all of which have the potential to induce inflammation. In addition, activation of PAR-2 can directly produce airway contraction and may facilitate hyperresponsiveness. In guinea pig airways, trypsin induces bronchoconstriction *in vivo*, which appears to depend on direct smooth muscle contraction and indirect mechanisms [35], one being a release of sensory neurokinins, as demonstrated in response to trypsin stimulation. In isolated human bronchi, activation of both PAR-1 [28] and PAR-2 causes a moderate contractile response that, at least in part, is mediated by a direct activation of smooth muscle cell receptors [22].

Another important aspect in the pathophysiology of asthma is the effect of PARs on resident cells and the consequences in terms of tissue repair and regeneration. PAR-1 and PAR-2 have been shown to stimulate lung fibroblasts and HASMC mitogenesis of both [15, 36–38]. PAR activation may also play a role in remodelling through the stimulated release of MMP-9 and procollagen from bronchial epithelial cells and lung fibroblasts, respectively [34]. Activation of PAR-1 and -2 on epithelial cells and fibroblasts has also been reported to stimulate the secretion of chemokines, including IL-8, granulocyte-macrophage colony-stimulating factor (GM-CSF), and eotaxin, as well as other pro-inflammatory mediators [39–42]. These results suggest that activation of PARs on airway cells can promote tissue growth and stimulate remodelling.

PAR MODULATION AND THERAPEUTIC PERSPECTIVES

Turning off the signal of PAR implicates several mechanisms which may be of importance in designing long-acting antagonists and agonists of PARs that may be therapeutically useful. Signals are attenuated by mechanisms that operate at the level of the agonist, the receptor and the G proteins and at various downstream steps of the signalling pathway. Some of these approaches have been initiated in asthma but would require further investigation to reach a clinical step.

AGONIST MODULATION

Agonist removal from the extracellular fluid is the earliest mechanism of attenuation. Pharmacological studies using protease inhibitors *in vivo* have yielded various result findings. The tryptase inhibitor APC366 failed to alter early asthmatic response or bronchial hyperresponsiveness in humans [43], whereas it blocked bronchial hyperresponsiveness, early and late responses after antigen challenge in allergic sheep [19]. In addition, the tryptase inhibitor MOL 6131 reduced bronchial inflammation (i.e. eosinophilia, peribronchial oedema, release of IL-4 and -13), but did not alter bronchial hyperresponsiveness in asthmatic mice [44].

PAR ANTAGONISTS

By using a *de novo* design approach, a series of potent heterocycle-based peptidomimetic antagonists of PAR-1 have been discovered and may have therapeutic potential for treating thrombosis and restenosis in humans. By contrast, other PAR antagonists are not yet available to be tested in asthma.

RWJ-56110 [45] and RWJ-58259 [46] are potent, selective PAR-1 antagonists, devoid of PAR-1 agonist and thrombin inhibitory activity: they bind to PAR-1, interfere with calcium mobilization and cellular functions associated with PAR-1, and do not affect PAR-2, -3, or -4. RWJ-56110 was determined to be a direct inhibitor of PAR-1 activation and internalization, without affecting PAR-1 N-terminal cleavage. At high concentrations of α-thrombin, RWJ-56110 fully blocks activation responses in human vascular cells, but not in human platelets, whereas, at high concentrations of TRAP-6, RWJ-56110 blocked activation responses in both cell types. RWJ-56110 and RWJ-58259 clearly interrupt the binding of a tethered ligand to its receptor. RWJ-58259 demonstrated antirestenotic activity in a rat balloon angioplasty model and antithrombotic activity in a monkey arterial injury model [47].

siRNA STRATEGY

RNAi is a highly conserved gene silencing mechanism that uses double-stranded RNA as a signal to trigger the degradation of homologous mRNA. It has been demonstrated that siRNA specifically suppresses the expression of various genes in different mammalian cell lines and this new tool for studying gene function in mammalian cells has then been used in primary somatic cells including T lymphocytes and endothelial cells [48, 49]. In the absence of conventional PAR-2 antagonists, we have applied the RNAi mechanism for gene silencing in HASMC in order to examine the function of PAR-2 [21]. The design of siRNA is a critical step for using the RNAi mechanism. Initially, Elbashir and co-workers defined different parameters including 21 nucleotide siRNA with overhanging 3' ends, a percentage of GC between 30 and 50% and a target localized in the open reading frame [50]. Since the activity of siRNA in mammalian cells is related to structural target accessibility, we have focused our attention to parts of PAR-2 mRNA with the highest probability to remain in a single strand manner, according to Zucker's mRNA secondary structure prediction software [51]. Using all these criteria, five siRNA directed against PAR-2 were synthesized *in vitro* (Table 5.2). siRNA nos. 1 and 3 significantly decreased protein and mRNA expression whereas siRNA no. 2 decreased protein expression but not mRNA levels. siRNA nos. 4 and 5 showed limited if any effect on PAR-2 expression. We focus our attention on siRNA no. 1 since it was the most potent in terms of mRNA levels and surface protein expression and we compared cells transfected with siRNA no. 1 with both cells transfected with two control siRNAs and untransfected cells. Regarding mRNA level or calcium response, cells transfected with the control siRNA no. 1-inv are indistinguishable from untransfected cells. The mechanisms of RNAi involve (i) 21–23-nt siRNAs homologous in sequence to the target gene, (ii) activation of the RNA inducing silencing complex (RISC) and (iii) target mRNA degradation [52]. Increasing the size of siRNA more than 29-nt, resulted in protein kinase R activation, non-specific mRNA degradation and apoptosis [50]. In addition, since the activation of RISC is saturable, the concentration of siRNA should be as low as possible. In our study, we used low amounts of 21-nt siRNA to avoid these non-specific effects.

As a consequence of its effect on PAR-2 expression, RNAi impaired PAR-2 mediated functional effects. Regarding the most selective PAR-2 agonist, the activating peptide

Table 5.2 PAR-2 siRNA sequences (adapted from [21])

siRNA nos.	Position	Sequence
1	321–341	5′-ACAGUCUUUUCUGUGGAUGUU-3′ 3′-UUUUGUCAGAAAAGACACCUAC 5′
2	463–483	5′-CUAAGAAGAAGCACCCUGCUU-3′ 3′-UUGAUUCUUCUUCGUGGGACG-5′
3	545–565	5′-GAUUGCCUAUCACAUACAUUU-3′ 3′-UUCUAACGGAUAGUGUAUGUA-5′
4	572–592	5′-CUGGAUUUAUGGGGAAGCUUU-3′ 3′-UUGACCUAAAUACCCCUUCGA-5′
5	626–646	5′-CAUGUACUGUUCCAUUCUCUU-3′ 3′-UUGUACAUGACAAGGUAAGAG-5′
Inverse no. 1	–	5′-ACAGUUCUUUCUGUGGAUGUU-3′ 3′-UUUUGUCAAGAAAGACACCUAC-5′
Scramble no. 1	–	5′-GUCUUAUCGGUUAUGGUACUU-3′ 3′-UUCAGAAUAGCCAAUACCAUG-5′

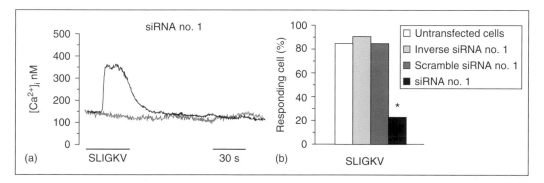

Figure 5.3 Effect of siRNA on HASMC calcium response assessed by microspectrofluorimetry. (a) Representative intracellular calcium response is presented following stimulation by 10^{-4} M SLIGKV-NH2 of untransfected cells (black) or cells transfected with siRNA sequence no. 1 (grey). (b) Percentage of responding cells according to experimental conditions. siRNA sequence no. 1 significantly decreased the mean $[Ca^{2+}]_i$ response when compared with controls (i.e. untransfected cells, cells transfected with an inverse or scramble sequence); $P < 0.05$ usng Chi^2 test.

SLIGKV, RNAi decreased the mean $[Ca^{2+}]_i$ response by approximately 50% (Figure 5.3) in agreement with the amplitude of the decrease in PAR-2 expression. However, this mean decrease was due to the coexistence of two cell populations following siRNA transfection: one population of fully responding cells and one population of non-responding cells, i.e. RNAi decreased the percentage of responding cells. It can therefore be concluded that, in our hands, RNAi was an all-or-none phenomenon. This result derived from functional data is supported by the analysis of the distribution of PAR-2 expression on HASMC showing the existence of both populations.

HASMC PAR-2 mediated calcium response results from receptor activation of pertussis toxin insensitive G protein, phopholipase C, and inositol 3-phosphate (IP3) formation leading to a calcium release from intracellular stores [4]. The RNAi effect of SLIGKV-induced calcium response is undoubtedly related to PAR-2 extinction since IP3 formation *via* activation of alternative PAR by means of trypsin and intracellular calcium release by means of caffeine remains unaltered by siRNA. Finally, the fact that the RNAi effect on tryptase-induced response is identical to that on SLIGKV provided molecular confirmation that tryptase-mediated effects are restricted to PAR-2 activation.

ATTENUATION OF PAR SIGNALLING

Although proteolysis is the physiological mechanism for PAR activation, proteases can also inactivate receptors. PAR cleavage may remove the tethered ligand before it is exposed and thus inactivates the receptor. Proteases may also cleave the tethered ligand after exposure and thereby terminate the signal. For example, it has been demonstrated that the cleavage of PAR by thrombin and trypsin renders cells unresponsive to proteases for long periods of time, until new intact receptors are expressed at the plasma membrane surface [53].

Attenuation of PAR signalling can also be obtained by PAR desensitization. Although homologous desensitization is mediated by agonist-dependent activation of the same receptor, heterologous desensitization may be caused by the activation of another receptor. Desensitization is associated with uncoupling of the activated receptor from its protein G by phosphorylation [54]. G protein receptor kinases mediate agonist-dependent phosphorylation and initiate homologous desensitization, whereas protein kinases C and A mediate agonist-independent phosphorylation and initiate heterogenous desensitization.

MODULATION OF PAR IN VIVO

The role of PAR-2 in allergic inflammation of the airways has been investigated *in vivo* using PAR-2$^{-/-}$ mice [32]. In a mouse model of asthma induced by ovalbumin, PAR-2 deficiency decreases about 90% of the ovalbumin-induced infiltration of eosinophils and lymphocytes in bronchoalveolar lavage fluid and is associated with a decrease in the infiltration of lung tissue by eosinophils [55]. This phenomenon is supported by findings reported by Schmidlin *et al.* [32] who observed that the deletion of PAR-2 diminished inflammatory cell infiltration into airways remarkably. These authors also showed that PAR-2 mRNA was readily detected in airway epithelial cells of wild-type mice. Therefore, it seems that PAR-2 expressed on epithelial cells participates in the infiltration of inflammatory cells. It is also reported in this study that bronchial eosinophilic inflammation in PAR-2$^{-/-}$ mice was caused by the insufficiency of eotaxin production in airway epithelial cells, suggesting that airway epithelial cells produce eotaxin when stimulated by PAR-2 activating peptide.

SUMMARY

PARs might be targets for novel drugs in many clinical situations that involve inflammation, such as asthma. The conventional approach for tackling inflammation is to inhibit this reaction with receptor antagonists. An alternative approach would be to develop receptor agonist drugs that activate constitutive anti-inflammatory responses that have to be overcome for inflammation to persist. In this respect, PAR modulation might be of interest since PAR-activating peptides or small-molecule mimetics could switch on anti-inflammatory mechanisms without the side-effects that endogenous enzymes might cause *via* other mechanisms. By activating endogenous anti-inflammatory cascades, unique treatments for chronic inflammatory diseases may be developed. However, stimulating PARs in airways may also trigger cellular growth and/or facilitate bronchial hyperresponsiveness. The development of PAR agonists activating endogenous anti-inflammatory pathways should thus take into account possible effects on airway smooth muscle and requires further definition of the effect of PAR agonists and antagonists *in vivo*.

REFERENCES

1. Cocks TM, Moffatt JD. Protease-activated receptors: sentries for inflammation? *Trends Pharmacol Sci* 2000; 21:103–108.
2. Reed CE, Kita H. The role of protease activation of inflammation in allergic respiratory diseases. *J Allergy Clin Immunol* 2004; 114:997–1008; quiz 9.
3. Vu TK, Hung DT, Wheaton VI, Coughlin SR. Molecular cloning of a functional thrombin receptor reveals a novel proteolytic mechanism of receptor activation. *Cell* 1991; 64:1057–1068.
4. Berger P, Tunon-De-Lara JM, Savineau JP, Marthan R. Selected contribution: tryptase-induced PAR-2-mediated Ca(2+) signalling in human airway smooth muscle cells. *J Appl Physiol* 2001; 91:995–1003.
5. Dery O, Corvera CU, Steinhoff M, Bunnett NW. Proteinase-activated receptors: novel mechanisms of signalling by serine proteases. *Am J Physiol* 1998; 274(pt 1):C1429–C1452.
6. Klages B, Brandt U, Simon MI, Schultz G, Offermanns S. Activation of G12/G13 results in shape change and Rho/Rho-kinase-mediated myosin light chain phosphorylation in mouse platelets. *J Cell Biol* 1999; 144:745–754.
7. Prenzel N, Zwick E, Daub H *et al*. EGF receptor transactivation by G-protein-coupled receptors requires metalloproteinase cleavage of proHB-EGF. *Nature* 1999; 402:884–888.
8. Lan RS, Knight DA, Stewart GA, Henry PJ. Role of PGE(2) in protease-activated receptor-1, -2 and -4 mediated relaxation in the mouse isolated trachea. *Br J Pharmacol* 2001; 132:93–100.
9. Yu Z, Ahmad S, Schwartz JL, Banville D, Shen SH. Protein-tyrosine phosphatase SHP2 is positively linked to proteinase-activated receptor 2-mediated mitogenic pathway. *J Biol Chem* 1997; 272: 7519–7524.
10. Pesci A, Foresi A, Bertorelli G, Chetta A, Oliveri D. Histochemical characteristics and degranulation of mast cells in epithelium and lamina propria of bronchial biopsies from asthmatic and normal subjects. *Am Rev Respir Dis* 1993; 147:684–689.
11. Brightling CE, Bradding P, Symon FA, Holgate ST, Wardlaw AJ, Pavord ID. Mast-cell infiltration of airway smooth muscle in asthma. *N Engl J Med* 2002; 346:1699–1705.
12. Berger P, Girodet PO, Begueret H *et al*. Tryptase-stimulated human airway smooth muscle cells induce cytokine synthesis and mast cell chemotaxis. *FASEB J* 2003; 17:2139–2141.
13. Brightling CE, Ammit AJ, Kaur D *et al*. The CXCL10/CXCR3 axis mediates human lung mast cell migration to asthmatic airway smooth muscle. *Am J Respir Crit Care Med* 2005; 171:1103–1108.
14. El-Shazly A, Berger P, Girodet PO *et al*. Fraktalkine produced by airway smooth muscle cells contributes to mast cell recruitment in asthma. *J Immunol* 2006; 176:1860–1868.
15. Berger P, Perng DW, Thabrew H *et al*. Tryptase and agonists of PAR-2 induce the proliferation of human airway smooth muscle cells. *J Appl Physiol* 2001; 91:1372–1379.
16. Brown JK, Jones CA, Rooney LA, Caughey GH, Hall IP. Tryptase's potent mitogenic effects in human airway smooth muscle cells are via nonproteolytic actions. *Am J Physiol Lung Cell Mol Physiol* 2002; 282:L197–L206.
17. Sekizawa K, Caughey GH, Lazarus SC, Gold WM, Nadel JA. Mast cell tryptase causes airway smooth muscle hyperresponsiveness in dogs. *J Clin Invest* 1989; 83:175–179.
18. Berger P, Compton SJ, Molimard M *et al*. Mast cell tryptase as a mediator of hyperresponsiveness in human isolated bronchi. *Clin Exp Allergy* 1999; 29:804–812.
19. Clark JM, Abraham WM, Fishman CE *et al*. Tryptase inhibitors block allergen-induced airway and inflammatory responses in allergic sheep. *Am J Respir Crit Care Med* 1995; 152(pt 1):2076–2083.
20. Knight DA, Lim S, Scaffidi AK *et al*. Protease-activated receptors in human airways: upregulation of PAR-2 in respiratory epithelium from patients with asthma. *J Allergy Clin Immunol* 2001; 108: 797–803.
21. Trian T, Girodet PO, Ousova O, Marthan R, Tunon-de-Lara JM, Berger P. RNA interference decreases PAR-2 expression and function in human airway smooth muscle cells. *Am J Respir Cell Mol Biol* 2006; 34:49–55.
22. Schmidlin F, Amadesi S, Vidil R *et al*. Expression and function of proteinase-activated receptor 2 in human bronchial smooth muscle. *Am J Respir Crit Care Med* 2001; 164:1276–1281.
23. Fiorucci S, Mencarelli A, Palazzetti B *et al*. Proteinase-activated receptor 2 is an anti-inflammatory signal for colonic lamina propria lymphocytes in a mouse model of colitis. *Proc Natl Acad Sci USA* 2001; 98:13936–13941.
24. Miike S, McWilliam AS, Kita H. Trypsin induces activation and inflammatory mediator release from human eosinophils through protease-activated receptor-2. *J Immunol* 2001; 167:6615–6622.

25. Naldini A, Sower L, Bocci V, Meyers B, Carney DH. Thrombin receptor expression and responsiveness of human monocytic cells to thrombin is linked to interferon-induced cellular differentiation. *J Cell Physiol* 1998; 177:76–84.

26. Cirino G, Cicala C, Bucci MR, Sorrentino L, Maraganore JM, Stone SR. Thrombin functions as an inflammatory mediator through activation of its receptor. *J Exp Med* 1996; 183:821–827.

27. Vergnolle N. Proteinase-activated receptor-2-activating peptides induce leukocyte rolling, adhesion, and extravasation in vivo. *J Immunol* 1999; 163:5064–5069.

28. Hauck RW, Schulz C, Schomig A, Hoffman RK, Panettieri RA Jr. α-thrombin stimulates contraction of human bronchial rings by activation of protease-activated receptors. *Am J Physiol* 1999; 277(pt 1): L22–L29.

29. Cocks TM, Moffatt JD. Protease-activated receptor-2 (PAR2) in the airways. *Pulm Pharmacol Ther* 2001; 14:183–191.

30. Cocks TM, Fong B, Chow JM *et al.* A protective role for protease-activated receptors in the airways. *Nature* 1999; 398:156–160.

31. Hollenberg MD, Saifeddine M, al-Ani B. Proteinase-activated receptor-2 in rat aorta: structural requirements for agonist activity of receptor-activating peptides. *Mol Pharmacol* 1996; 49:229–233.

32. Schmidlin F, Amadesi S, Dabbagh K *et al.* Protease-activated receptor 2 mediates eosinophil infiltration and hyperreactivity in allergic inflammation of the airway. *J Immunol* 2002; 169:5315–5321.

33. Asokananthan N, Graham PT, Fink J *et al.* Activation of protease-activated receptor (PAR)-1, PAR-2, and PAR-4 stimulates IL-6, IL-8, and prostaglandin E2 release from human respiratory epithelial cells. *J Immunol* 2002; 168:3577–3585.

34. Vliagoftis H, Schwingshackl A, Milne CD *et al.* Proteinase-activated receptor-2-mediated matrix metalloproteinase-9 release from airway epithelial cells. *J Allergy Clin Immunol* 2000; 106:537–545.

35. Ricciardolo FL, Steinhoff M, Amadesi S *et al.* Presence and bronchomotor activity of protease-activated receptor-2 in guinea pig airways. *Am J Respir Crit Care Med* 2000; 161:1672–1680.

36. Akers IA, Parsons M, Hill MR *et al.* Mast cell tryptase stimulates human lung fibroblast proliferation via protease-activated receptor-2. *Am J Physiol Lung Cell Mol Physiol* 2000; 278:L193–L201.

37. Chambers LS, Black JL, Poronnik P, Johnson PR. Functional effects of protease-activated receptor-2 stimulation on human airway smooth muscle. *Am J Physiol Lung Cell Mol Physiol* 2001; 281:L1369–L1378.

38. Panettieri RA Jr, Hall IP, Maki CS, Murray RK. α-thrombin increases cytosolic calcium and induces human airway smooth muscle cell proliferation. *Am J Respir Cell Mol Biol* 1995; 13:205–216.

39. Gordon JR, Zhang X, Stevenson K, Cosford K. Thrombin induces IL-6 but not TNFα secretion by mouse mast cells: threshold-level thrombin receptor and very low level FcεRI signalling synergistically enhance IL-6 secretion. *Cell Immunol* 2000; 205:128–135.

40. Ludwicka-Bradley A, Bogatkevich G, Silver RM. Thrombin-mediated cellular events in pulmonary fibrosis associated with systemic sclerosis (scleroderma). *Clin Exp Rheumatol* 2004; 22(suppl 33):S38–S46.

41. Sun G, Stacey MA, Schmidt M, Mori L, Mattoli S. Interaction of mite allergens Der p3 and Der p9 with protease-activated receptor-2 expressed by lung epithelial cells. *J Immunol* 2001; 167:1014–1021.

42. Vliagoftis H, Befus AD, Hollenberg MD, Moqbel R. Airway epithelial cells release eosinophil survival-promoting factors (GM-CSF) after stimulation of proteinase-activated receptor 2. *J Allergy Clin Immunol* 2001; 107:679–685.

43. Krishna MT, Chauhan A, Little L *et al.* Inhibition of mast cell tryptase by inhaled APC 366 attenuates allergen-induced late-phase airway obstruction in asthma. *J Allergy Clin Immunol* 2001; 107:1039–1045.

44. Oh SW, Pae CI, Lee DK *et al.* Tryptase inhibition blocks airway inflammation in a mouse asthma model. *J Immunol* 2002; 168:1992–2000.

45. Andrade-Gordon P, Maryanoff BE, Derian CK *et al.* Design, synthesis, and biological characterization of a peptide-mimetic antagonist for a tethered-ligand receptor. *Proc Natl Acad Sci USA* 1999; 96: 12257–12262.

46. Damiano BP, Derian CK, Maryanoff BE, Zhang HC, Gordon PA. RWJ-58259: a selective antagonist of protease activated receptor-1. *Cardiovasc Drug Rev* 2003; 21:313–326.

47. Maryanoff BE, Zhang HC, Andrade-Gordon P, Derian CK. Discovery of potent peptide-mimetic antagonists for the human thrombin receptor, protease-activated receptor-1 (PAR-1). *Curr Med Chem Cardiovasc Hematol Agents* 2003; 1:13–36.

48. Iyer S, Ferreri DM, DeCocco NC, Minnear FL, Vincent PA. VE-cadherin-p120 interaction is required for maintenance of endothelial barrier function. *Am J Physiol Lung Cell Mol Physiol* 2004; 286:L1143–L1153.

49. McManus MT, Haines BB, Dillon CP *et al.* Small interfering RNA-mediated gene silencing in T lymphocytes. *J Immunol* 2002; 169:5754–5760.

50. Elbashir SM, Harborth J, Weber K, Tuschl T. Analysis of gene function in somatic mammalian cells using small interfering RNAs. *Methods* 2002; 26:199–213.

51. Zuker M. Mfold web server for nucleic acid folding and hybridization prediction. *Nucleic Acids Res* 2003; 31:3406–3415.

52. Elbashir SM, Harborth J, Lendeckel W, Yalcin A, Weber K, Tuschl T. Duplexes of 21-nucleotide RNAs mediate RNA interference in cultured mammalian cells. *Nature* 2001; 411:494–498.

53. Renesto P, Si-Tahar M, Moniatte M *et al*. Specific inhibition of thrombin-induced cell activation by the neutrophil proteinases elastase, cathepsin G, and proteinase 3: evidence for distinct cleavage sites within the aminoterminal domain of the thrombin receptor. *Blood* 1997; 89:1944–1953.

54. Bohm SK, Grady EF, Bunnett NW. Regulatory mechanisms that modulate signalling by G-protein-coupled receptors. *Biochem J* 1997; 322(pt 1):1–18.

55. Takizawa T, Tamiya M, Hara T *et al*. Abrogation of bronchial eosinophilic inflammation and attenuated eotaxin content in protease-activated receptor 2-deficient mice. *J Pharmacol Sci* 2005; 98:99–102.

6

Nitric oxide synthase as a therapeutic target in asthma

F. L. M. Ricciardolo, G. Folkerts

INTRODUCTION

Nitric oxide (NO) is a diatomic free reactive radical endogenously formed in the human lung [1]. This inorganic gas is synthesized by a diverse range of cells in virtually every vertebrate organ system from the semi-essential amino acid L-arginine by different stereo-specific enzymes called NO synthases (NOS) [2].

Endogenous NO plays a key role in physiological regulation of airway functions and is implicated in various airway diseases such as asthma. Recently, new evidence has revealed the intimate mechanisms able to modulate the expression and the activity of the different NOS isoforms releasing endogenous NO with various effects in the airways. The pharmacological regulation of the various NOS isoforms in asthma may provide new therapeutic approaches in the future.

Moreover, NO has been detected in the exhaled air of animals and human beings [3] and the NO concentrations are changed in different inflammatory diseases of the airways such as asthma [4]. Exhaled NO, mainly derived from the pro-inflammatory inducible isoform of NOS, is detectable by non-invasive methods and it can therefore be a clinical marker of airway inflammation in asthma.

NITRIC OXIDE SYNTHASES

NO is produced by a wide variety of residential and inflammatory cells in the airways [1]. NO itself is generated *via* a five-electron oxidation of the amino acid L-arginine by the enzyme NOS (Figure 6.1). The reaction is both oxygen- and nicotinamide adenine dinucleotide phosphate (NADPH)-dependent and yields the co-product L-citrulline in addition to nitroxyl (NO^-) in a 1:1 stoichiometry [1]. NOS functionally exists in three distinct isoforms: (1) constitutive neuronal NOS (NOS-I or nNOS); (2) inducible NOS (NOS-II or iNOS); (3) constitutive endothelial NOS (NOS-III or eNOS). Protein purification and molecular cloning approaches have identified the three distinct isoforms of NOS. nNOS, iNOS and eNOS, all expressed in the airways, are products of distinct genes located on different human chromosomes (12, 17 and 7 chromosomes, respectively) [5–7].

Fabio L.M. Ricciardolo, MD, PhD, Consultant Pneumologist, Unit of Pneumology, IRCCS Gaslini Institute, Genoa, Italy

Gert Folkerts, PhD, Department of Pharmacology and Pathophysiology, Faculty of Pharmaceutical Sciences, Utrecht University, Utrecht, The Netherlands

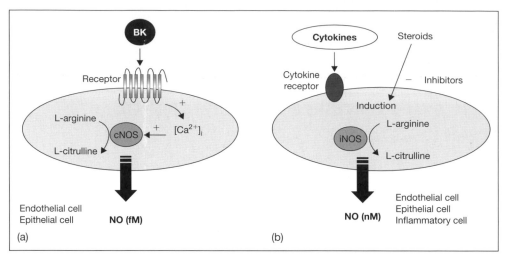

Figure 6.1 NO synthesis by the two functional NOS. L-arginine is transported into the cell *via* the CAT system and NOS converts L-arginine in two steps to NO and L-citrulline with N^G-hydroxy-L-arginine as an intermediate. Constitutive NOS (cNOS) is activated by an increase in intracellular Ca^{2+} concentrations upon receptor stimulation. Expression of iNOS are caused by a variety of stimuli that activate tyrosine kinase with subsequent activation of nuclear transcription factor NF-κB *via* phosphorylation and degradadtion of inhibitory (I)κB. NF-κB will accordingly be translocated to the nucleus and this will lead to mRNA transcription of the iNOS gene (see text).

NOS is structurally divided into two major domains, the reductase and oxygenase domains [1]. The C-terminal region possesses consensus sequences for flavin adenine dinucleotide (FAD), flavin mononucleotide (FMN), and NADPH binding sites, and exhibiting close sequence homology to another mammalian enzyme, cytochrome P-450 reductase, it is referred to as the reductase domain. The N-terminal region, termed oxygenase domain, is thought to function as haeme, tetrahydrobiopterin (H_4B) and L-arginine binding sites. NADPH acts as the source of electrons for oxygen activation and substrate oxidation. It is also believed that FAD and FMN play a role in shuttling electrons from NADPH to the iron haeme. Thus, the haeme component of NOS represents the catalytic centre, responsible for binding and reducing molecular oxygen and subsequent oxidation of substrate. Linking the reductase and oxygenase domains is a consensus sequence representative of a calmodulin binding site. The function of calmodulin is to transfer electrons between flavins and haeme moiety and to couple the reductase and oxygenase domains [1].

Functionally, NOS exists in constitutive (cNOS) and inducible (iNOS) forms [8]. cNOS is a Ca^{2+}- and calmodulin-dependent enzyme and releases, within seconds, fM or pM concentrations of NO upon receptor stimulation by selective agonists (Figure 6.1) [8]. iNOS isoform is regulated at a pre-translational level and can be induced by pro-inflammatory cytokines, such as tumour necrosis factor-α (TNFα), interferon-γ (INFγ) and interleukin (IL)-1 β [9]. iNOS releases large quantities (nM concentrations) of pro-inflammatory NO several hours after exposure, which may continue in a sustained manner (hours or days) (Figure 6.1).

The cellular synthesis of the three isoforms is dynamically regulated. A major part of iNOS regulation occurs at a pre-translational step such as transcription or mRNA stability [9]. iNOS is constitutively expressed in human airway epithelium and this unusual expression was lost when human airway epithelium was cultured [10]. An autocrine mechanism of induction and maintenance of iNOS has been identified in human airway epithelial cells through the synthesis and secretion of a soluble mediator [11]. Several lines of experimentation have established that transcriptional control mechanisms form an important basis for regulation of this isoform. Induction of macrophage iNOS mRNA by lipopolysacharide (LPS) plus IFNγ reflects increased iNOS gene transcription without changes in iNOS mRNA stability [9]. On the other hand, transforming growth factor β (TGFβ) suppresses macrophage iNOS expression *via* decreased iNOS mRNA stability and translational efficiency and by decreased stability of iNOS protein, but TGFβ does not alter iNOS transcription [9]. Availability of molecular clones corresponding to the mouse iNOS promoter allowed, through the analysis of controlled deletions within the promoter region, the characterization of two major 5′ flanking regulatory regions, one LPS-sensitive and the other IFNγ-sensitive, the latter possessing functional characteristics of an enhancer [12]. The LPS-sensitive region contains a binding site for nuclear factor-κB (NF-κB), a transcription factor that has been implicated in the activation of various pro-inflammatory genes. After specific receptor (CD14) stimulation, LPS activates the MAP kinase pathway with subsequent activation of NF-κB through phosphorylation and degradation of IκB (Figure 6.1) [13]. An upstream site contains enhancer regions with binding sites for a γ-activated site (GAS) element and an IRF-1 specific response element (ISRE) that account for IFNγ induction [14]. IFNγ is crucial for induction of iNOS expression in airway epithelial cells *in vitro* [15]. IFNγ signalling to gene expression begins with a specific receptor interaction followed by the Janus kinase (JAK)-STAT1 pathway which involves a tyrosine phosphorylation cascade [16]. In fact, pre-treatment with genistein, a tyrosine kinase inhibitor, prevents IFNγ induction of iNOS expression in airway epithelial cells [17]. STAT1 is also able to activate another transcription factor, IRF-1. Both STAT1 and IRF-1 interact with the response elements GAS and ISRE in the iNOS promoter regions [13, 14].

Recent evidence suggests that the expression of nNOS and eNOS can also be regulated under various conditions. nNOS mRNA transcripts and/or protein have been detected in specific neurons of the central and peripheral nervous systems and in non-neuronal cell types such as airway epithelial cells [18]. The subcellular localization of nNOS protein varies among the cell types studied. In neurons, both soluble and particulate protein is found. nNOS expression can be dynamically regulated by various physiological and pathological conditions [18]. nNOS mRNA upregulation seems to represent a general response of neuronal cells to stress induced by a large array of physical, chemical and biological agents such as heat, electrical stimulation, light exposure and allergic substances. Enhanced nNOS expression is often associated with co-induction of transcription factors such as c-jun and c-fos [1].

While iNOS has been characterized as a soluble (cytosolic) protein, eNOS is targeted to Golgi membranes and plasmalemmal caveolae (small invaginations in the plasma membrane characterized by the presence of the transmembrane protein caveolin). This complex process is probably dependent on myristoylation, palmitoylation, and tyrosine phosphorylation of the enzyme as well as protein–protein interactions with caveolins [19]. In endothelial cells, it has been demonstrated that the association between eNOS and caveolin suppresses eNOS activity. After agonist activation the increase in $[Ca^{2+}]_i$ promotes calmodulin binding to eNOS and the dissociation of caveolin from eNOS. eNOS-calmodulin complex synthesizes NO until $[Ca^{2+}]_i$ decreases and then the inhibitory eNOS-caveolin complex reforms [19]. Interestingly, oestrogen upregulates and activates eNOS in endothelial cells and in H441 human airway epithelial cells [20].

LOCALIZATION OF NOS IN THE AIRWAYS

eNOS (NOS III)

eNOS is constitutively expressed in human bronchial epithelium [21] and in type II human alveolar epithelial cells [22]. Immunoreactivity for eNOS is also localized in the epithelium of human nasal mucosa [23]. Ultra-structural studies revealed that eNOS is localized at the basal membrane of ciliary micro-tubules [24], where it is thought to contribute to the regulation of ciliary beat frequency [25].

nNOS (NOS I)

NOS I is localized in airway nerves of humans [26]. In human airways, nerve fibres containing nNOS have been shown both by immunohistochemistry and NADPH-diaphorase histochemistry [26]. These nerve fibres are present in the airway smooth muscle (SM), where NO is the major mediator for the neural SM relaxation [27]. The density of these nerve fibres decreases from trachea to small bronchi [26] which is associated with a reduced neural bronchodilatation [28] mediated by the inhibitory non-adrenergic, non-cholinergic (iNANC) system [29]. Co-localization with vasoactive intestinal peptide (VIP) is frequently observed [30]. In human airways, NOS-containing nerve fibres are present around submucosal glands [26].

The cell bodies of these neurons innervating human airways are localized predominantly in the local parasympathetic ganglia [31]. Additional sources of NOS immunoreactive nerve fibres are found in vagal sensory and sympathetic ganglia [31]. In sensory neurons, NO could act as a neuromediator both at the central ending and the periphery [29].

iNOS (NOS II)

iNOS (NOS II) has been identified in lungs of rats after endotoxin treatment [32]. In macrophages it has been revealed by cloning and sequencing that iNOS is expressed *de novo* at the transcriptional level [33]. It is now clear that this isoform is not only localized to macrophages [34], but it can be induced in many different cells [35]. In the respiratory tract alone, expression of iNOS has been reported in alveolar type II epithelial cells [36], lung fibroblasts [37], airway and vascular SM cells [38], airway respiratory epithelial cells [39], mast cells, endothelial cells, neutrophils and chondrocytes [1]. The stimuli that cause transcriptional activation of iNOS in these cells vary widely and include endogenous mediators (such as chemokines and cytokines) as well as exogenous factors such as bacterial toxins, virus infection, allergens, environmental pollutants (ozone, oxidative stress, silica), hypoxia, tumours, etc. [40]. The expression of iNOS in the lung can be prevented by glucocorticoids [41] presumably reducing the inflammatory signals that lead to the induction of iNOS.

L-ARGININE AS NOS SUBSTRATE

L-arginine is an essential amino acid, which is supplied by the diet and actively transported into the cell *via* cationic amino acid transporter (CAT). L-arginine is the physiological substrate for NOS and L-arginine availability could determine cellular rates of NO production.

A high-affinity carrier resembling the CAT system y^+ is likely to be responsible for the transcellular transport of arginine with minor roles being played by systems $b^{0,+}$, $B^{0,+}$, and y^+L [42]. The physiological hallmarks of system y^+ are the high affinity for amino acids with a positively charged side chain, its independence from the concentration of extracellular Na^+, and the *trans*-stimulation of arginine transport by the other cationic amino acids L-lysine and L-ornithine. This system has been detected in many cells, among them macrophages, endothelial cells, platelets and vascular SM cells [42]. System y^+ activity is mediated by the CAT family that is composed of four isoforms, CAT-1, CAT-2A, CAT-2B, and CAT-3 [43].

L-arginine transport in tissues and many different cell types, such as vascular SM cells and macrophages, can be stimulated by LPS, but is hardly affected by tumour necrosis factor-α, interleukin-1α or interferon-γ [43]. These findings suggest that induction of iNOS and L-arginine transporter activity are dependent on the stimulus used, with an adequate combination of cytokines and/or LPS being responsible for full activation of one or both pathways. Dexamethasone selectively inhibits the production of NO produced by iNOS whilst having no effect on transport, indicating that the gene for the L-arginine transporter is not sensitive to regulation by glucocorticoids [44]. Oral administration of L-arginine to man is associated with an increased concentration of NO in exhaled air and was associated with an increase in the concentration of L-arginine and nitrate in plasma [45]. These results suggest that an increase in the amount of substrate for NO can increase the formation of endogenous NO.

Arginine can be metabolized by two groups of enzymes. As mentioned above, arginine can be converted by NOS to citrulline but can also be catabolized by arginase. Arginase exists in two isoforms, liver-type arginase I and non-hepatic type arginase II [46]. Arginase I is localized in cytosol, and arginase II is located in the mitochondrial matrix. Arginase I, but not arginase II, is co-induced with iNOS in rat peritoneal macrophages and *in vivo* in rat lung after LPS treatment. Arginase can be induced in the lungs of rats after hyperoxia [47]. Allergy is considered to be a T helper (Th)2-mediated disease and indeed arginase activity is increased 3.5-fold in the lungs of guinea pigs after ovalbumin sensitization and challenge [48]. Meurs *et al.* [49] hypothesized that the corresponding airway hyperresponsiveness in these animals is caused by a NO deficiency due to the increased arginase activity. Indeed, pre-treatment of the tissues with the arginase inhibitor, N^{ω}-hydroxy-nor-L-arginine (nor-NOHA: an intermediate in NO biosynthesis) suppressed the allergen-induced airway hyperresponsiveness [48, 50]. Further, Zimmermann *et al.* demonstrated in animal experiments as well as in asthmatic patients that arginase was upregulated in the airways [51, 52]. Futhermore, arginase activity is increased and arginine bioavailability is decreased in the serum of asthmatics [53].

Therefore, a delicate balance between the beneficial and harmful pathophysiological effects of NO exists in the airways, which might be regulated by arginine metabolism.

MECHANISMS OF NO BIOACTIVITY

NO itself has a short half-life *in vivo* (1–5 s) because of its reactivity with transition metals (such as iron bound within haemoglobin) [54] and a broad spectrum of other biological compounds including oxygen and superoxide radicals. NO may be formed and/or bioactivated as nitroxyl (NO^{-}) or nitrosonium (NO^{+}). These chemical species have short half-lives in aqueous solution (<1 s), but are stabilized in biological complexes with thiols ($RS^{-}...^{+}NO$), nitrite ($O_2N^{-}...^{+}NO$) and other targets and intermediates [55]. NO is an ubiquitous messenger molecule that affects various biological functions, either at low concentrations as a signal in many physiological processes such as blood flow regulation, and non-adrenergic non-cholinergic neurotransmission, or at high concentrations as cytotoxic and cytostatic defensive mechanisms against pathogens [2].

Reactions of NO ultimately lead to the nitration (addition of $-NO_2$), nitrosation (addition of $-NO^{+}$), nitrosylation ($-NO$) of most classes of biomolecules. One of the best known interactions of NO leading to cell signalling is the reversible covalent binding, nitrosylation, with the ferrous haem in soluble guanylyl cyclase. Another aspect of NO signalling is the role of S-nitrosothiols (SNOs) that appear to be important molecules signalling 'NO' bioactivity in the lung. SNOs are products of NOS activation that are present in the airway lining fluid in μM concentrations, stored in specific cellular compartments to achieve bioactivity and metabolically regulated to deliver bioactivities both through transnitrosation reactions and through release of NO.

NO bioactivities are broadly classified as NO-mediated/cyclic GMP-dependent and cyclic guanosine monophosphate (cGMP)-independent. Many bioactivities, such as airway SM relaxation, appear to use both.

Chemical features of NO radical include its rapid diffusion from the point of synthesis, the ability to permeate cell membranes, the interactions with intracellular molecular sites within both generating and target cells and its intrinsic instability, all properties that eliminate the need for extracellular NO receptors or targeted NO degradation. The best-characterized target site for NO is the iron bound in the haeme component of soluble guanylyl cyclase stimulating conversion of GTP to cGMP and mediating the biological effects attributed to eNOS-derived NO [56]. Subsequently, cGMP exerts most of the intracellular actions by coupling to cGMP-dependent protein kinase (PKG). It is generally accepted that cGMP triggers relaxation of SM by activating two molecular mechanisms: reduction of intracellular Ca^{2+} ($[Ca^{2+}]_i$), and reduction of the sensitivity of the contractile system to the Ca^{2+}. The former is due to the ability of activated PKG to phosphorylate several key target proteins with the final effect of $[Ca^{2+}]_i$ reduction. In particular, PKG may stimulate Ca^{2+}-activated K^+ channels (K_{Ca}), inhibit membrane Ca^{2+} channel activity, activate Ca^{2+}/ATPase pump in the plasma membrane and in the sarcoplasmatic reticulum and inhibit inositol triphosphate receptor and generation [57]. The mechanism of the cGMP-induced Ca^{2+} desensitization is mainly ascribed to the stimulation of myosin light chain phosphatase activity *via* inhibition of RhoA-dependent pathway [58].

In addition, NO mediates other actions that are independent of guanylyl cyclase and cGMP. The high level of NO released by iNOS has an effect as immune effector molecule in killing tumour cells [59], in halting viral replication [60] and in eliminating various pathogens. In fact, NO has been reported to inhibit the growth of or kill a number of fungi, parasites, and bacteria including *Mycobacterium tuberculosis* [61].

Pulmonary SNO bioactivities are those in which functional protein modification is caused by NO transfer to a cysteine thiol. Specificity of this signalling is achieved by regulation of synthesis, compartmentalization, compositional balance and catabolism. S-nitrosothiol synthesis may be regulated following NOS activation by proteins such as ceruloplasmin, haemoglobin and albumin [62], and/or NOS itself [63]. Specific compartments of relevance are, e.g., the mitochondrial intermembrane space, where S-nitrosylated caspases are sequestered before being released into the reducing environment of the cytosol and thereby activated by reductive cleavage of the SNO bond [64]. Compositional specificity is reflected in the requirement of S-nitrosoglutathione to be cleaved to S-nitrosocysteineylglycine – and thereby activated for intracellular transport – by gamma glutamyl transpeptidase [65].

Interaction of NO with many molecular targets may also represent a pathway for its breakdown and inactivation. The most important interaction is probably its reaction with super oxide anion (O_2^-) to yield peroxynitrite anion ($ONOO^-$), which is a potent cytotoxic molecule [66].

NITRIC OXIDE AND OXIDATIVE STRESS: 'NITROSATIVE STRESS'

Reactive oxygen species (ROS) are generated by various enzymatic reactions and chemical processes or they can be directly inhaled. NO can interact with ROS to form other reactive nitrogen species (RNS) [66]. ROS, NO and RNS are essential in many physiological reactions and are important for the killing of invading micro-organisms. However, when airway cells and tissues are exposed to oxidative stress elicited by environmental pollutants, infections, inflammatory reactions or decreased levels of anti-oxidants, enhanced levels of ROS and RNS can have a variety of deleterious effects within the airways, thereby inducing several pathophysiological conditions. ROS and RNS can damage DNA, lipids, proteins and carbohydrates leading to impaired cellular functions and enhanced inflammatory reactions. In this way, ROS and RNS play a prominent role in the pathogenesis of various lung disorders such as asthma [66–68].

Because NO and super oxide are free radicals, both molecules rapidly react with many different molecules in a biological environment. Enhanced cytotoxicity is possible when NO and super oxide are released simultaneously, which is a likely event during inflammatory responses. Many of the products formed by the interaction of super oxide and NO are even more reactive than their precursors. The most direct interaction between NO and super oxide is their rapid iso-stoichiometric reaction to form the potent oxidant peroxynitrite [69]. The interaction between NO and super oxide may generate other RNS. Besides peroxynitrite formation, NO-derived nitrite can be utilized in the myeloperoxidase pathway leading to NO_2Cl and NO_2^* [70].

ROS is a collective term that includes a large variety of free oxygen radicals (e.g. super oxide anion and hydroxyl radicals) but also derivatives of oxygen that do not contain unpaired electrons (e.g. hydrogen peroxide, hypochlorous acid, peroxynitrite and ozone). The univalent reduction of oxygen to super oxide anion is the first step in the formation of ROS. These compounds can either spontaneously or enzymatically dismutase to hydrogen peroxide. Granulocytes contain peroxidases (myeloperoxidase and eosinophil peroxidase [EPO]) that are able to catalyse the reaction of hydrogen peroxide with halides leading to the formation of hypohalides (e.g. hypochlorous acid) [71].

Formation of ROS takes place constantly in every cell during normal metabolic processes. Cellular sites for production of ROS include mitochondria, microsomes and enzymes (e.g. xanthine oxidase, P450 mono-oxygenase, cyclo-oxygenase, lipoxygenase, indole amine dioxygenase, monoamine oxidase) [72]. Activated phagocytic cells (neutrophils, eosinophils, monocytes and macrophages) produce large amounts of ROS. These cells are stimulated when encountering inhaled particles, micro-organisms or other mediators that lead to the activation of the membrane-bound NADPH-oxidase complex and the generation of the super oxide anion [71, 73].

Besides the generation of reactive species *via* cellular pathways, formation of ROS and RNS in the lungs can also take place after inhalation of exogenous compounds like ozone, nitrogen dioxide, cigarette smoke and other chemicals and dust particles [72, 74]. In addition, such exposures lead to depletion of endogenous anti-oxidants that are present in the epithelial lining fluid.

Due to the complex chemistry and often short half-life of RNS, the exact metabolic fate *in vivo* remains unclear. Nonetheless, some stable end-products of RNS are detectable in body fluids and tissues. Firstly, NO decomposes into nitrite and nitrate and these metabolites can be measured in plasma [75]. Furthermore, 3-nitrotyrosine residues have been found in tissue samples by the use of immunohistochemistry [76], but also in biological fluids [77]. 3-nitrotyrosine is readily formed by a NO-independent process mediated by myeloperoxidase, with hydrogen peroxide and nitrite as substrates [70]. Moreover, EPO is an even stronger promoter of 3-nitrotyrosine formation *via* this pathway [78, 79].

Nitrite and nitrate levels in plasma, for example, can reflect dietary intake rather than NO metabolism *in vivo* [80]. Moreover, NO is also formed enzyme-independently from nitrite under acidic conditions [81]. Hunt *et al.* [82] showed that the pH in the airways drops dramatically during an acute asthma attack, which facilitates the conversion of nitrite to NO. Hence, increased NO concentrations in the exhaled air of asthmatic patients may reflect nitrite conversion rather than NOS activity.

Enzymes and chemicals are present within the airway cells and in the epithelial lining fluid of the airways to protect against the toxicity of generated ROS and RNS. The major enzymatic systems present in the airways are manganese and copper–zinc super oxide dismutases, which rapidly convert the super oxide anion to hydrogen peroxide, catalase that converts hydrogen peroxide into oxygen and water and the glutathione redox system (GSH-peroxidase and GSH-reductase) that inactivates NO, hydrogen peroxide and other hydroperoxides [67, 83, 84]. The epithelial lining fluid of the respiratory tract contains large amounts of glutathione and more than 95% of this glutathione is in the reduced form [85].

The effects of RNS, once formed *in vivo*, on tissues, cells and biomolecules are diverse. Important targets of RNS in proteins are, for example, tyrosine residues [86], thiols [1] and haeme groups [87]. Furthermore, RNS alter lipid oxidation pathways [88], cause DNA damage [89] and inhibit mitochondrial respiration [90]. Exposure of cells to RNS leads to both apoptosis and necrosis dependent on the severity of cell damage [79]. Mitogen-activated protein kinases (MAPK) may mediate signal transduction pathways induced by RNS in lung epithelial cells leading to cell death [91].

It has been shown that 3-NT, 3-bromotyrosine and 3-chlorotyrosine, markers of protein nitration and EPO- and myeloperoxidase-catalyzed oxidation, respectively, are dramatically increased in the broncoalveolar lavage of severe asthmatics compared to non-asthmatic subjects [92]. In the bronchial tissues from individuals who died of asthma the most intense 3-NT immunostaining were in epitopes that co-localized with eosinophils suggesting a major role for eosinophils as a source of the nitrating process in asthma.

NO AS INFLAMMATORY MARKER IN ASTHMA

NO AND Th2-MEDIATED INFLAMMATION IN ASTHMA

NO, derived from airway epithelial cells, macrophages and Th1 cells, plays an important role in amplifying and perpetuating the Th2-cell-mediated inflammatory response, both in allergic and non-allergic asthma. iNOS may be induced in epithelial cells by exposure to pro-inflammatory cytokines such as TNFα and IL-1β secreted by macrophages, and IFNγ secreted by Th1 cells. It is possible that viral infections may also induce iNOS in airway epithelial cells, augmenting the secretion of NO during asthma exacerbations. Using an allergic animal model, it has been shown that the manifestations of allergic airway disease, including infiltration of inflammatory cells (eosinophils), microvascular leakage and airway occlusion are markedly less severe in the iNOS$^{-/-}$ mutants than in wild-type animals [93]. Interestingly, the suppression of allergic inflammation was accompanied by marked increases in T cell production of IFNγ but not by reduction in the secretion of either IL-4 or IL-5. The markedly enhanced production of IFNγ in iNOS$^{-/-}$ mice was apparently responsible for the suppression of both eosinophils and disease, as *in vivo* depletion of this factor restored allergic pathology in these animals [93]. Thus, iNOS promotes allergic inflammation in airways *via* downregulation of IFNγ activity and suggests that inhibitors of this molecule may represent a worthwhile therapeutic strategy for allergic diseases including asthma.

In addition, NO has been reported to promote the production of chemotactic factors (chemokines) for eosinophils in mice [94], suggesting the possibility that NO acts as part of a positive feedback loop in which inflammatory cells produce NO and thereby promote their further recruitment through the action of chemokines.

Recent studies also demonstrated that NO inhibits macrophage-derived IL-12 release, which is a major inducer of Th1 cells, preventing the excessive amplification of Th1 cells [95], and that NO-generating agents increased the secretion of IL-4 in Th2 clones [96]. This suggests that, despite the complex feedback network regulating NO production, the enhanced IL-4 expression would lead to the expansion of Th2 cells once NO is generated.

EXHALED NO

Although bronchial biopsies remain the gold standard to understanding and treating asthma, there is a preference for non-invasive techniques such as exhaled NO in monitoring inflammation in asthma. Exhaled NO measurements are easy to perform and are repeatable. Given the strong correlations between exhaled NO and bronchial biopsy and induced sputum eosinophilia NO may now be advocated as a surrogate for these tests [97].

NO is detectable in exhaled air of humans as measured by chemiluminescence analysers [3]. The measurement of exhaled NO is critically dependent on expiratory flow [98], which requires careful standardization of the measurement. Such standardization was accomplished by international guidelines on the methods of measurement of exhaled NO, both for adults and in children [99, 100].

NO production and expiratory NO concentrations can be predicted by a two-compartment model of the lung, consisting of a non-expansible compartment representing the conducting airways and an expansible compartment representing the respiratory bronchioles and alveoli

[101]. The model predicts that both compartments contribute to NO in the exhaled breath, and that the relative contributions of airways and parenchyma can be separated by analysis of the relationship between exhaled NO output (nl/s) against expiratory flow rate (ml/s) [101, 102]. Interestingly, such analysis may indeed allow the discrimination of airways diseases, such as asthma, from alveolitis [103] or liver cirrhosis [104] in patients with elevated levels of exhaled NO.

In atopic asthma exhaled NO is heightened in comparison with healthy controls [105, 106]. In asthma the increased levels of exhaled NO have a predominant lower airway origin [107, 108]; and appear to be associated with increased expression of corticosteroid-sensitive iNOS [76]. Recent studies showed that exhaled NO levels in asthma are almost suppressed by the novel selective iNOS inhibitor SC-51 [109]. Thus, NOS-II is the most important source of NO detected in the exhaled air of asthmatics. Furthermore, exhaled NO may reflect disease severity [110] and, to a greater extent, clinical control of asthma [111] particularly during exacerbations [112].

Exhaled NO has been used to monitor asthma exacerbations, both spontaneous [113] and induced by steroid reduction [114], and the effect of anti-inflammatory treatment in asthma [110]. Asthma treatment with corticosteroids results in a reduction of expired NO levels due to both reducing effects of steroids on the underlying airways inflammation in asthma and inhibitory effects on iNOS expression itself. Oral and inhaled corticosteroids have been shown to result in a rapid (after 6 h following a single corticosteroid treatment) [114] and dose-dependent reduction [115, 116]. In patients with more severe persistent asthma, airway inflammatory processes may overcome this steroid-sensitivity of NO, leading to increased levels of exhaled NO even during treatment with high doses of oral or inhaled corticosteroids [114].

During the last few years several studies have been performed in order to assess the relationship between levels of exhaled NO and other markers of airway inflammation. Exhaled NO is associated with eosinophilic inflammation as determined in blood [117], urine [118], bronchoalveolar lavage [119] and sputum [120] in asthmatics with varying disease severity. A significant relationship has also been shown between exhaled NO and mucosal eosinophil numbers in bronchial biopsies from children with difficult asthma [121] and from atopic adult asthmatics after allergen challenge. This indicates that exhaled NO is a novel non-invasive biomarker reflecting airway eosinophilic inflammation in asthma. High production of endogenous NO such as in acute asthma may result in a deleterious effect, and may be involved in the orchestration of eosinophilic inflammation that characterizes asthma.

THERAPEUTIC EFFECTS FOR NO RELEASE IN ASTHMA

AIRWAY CONTRACTIONS

Nijkamp *et al.* [122] showed in guinea pigs that aerosolized NOS inhibitors enhanced bronchoconstriction induced by increasing intravenous doses of histamine *in vivo*, suggesting a modulator role for endogenous NO in airway reactivity. Recently, similar results were found in mice, in which the endogenous NO were modulated by IL-10 and related to airway responsiveness [123]. Furthermore, Ricciardolo *et al.* [124] found an L-arginine/NO-dependent modulation of bradykinin-induced bronchoconstriction in guinea pigs that originates independently from the simultaneous activation of the excitatory neural component: postganglionic cholinergic nerves and capsaicin-sensitive afferent nerves. Furthermore, it has been shown that eNOS$^{-/-}$ mice were more hyperresponsive to inhaled methacholine and less sensitive to NOS inhibitor compared to wild-type mice demonstrating that NO derived from eNOS plays a physiological role in controlling airway reactivity [125]. We showed that airway hyperresponsiveness to methacholine was completely abolished in eNOS overexpressing, ovalbumin-challenged mice compared to control mice in conjunction with a decrease in the number of lymphocytes and eosinophils in the bronchoalveolar lavage (BAL) fluid [126]. Recently, similar findings were published in mice where iNOS was upregulated by doxycycline [127] or nNOS was activated by oestrogen [128].

The functional importance of epithelium in airway reactivity is now generally accepted. Experimental evidence has shown that airway epithelium is the source of NO as modulator of bronchomotor tone. Treatment of guinea pig trachea *in vitro* with an inactivator of guanylyl cyclase caused a 5-fold increase in the sensitivity to histamine contractile response indicating the involvement of NO/cGMP pathway in the development of airway hyperresponsiveness [129]. The electrochemical detection of bradykinin-induced NO release in guinea pig airways was fast (duration ~2 s), mainly dependent on the epithelium and absent in Ca^{2+}-free medium, suggesting that a Ca^{2+}-dependent eNOS pathway seems to be involved in the endogenous release of bronchoprotective NO [130].

Cationic proteins inhibit L-arginine uptake in rat alveolar macrophages and tracheal epithelial cells, suggesting that polycationic peptides released by activated eosinophils in the inflamed airways may contribute to the deficiency of bronchoprotective eNOS-derived NO [131]. Indeed, polycation-induced airway hyperreactivity to methacholine is dependent on the deficiency of endogenous NO [132]. In a further study, these authors found that endogenous arginase activity potentiates methacholine-induced airway constriction by inhibition of NO production in naive guinea pig, presumably by competition with eNOS for the common substrate L-arginine [133]. In a recent and elegant study Ten Broeke *et al.* [134] showed that calcium-like peptides (CALP1 and CALP2) targeting calcium-binding EF hand motif of calcium sensors (calmodulin and calcium channels) may have a role in regulating airway responsiveness by controlling $[Ca^{2+}]_i$ and, consequently, modulating the activity of eNOS. In fact CALP2 inhibition of CALP1-induced airway hyperresponsiveness was Ca^{2+}-epithelium-dependent and NO-mediated [135]. Interestingly, they found that bradykinin-induced $[Ca^{2+}]_i$ increase in epithelial cells was markedly higher after incubation with CALP2. Thus, CALP2, which acts as calmodulin antagonist, selectively increases $[Ca^{2+}]$ in epithelial cells resulting in the release of NO from the epithelium with the subsequent relaxation of the SM. On the other hand, CALP1, which acts as calmodulin agonist, decreases $[Ca^{2+}]$ in epithelial cells and therefore NO production is diminished leading to airway SM contraction (Figure 6.2) [135].

In allergen-challenged guinea pigs, the enhanced contractile response to agonists in tracheal preparations after early reaction was not augmented by NOS inhibition as shown in naive animals suggesting an impairment of protective NO [136]. In a further study, the same authors showed that L-arginine administration reduced methacholine-induced contraction in isolated perfused tracheae from guinea pigs indicating that limitation of the substrate may underlie the reduced eNOS activity and the excessive contractile response [137]. Finally, it has also been demonstrated that increased arginase activity contributes to allergen-induced deficiency of eNOS-derived NO and airway hyperresponsiveness after early allergen reaction in guinea pigs, presumably by direct competition with eNOS for L-arginine [48].

Different groups of investigators have shown that acute bronchoconstriction induced by allergen inhalation is potentiated by NOS inhibitors in sensitized guinea pigs *in vivo*, suggesting a modulation by endogenous protective NO on early asthmatic reaction in animal models [138–140]. Other *in vivo* studies in guinea pigs have shown that the enhanced airway reactivity induced by allergen (6 h after exposure) is not further potentiated by pre-treatment with NOS inhibitors [141, 142] and that virus-induced airway reactivity is completely blocked by low doses of inhaled L-arginine [143], suggesting that allergen- or virus-induced airway hyperreactivity is due to the impairment of endogenous release of protective NO.

AIRWAY HYPERRESPONSIVENESS

Recently, in order to examine the possible involvement of the eNOS gene as the genetic basis of bronchial asthma, it has been investigated whether there was any association

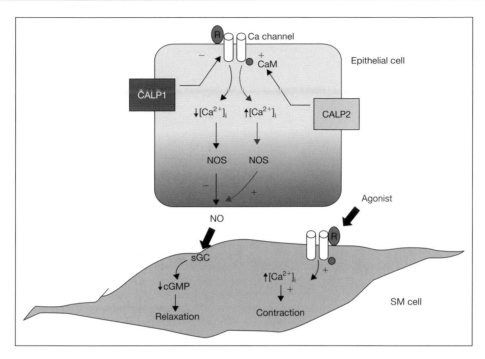

Figure 6.2 Diagram of the hypothesized action of CALP1 and CALP2 on airway epithelial cell modulating SM contraction. Calcium influx in the SM after agonist stimulation leads to a contraction, whilst calcium influx in the epithelial cells (EC) after agonist stimulation (e.g. bradykinin) results in the production of NO leading to relaxation of the SM ('biochemical antagonism'). In asthma epithelial damage and/or impaired NO synthesis may provoke enhanced SM contraction (see text). CALP2 selectively increases $[Ca^{2+}]_i$ in epithelial cells resulting in the release of NO from the epithelium and subsequent SM relaxation. On the other hand, CALP1 decreases $[Ca^{2+}]_i$ in epithelial cells and subsequently NO production is reduced leading to increased airway hyperresponsiveness. Ca = Calcium channel; $[Ca^{2+}]_i$ = intracellular calcium concentration; CaM = calmodulin; R = receptor; sGC = soluble guanylate cyclase; SM = smooth muscle.

between bronchial asthma and polymorphisms of the *eNOS* gene. The study by Lee *et al.* [144] revealed that the distribution of one genotype (bb) of eNOS was significantly higher in the asthma group than in the control population, but the eNOS genotype distribution did not differ significantly among groups of patients with different severities of asthma. In addition, as mentioned above, a recent analysis has demonstrated an association between a missense sequence variant in the *eNOS* gene and exhaled NO levels in asthma, in the absence of associations of this mutation with the level of airways obstruction or its reversibility in these patients [145]. Therefore, all of these results suggest that polymorphisms of the eNOS gene may be associated with the development of asthma, but the severity of asthma may not be influenced by polymorphisms of *eNOS* gene. *nNOS* gene polymorphism has also been associated with asthma [146]. More recently, it has been shown that *nNOS* gene polymorphism is associated with atopy [147] and immunoglobulin (Ig)E levels [148].

Allergen and viral infection are also called inducers of airway hyperresponsiveness since they are able to increase naive reactivity in animal and human asthma [149, 150]. Increased airway hyperresponsiveness to bradykinin, induced by allergen exposure in asthma, is due to impaired production of bronchoprotective NO, a phenomenon that is associated with downregulation of eNOS and upregulation of iNOS within the airway epithelium [151]. The latter findings underscore the relevance of bronchoprotection by endogenous NO to limit airway hyperresponsiveness in asthma and warrant the development of treatment strategies to restore eNOS activity during exacerbations [151].

Clinical researchers investigated the capability of endogenous NO to affect airway hyperresponsiveness in asthma. Ricciardolo *et al.* [152], for the first time, performed a randomized double-blind, placebo-controlled study of the effect of NOS inhibition in bradykinin-induced asthma. The authors described a potentiation of bradykinin- and methacholine-induced airway hyperresponsiveness (AHR) after pre-treatment with the NOS inhibitor, suggesting a bronchoprotective role for endogenous NO in mild asthma. Furthermore, they found that this potentiation was much greater in AHR to bradykinin in comparison to methacholine, indicating that a mediator-specific response is involved. In a further study, the same group revealed an impairment of NOS inhibition on AHR to bradykinin in severe asthma, possibly due to the reduction or absence of eNOS in the airway of severe asthmatic patients [153]. Following these observations, it has also been discovered that severe asthmatics treated with a higher dose of corticosteroids than in the previous study are less hyperresponsive to bradykinin, but that the pre-treatment with NOS inhibitor markedly enhanced AHR to bradykinin as shown in mild asthma [154]. This suggests an effect of high doses of corticosteroids in renewing eNOS activity by suppression of iNOS expression. A similar mode of action cannot be excluded for montelukast as well [155]. On the other hand, the corticoid-induced suppression of iNOS expression in airway epithelium may also result in a decreased inflammatory response and hence in suppression of AHR [156]. Moreover, NO will not suppress AHR under all conditions, since oral L-arginine did not influence AHR to histamine as reflected by PC_{20}, although the dose–response slope was slightly reduced in patients with asthma [157]. Recently, Redington [158] reviewed the therapeutical potential for NO in asthma and chronic obstructive pulmonary disease (COPD) in an excellent review.

AIRWAY REMODELLING

Airway SM hypertrophy and hyperplasia, features of airway remodelling, are important determinants of airway hyperresponsiveness in asthma. *In vitro* studies have recently demonstrated that DNA synthesis and proliferation of human airway SM cells (HASMC) are reduced by exogenous administration of NO donors [159, 160]. More recently, it has been demonstrated that NO inhibited HASMC proliferation in G1 phase *via* cGMP-dependent pathway, but the inhibition of HASMC proliferation in S phase was due to cGMP-independent inhibition of ribonucleotide reductase [161]. These newly discovered antiproliferative effects of NO on airway SM might become an important clue for future strategies to prevent airway remodelling in chronic asthma and COPD.

SUMMARY

It is of great therapeutic value that appropriate pharmacological treatments are made available to either promote or inhibit NO production since both excess tissue NO and its deficiency have been implicated in the development of several disease states, a typical example being asthma.

The discovery of the delicate role of endogenous NO in the homeostasis of various cellular functions and the dynamic behaviour of the airways, has led to a new, rapidly progressing area of physiological science that has direct bearing on our understanding of multiple airway diseases. Moreover, there are novel opportunities for modulating NO-synthesis aimed at restoring the balance between the protective and deleterious effects of NO. This is potentially beneficial in both airway and alveolar diseases. Such interventions might be targeted in various ways, e.g. by using selective NOS inhibitors, NO donors, inhalation of NO. Pharmaceutical industries try to modulate the expression of the different NOS enzymes. The development of gene transfer therapy selectively for NOS isoforms could open a new horizon in the treatment of bronchial asthma. Recombinant adenovirus overexpressing eNOS or nNOS may have potentially protective effects in asthmatic airways including neuromodulation by mediating inhibitory non-cholinergic non-adrenergic nerve activity, SM relaxation and reduction in airway hyperresponsiveness.

REFERENCES

1. Ricciardolo FLM, Sterk PJ, Gaston B et al. Nitric oxide in health and disease of the respiratory system. *Physiol Rev* 2004; 84:731–765.
2. Moncada S, Palmer RMJ, Higgs EA. Nitric oxide: physiology, pathophysiology, and pharmacology. *Pharmacol Rev* 1991; 43:109–142.
3. Gustafsson LE, Leone AM, Persson MG et al. Endogenous nitric oxide is present in the exhaled air of rabbits, guinea pigs and humans. *Biochem Biophys Res Commun* 1991; 181:852–857.
4. Alving K, Weitzberg E, Lundberg JM. Increased amount of nitric oxide in exhaled air of asthmatics. *Eur Respir J* 1993; 6:1368–1370.
5. Kobzik L, Bredt DS, Lowenstein CJ et al. Nitric oxide synthase in human and rat lung: immunocytochemical and histochemical localization. *Am J Respir Cell Mol Biol* 1993; 9:371–377.
6. Hamid Q, Springall DR, Riveros-Moreno V et al. Induction of nitric oxide synthase in asthma. *Lancet* 1993; 342:1510–1513.
7. Fischer A, Mundel P, Mayer B et al. Nitric oxide synthase in guinea pig lower airway innervation. *Neurosci Lett* 1993; 149:157–160.
8. Förstermann U, Schmidt HH, Pollock JS et al. Isoforms of nitric oxide synthase: characterization and purification from different cell types. *Biochem Pharmacol* 1991; 42:1849–1857.
9. Morris SM, Billiar T. New insights into the regulation of inducible nitric oxide synthesis. *Am J Physiol* 1994; 266:E829–E839.
10. Guo FH, DeRaeve HR, Rice TW et al. Continuous nitric oxide synthesis by inducible nitric oxide synthase in normal human airway epithelium in vivo. *Proc Natl Acad Sci USA* 1995; 92:7809–7813.
11. Uetani K, Thomassen MJ, Erzurum SC. Nitric oxide synthase 2 through an autocrine loop via respiratory epithelial cell-derived mediator. *Am J Physiol Lung Cell Mol Physiol* 2001; 280:L1179–L1188.
12. Robbins RA, Springall DR, Warren JB et al. Inducible nitric oxide synthase is increased in murine lung epithelial cells by cytokine stimulation. *Biochem Biophys Res Commun* 1994; 198:1027–1033.
13. Lyons C. Emerging roles of nitric oxide in inflammation. *Hosp Pract* 1996; 31:77–80.
14. Pitt BR, St Croix CM. Complex regulation of iNOS in lung. *Am J Respir Cell Mol Biol* 2002; 26:6–9.
15. Guo FH, Uetani K, Haque SJ et al. Interferon γ and interleukin 4 stimulate prolonged expression of inducible nitric oxide synthase in human airway epithelium through synthesis of soluble mediators. *J Clin Invest* 1997; 100:829–838.
16. Haque SJ, Williams BR. Signal transduction in the interferon system. *Semin Oncol* 1998; 25:14–22.
17. Guo FH, Comhair SA, Zheng S et al. Molecular mechanisms of increased nitric oxide (NO) in asthma: evidence for trascriptional and post-translational regulation of NO synthesis. *J Immunol* 2000; 164:5970–5980.
18. Forstermann U, Boissel JP, Kleinert H. Expressional control of the 'constitutive' isoforms of nitric oxide synthase (NOS I and eNOS). *FASEB J* 1998; 12:773–790.
19. Michel T, Feron O. Nitric oxide synthases: which, where, how, and why? *J Clin Invest* 1997; 100:2146–2152.
20. Kirsch EA, Yuhanna IS, Chen Z et al. Estrogen acutely stimulates endothelial nitric oxide synthase in H441 human airway epithelial cells. *Am J Respir Cell Mol Biol* 1999; 20:658–666.
21. Shaul P, North AJ, Wu LC et al. Endothelial nitric oxide synthase is expressed in cultured human bronchiolar epithelium. *J Clin Invest* 1994; 94:2231–2236.
22. Pechkovsky DV, Zissel G, Goldmann T et al. Pattern of NOS2 and NOS3 mRNA expression in human A549 cells and primary cultured AEC II. *Am J Physiol Lung Cell Mol Physiol* 2002; 282:L684–L692.
23. Kawamoto H, Takumida M, Takeno S et al. Localization of nitric oxide synthase in human nasal mucosa with nasal allergy. *Acta Otolaryngol* 1998; 539:65–70.
24. Xue C, Botkin SJ, Johns RA. Localization of endothelial NOS at the basel microtubule membrane in ciliated epithelium of rat lung. *J Hist Cytochem* 1996; 44:463–471.
25. Jain B, Rubinstein I, Robbins RA et al. Modulation of airway epithelial cell ciliary beat frequency by nitric oxide. *Biochem Biophys Res Commun* 1993; 191:83–88.

26. Fischer A, Hoffmann B. Nitric oxide synthase in neurons and nerve fibers of lower airways and in vagal sensory ganglia of man. *Am J Respir Crit Care Med* 1996; 154:209–216.

27. Belvisi MG, Stretton CD, Yacoub M *et al*. Nitric oxide is the endogenous neurotransmitter of bronchidilator nerves in humans. *Eur J Pharmacol* 1992; 210:221–222.

28. Ellis JL, Undem BJ. Inhibition by L-N^G-nitro-L-arginine of nonadrenergic-noncholinergic-mediated relaxations of human isolated central and peripheral airways. *Am Rev Respir Dis* 1992; 146: 1543–1547.

29. Widdicombe J. Autonomic regulation. i-NANC/e-NANC. *Am J Respir Crit Care Med* 1998; 158:S171–S175.

30. Kummer W, Fischer A, Mundel P *et al*. Nitric oxide synthase in VIP-containing vasodilator nerve fibres in the guinea pig. *Neuro Rep* 1992; 3:653–655.

31. Fischer A, Mayer B, Kummer W. Nitric oxide synthase in vagal sensory and sympathetic neurons innervating the guinea-pig trachea. *J Auton Nerv Syst* 1996; 56:157–160.

32. Knowles RG, Merrett M, Salter M *et al*. Differential induction of brain, lung and liver nitric oxide synthase by endotoxin in rat. *Biochem J* 1990; 270:833–836.

33. Xie Q, Cho HJ, Calaycay J *et al*. Cloning and characterization of inducible nitric oxide synthase from mouse macrophages. *Science* 1992; 256:225–228.

34. Pechkovsky DV, Zissel G, Stamme C *et al*. Human alveolar epithelial cells induce nitric oxide synthase-2 expression in alveolar macrophages. *Eur Respir J* 2002; 19:672–683.

35. Fischer A, Folkerts G, Geppetti P *et al*. Mediators of asthma: nitric oxide. *Pulm Pharmacol Ther* 2002; 15:73–81.

36. Warner RL, Paine R, Christensen PJ *et al*. Lung sources and cytokine requirements for in vivo expression of inducible nitic oxide synthase. *Am J Respir Cell Mol Biol* 1995; 12:649–661.

37. Romanska HM, Polak JM, Coleman RA *et al*. iNOS gene upregulation is associated with the early proliferative response of human lung fibroblasts to cytokine stimulation. *J Pathol* 2002; 197:372–379.

38. Griffith MJ, Liu S, Curzen NP *et al*. In vivo treatment with endotoxin induces nitric oxide synthase in rat main pulmonary artery. *Am J Physiol – Lung Cell Mol Physiol* 1995; 268:L509-L518.

39. Watkins DN, Peroni DJ, Basclain KA *et al*. Expression and activity of nitric oxide synthases in human airway epithelium. *Am J Respir Cell Mol Biol* 1997; 16:629–639.

40. Yan ZQ, Hansson GK, Skoogh BE *et al*. Induction of nitric oxide synthase in a model of allergic occupational asthma. *Allergy* 1995; 50:760–764.

41. Haddad EB, Liu SF, Salmon M *et al*. Expression of inducible nitric oxide synthase mRNA in Brown Norway rats exposed to ozone: effect of dexamethasone. *Eur J Pharmacol* 1995; 293:287–290.

42. Deves R, Boyd C. Transporters for cationic amino acids in animal cells: discovery, structure, and function. *Physiol Rev* 1998; 78:487–545.

43. Mori M, Gotoh T. Regulation of nitric oxide production by arginine metabolic enzymes. *Biochem Biophys Res Commun* 2000; 275:715–719.

44. Wileman SM, Mann GE, Baydoun AR. Induction of L-arginine transport and nitric oxide synthase in vascular smooth muscle cells: synergistic actions of pro-inflammatory cytokines and bacterial lipopolysaccharide. *Br J Pharmacol* 1995; 116:3243–3250.

45. Sapienza A, Kharitonov SA, Horvath I *et al*. Effect of inhaled L-arginine on exhaled nitric oxide in normal and asthmatic subjects. *Thorax* 1998; 53:172–175.

46. Ricciardolo FLM, Zaagsma J, Meurs H. The therapeutic potential of drugs targeting the arginase pathway in asthma. *Expert Opin Investig Drugs* 2005; 14:1221–1231.

47. Que L, Kantrow S, Jenkinson C *et al*. Induction of arginase isoforms in the lung during hyperoxia. *Am J Physiol* 1998; 275:L96–L102.

48. Meurs H, McKay S, Maarsingh H *et al*. Increased arginase activity underlies allergen-induced deficiency of cNOS-derived nitric oxide and airway hyperresponsiveness. *B J Pharmacol* 2002; 136:391–398.

49. Meurs H, Maarsingh H, Zaagsma J. Arginase and asthma: novel insights into nitric oxide homeostasis and airway responsiveness. *Trends Pharmacol Sci* 2003; 24:450–455.

50. Buga G, Singh R, Pervin S *et al*. Arginase activity in endothelial cells: inhibition by N^G-hydroxy-L-arginine during high-output NO production. *Am J Physiol* 1996; 271:H1988–H1998.

51. Zimmermann N, King NE, Laporte J *et al*. Dissection of experimental asthma with DNA microarray analysis indentifies arginase in asthma pathogenesis. *J Clin Invest* 2003; 111:1863–1874.

52. King NE, Rothenberg ME, Zimmermann N. Arginine in asthma and lung inflammation. *J Nutr* 2004; 134:2830S–2836S.

53. Morris CR, Poljakovic M, Lavrisha L et al. Decreased arginine biovailability and increased serum arginase activity in asthma. Am J Respir Crit Care Med 2004; 170:148–153.
54. Thomas DD, Liu X, Kantrow SP et al. The biological lifetime of nitric oxide: implications for the perivascular dynamics of NO and O_2. Proc Natl Acad Sci USA 2001; 98:355–360.
55. Stamler JS, Singel DJ, Loscalzo J. Biochemistry of nitric oxide and its redox-activated forms. Science 1992; 258:1898–1902.
56. Ignarro L, Kadowitz P. The pharmacological and physiological role of cyclic GMP in vascular smooth muscle relaxation. Ann Rev Pharmacol Toxicol 1985; 25:171–191.
57. Carvajal JA, Germain AM, Huidobro-Toro JP et al. Molecular mechanism of cGMP-mediated smooth muscle relaxation. J Cell Physiol 2000; 184:409–420.
58. Sauzeau V, Le Jeune H, Cario-Toumaniantz C et al. Cyclic GMP-dependent protein kinase signaling pathway inhibits Rho-induced Ca^{2+} sensitization of contraction in vascular smooth muscle. J Biol Chem 2000; 275:21722–21729.
59. Hibbs JB, Taintor RR, Vavrin Z et al. Nitric oxide: a cytotoxic activated macrophages effector molecule. Biochem Biophys Res Commun 1988; 157:87–94.
60. Karupiah G, Xie QW, Buller RM et al. Inhibition of viral replication by interferon-gamma induced nitric oxide synthase. Science 1993; 261:1445–1448.
61. Denis M. Interferon-gamma-treated murine macrophages inhibit growth of tubercle bacilli via the generation of reactive nitrogen intermediates. Cell Immunol 1991; 132:150–157.
62. Rafikova O, Rafikova R, Nudler E. Catalysis of S-nitrosothiols formation by serum albumin: the mechanism and implication in vascular control. Proc Natl Acad Sci USA 2002; 59:5913–5918.
63. Gow A, Chen Q, Hess D et al. Basal and stimulated protein S-nitrosylation in multiple cell types and tissues. J Biol Chem 2002; 277:9637–9640.
64. Mannick J, Schonhoff C, Papeta N et al. S-nitrosylation of mitochondrial caspases. J Cell Biol 2001; 154:1111–1116.
65. Lipton A, Johnson M, Macdonald T et al. Nitrosothiols signal the ventilatory response to hypoxia. Nature 2001; 413:171–174.
66. Ricciardolo FLM, Di Stefano A, Sabatini F et al. Reactive nitrogen species in the respiratory tract. Eur J Pharmacol 2006; 533;240–252.
67. Repine J, Bast A, Lankhorst I et al. Oxidative stress in chronic obstructive pulmonary disease. Am J Respir Crit Care Med 1997; 156:341–357.
68. Bowler RP, Crapo JD. Oxidative stress in allergic respiratory diseases. J Allergy Clin Immunol 2002; 110:349–356.
69. Muijsers RBR, Folkerts G, Henricks PAJ et al. Peroxynitrite: a two faced metabolite of nitric oxide. Life Sci 1997; 60:1833–1845.
70. Eiserich J, Hristova M, Cross C et al. Formation of nitric oxide-derived inflammatory oxidants by myeloperoxidase in neutrophils. Nature 1998; 391:393–397.
71. Babior BM. Oxygen-dependent microbial killing by phagocytes. N Engl J Med 1978; 298:659–688.
72. Vallyathan V, Shi X. The role of oxygen free radicals in occupational and environmental lung diseases. Environ Health Perspect 1997; 105:165–177.
73. Henricks PAJ, Verhoef J, Nijkamp FP. Modulation of phagocytic cell function. Vet Res Commun 1986; 10:165–188.
74. Krishna M, Chauhan A, Frew A et al. Toxicological mechanisms underlying oxidant pollutant-induced airway injury. Rev Environ Health 1998; 13:59–71.
75. Kelm M. NO metabolism and breakdown. Biochim Biophys Acta 1999; 1411:273–289.
76. Saleh D, Ernst P, Lim S et al. Increased formation of the potent oxidant peroxynitrite in the airways of asthmatic patients is associated with induction of nitric oxide synthase: effect of inhaled glucocorticoid. FASEB J 1998; 12:929–937.
77. Ohshima H, Celam I, Chazotte L et al. Analysis of 3-nitrotyrosine in biological fluids and protein hydrolyzates by high-performance liquid chromatography using a postseparation, on-line reduction column and electrochemical detection: results with various nitrating agents. Nitric Oxide 1999; 3:132–141.
78. Wu W, Chen Y, Hazen SL. Eosinophil peroxidase nitrates protein tyrosyl residues. Implications for oxidative damage by nitrating intermediates in eosinophilic inflammatory disorders. J Biol Chem 1999; 274:25933–25944.
79. Murphy M. Nitric oxide and cell death. Biochim Biophys Acta 1999; 1411:401–414.

80. Ahren C, Jungersten L, Sandberg T. Plasma nitrate as an index of nitric oxide formation in patients with acute infectious diseases. *Scand J Infect Dis* 1999; 31:405–407.

81. Zweier JL, Samouilov A, Kuppusamy P. Non-enzymatic NO synthesis in biological systems. *Biochim Biophys Acta* 1999; 1411:250–262.

82. Hunt JF, Fang K, Malik R *et al*. Endogenous airway acidification. Implications for asthma pathophysiology. *Am J Respir Crit Care Med* 2000; 161:694–699.

83. Cantin A, Fells G, Hubbard R *et al*. Antioxidant macromolecules in the epithelial lining fluid of the normal human lower respiratory tract. *J Clin Invest* 1990; 86:962–971.

84. Pietarinen-Runtti P, Lakari E, Raivio K *et al*. Expression of antioxidant enzymes in human inflammatory cells. *Am J Physiol* 2000; 279:C118–C125.

85. Cantin A, North S, Hubbard R *et al*. Normal alveolar epithelial lining fluid contains high levels of glutathione. *J Appl Physiol* 1987; 63:152–157.

86. Van der Vliet A, Eiserich JP, Shigenaga MK *et al*. Reactive nitrogen species and tyrosine nitration in the respiratory tract: epiphenomena or a pathobiologic mechanism of disease? *Am J Respir Crit Care Med* 1999; 160:1–9.

87. Fang FC. Perspectives series: host/pathogen interactions. Mechanisms of nitric oxide-related antimicrobial activity. *J Clin Invest* 1997; 99:2818–2825.

88. O'Donnell VB, Eiserich JP, Bloodsworth A *et al*. Nitration of unsaturated fatty acids by nitric oxide-derived reactive species. *Methods Enzymol* 1999; 301:454–470.

89. Zingarelli B, O'Connor M, Wong H *et al*. Peroxynitrite-mediated DNA strand breakage activates poly-adenosine diphosphate ribosyl synthetase and causes cellular energy depletion in macrophages stimulated with bacterial lipopolysaccharide. *J Immunol* 1996; 156:350–358.

90. Packer MA, Murphy MP. Peroxynitrite formed by simultaneous nitric oxide and superoxide generation causes cyclosporin-A-sensitive mitochondrial calcium efflux and depolarization. *Eur J Biochem* 1995; 234:231–239.

91. Nabeyrat E, Jones G, Fenwick P *et al*. Mitogen-activated protein kinases mediate peroxynitrite-induced cell death in human bronchial epithelial cells. *Am J Physiol* 2003; 284:L1112–L1120.

92. MacPherson JC, Comhair SA, Erzurum SC *et al*. Eosinophils are a major source of nitric oxide-derived oxidants in severe asthma: characterization of pathways available to eosinophils for generating reactive nitrogen species. *J Immunol* 2001; 166:5763–5772.

93. Xiong Y, Karupiah G, Hogan S *et al*. Inhibition of allergic airway inflammation in mice lacking nitric oxide synthase 2. *J Immunol* 1999; 162:445–452.

94. Trifilieff A, Fujitani Y, Mentz F *et al*. Inducible nitric oxide synthase inhibitors suppress airway inflammation in mice through down-regulation of chemokine expression. *J Immunol* 2000; 165:1526–1533.

95. Huang FP, Niedbala W, Wei XQ *et al*. Nitric oxide regulates Th1 cell development through the inhibition of IL-12 synthesis by macrophages. *Eur J Immunol* 1998; 28:4062–4070.

96. Chang RH, Feng MH, Liu WH *et al*. Nitric oxide increased interleukin-4 expression in T lymphocytes. *Immunology* 1997; 90:364–369.

97. Smith AD, Taylor DR. Is exhaled nitric oxide measurement a useful clinical test in asthma? *Curr Opin Allergy Clin Immunol* 2005; 5:49–56.

98. Phillips CR, Giraud GD, Holden WE. Exhaled nitric oxide during exercise: site of release and modulation by ventilation and blood flow. *J Appl Physiol* 1996; 80:1865–1871.

99. Kharitonov S, Alving K, Barnes PJ. Exhaled and nasal nitric oxide measurements: recommendations. *Eur Respir J* 1997; 10:1683–1693.

100. Baraldi E, de Jongste JC, The ERS/ATS Task Force. Measurement of exhaled nitric oxide in children. *Eur Respir J* 2002; 20:223–237.

101. Tsoukias NM, George SC. A two-compartment model of pulmonary nitric oxide exchange dynamics. *J Appl Physiol* 1998; 85:653–666.

102. Sylvester JT, Permutt S. Exhaled NO: first, hold your breath. *J Appl Physiol* 2001; 91:474–476.

103. Lehtimaki L, Kankaanranta H, Saarelainen S *et al*. Extended exhaled NO measurement differentiates between alveolar and bronchial inflammation. *Am J Respir Crit Care Med* 2001; 163:1557–1561.

104. Delclaux C, Mahut B, Zerah-Lancner F *et al*. Increased nitric oxide output from alveolar origin during liver cirrhosis versus bronchial source during asthma. *Am J Respir Crit Care Med* 2002; 165:332–337.

105. Kharitonov SA, Yates D, Robbins RA *et al*. Increased nitric oxide in exhaled air of asthmatic patients. *Lancet* 1994; 343:133–135.

106. Gratziou C, Lignos M, Dassiou M et al. Influence of atopy on exhaled nitric oxide in patients with stable asthma and rhinitis. Eur Respir J 1999; 14:897–901.

107. Kharitonov SA, O'Connor BJ, Evans DJ et al. Allergen-induced late asthmatic reactions are associated with elevation of exhaled nitric oxide. Am J Respir Crit Care Med 1995; 151:1894–1899.

108. Massaro AF, Mehta S, Lilly CM et al. Elevated nitric oxide concentrations in isolated lower airway gas of asthmatic subjects. Am J Respir Crit Care Med 1996; 153:1510–1514.

109. Hansel TT, Kharitonov SA, Donnelly LE et al. A selective inhibitor of inducible nitric oxide synthase inhibits exhaled breath nitric oxide in healthy volunteers and asthmatics. FASEB J 2003; 17:1298–1300.

110. Kharitonov SA, Yates DH, Barnes PJ. Inhaled glucocorticoids decrease nitric oxide in exhaled air of asthmatic patients. Am J Respir Crit Care Med 1996; 153:454–457.

111. Sippel JM, Holden WE, Tilles SA et al. Exhaled nitric oxide levels correlate with measures of disease control in asthma. J Allergy Clin Immunol 2000; 106:645–650.

112. de Gouw HWFM, Grunberg K, Schot R et al. Relationship between exhaled nitric oxide and airway hyperresponsiveness following experimental rhinovirus infection in asthmatic subjects. Eur Respir J 1998; 11:126–132.

113. Massaro AF, Gaston B, Kita D et al. Expired nitric oxide levels during treatment of acute asthma. Am J Respir Crit Care Med 1995; 152:800–803.

114. Kharitonov SA, Yates DH, Chung KF et al. Changes in the dose of inhaled steroid affect exhaled nitric oxide levels in asthmatic patients. Eur Respir J 1996; 9:196–201.

115. Jatakanon A, Kharitonov S, Lim S et al. Effect of differing doses of inhaled budesonide on markers of airway inflammation in patients with mild asthma. Thorax 1999; 54:108–114.

116. Van Rensen EL, Straathof KC, Veselic-Charvat MA et al. Effect of inhaled steroids on airway hyperresponsiveness, sputum eosinophils, and exhaled nitric oxide levels in patients with asthma. Thorax 1999; 54:403–408.

117. Silvestri M, Spallarossa D, Frangova Yourukova V et al. Orally exhaled nitric oxide levels are related to the degree of blood eosinophilia in atopic children with mild-intermittent asthma. Eur Respir J 1999; 13:321–326.

118. Mattes J, Storm van's Gravesande K, Reining U et al. NO in exhaled air is correlated with markers of eosinophilic airway inflammation in corticosteroid-dependent childhood asthma. Eur Respir J 1999; 13:1391–1395.

119. Lim S, Jatakanon A, John M et al. Effect of inhaled budesonide on lung function and airway inflammation. Am J Respir Crit Care Med 1999; 159:22–30.

120. Gibson PG, Henry RL, Thomas P. Non invasive assessment of airway inflammation in children: induced sputum, exhaled nitric oxide, and breath condensate. Eur Respir J 2000; 16:1008–1015.

121. Payne DN, Adcock IM, Wilson NM et al. Relationship between exhaled nitric oxide and mucosal eosinophilic inflammation in children with difficult asthma, after treatment with oral prednisolone. Am J Respir Crit Care Med 2001; 164:1376–1381.

122. Nijkamp FP, Van der Linde HJ, Folkerts G. Nitric oxide synthesis inhibitors induce airway hyperresponsiveness in the guinea pig in vivo and in vitro. Am Rev Respir Dis 1993; 148:727–734.

123. Ameredes BT, Sethi JM, Liu HL et al. Enhanced nitric oxide production associated with airway hyporesponsiveness in the absence of IL-10. Am J Physiol Lung Cell Mol Physiol 2004; 288:868–873.

124. Ricciardolo FLM, Nadel JA, Yoishihara S et al. Evidence for reduction of bradykinin-induced bronchoconstriction in guinea pigs by release of nitric oxide. Br J Pharmacol 1994; 113:1147–1152.

125. Feletou M, Lonchampt M, Coge F et al. Regulation of murine airway responsiveness by endothelial nitric oxide synthase. Am J Physiol 2001; 281:L258–L267.

126. Ten Broeke R, Folkerts R, De Crom R et al. Overexpression of eNOS suppresses asthmatic features in a mouse model of allergic asthma (Abstract). Eur Respir J 2002; 20:28s.

127. Hjoberg J, Shore S, Kobzik L et al. Expression of nitric oxide synthase-2 in the lungs decreases airway resistance and responsiveness. J Appl Physiol 2004; 97:249–259.

128. Dimitropoulou C, White RE, Ownby DR et al. Estrogen reduces carbachol-induced constriction of asthmatic airways by stimulating large-conductance voltage and calcium-dependent potassium channels. Am J Respir Cell Mol Biol 2005; 32:239–247.

129. Sadeghi-Hashjin G, Folkerts G, Henricks PAJ et al. Relaxation of guinea-pig trachea by sodium nitroprusside: cyclic GMP and nitric oxide not involved. Br J Pharmacol 1996; 118:466–470.

130. Ricciardolo F, Vergnani L, Wiegand S et al. Detection of bradykinin-induced nitric oxide release in the airways of guinea pigs by porphirinic microsensor. Am J Respir Cell Mol Biol 2000; 22:97–104.

131. Hammermann R, Hirschmann J, Hey C *et al*. Cationic proteins inhibit L-arginine uptake in rat alveolar macrophages and tracheal epithelial cells. Implications for nitric oxide synthesis. *Am J Respir Cell Mol Biol* 1999; 21:155–162.

132. Meurs H, Schuurman, Duyvendak M *et al*. Deficiency of nitric oxide in polycation-induced airway hyperreactivity. *Br J Pharmacol* 1999; 126:559–562.

133. Meurs H, Hamer M, Pethe S *et al*. Modulation of cholinergic airway reactivity and nitric oxide production by endogenous arginase activity. *Br J Pharmacol* 2000; 130:1793–1798.

134. Ten Broeke R, Folkerts G, Leusink-Muis T *et al*. Calcium sensors as new therapeutic targets for airway hyperresponsiveness and asthma. *FASEB J* 2001; 15:1831–1833.

135. Ten Broeke R, Blalock JE, Nijkamp FP *et al*. Calcium sensors as new therapeutic targets for asthma and chronic obstructive pulmonary disease. *Clin Exp Allergy* 2004; 34:170–176.

136. De Boer J, Meurs H, Coers W *et al*. Deficiency of nitric oxide in allergen-induced airway hyperreactivity to contractile agonists after the early asthmatic reaction: an ex vivo study. *Br J Pharmacol* 1996; 119:1109–1116.

137. De Boer J, Duyvendak M, Schuurman F *et al*. Role of L-arginine in the deficiency of nitric oxide and airway hyperreactivity after the allergen-induced early asthmatic reaction in guinea-pigs. *Br J Pharmacol* 1999; 128:1114–1120.

138. Persson MG, Friberg SG, Hedqvist P *et al*. Endogenous nitric oxide counteracts antigen-induced bronchoconstriction. *Eur J Pharmacol* 1993; 249:R7–R8.

139. Persson MG, Friberg SG, Gustafsson LE *et al*. The promotion of patent airways and inhibition of antigen-induced bronchial obstruction by endogenous nitric oxide. *Br J Pharmacol* 1995; 116:2957–2962.

140. Mehta S, Lilly C, Rollenhagen J *et al*. Acute and chronic effects of allergic airway inflammation on pulmonary nitric oxide production. *Am J Physiol* 1997; 272:L124–L131.

141. Schuiling M, Meurs H, Zuidhof A *et al*. Dual action of iNOS-derived nitric oxide in allergen-induced airway hyperreactivity in conscious, unrestrained guinea pigs. *Am J Respir Crit Care Med* 1998; 158:1442–1449.

142. Schuiling M, Zuidhof A, Bonouvrie M *et al*. Role of nitric oxide in the development and partial reversal of allergen-induced airway hyperreactivity in conscious, unrestrained guinea-pigs. *Brit J Pharmacol* 1998; 123:1450–1456.

143. Folkerts, Linde HJ, Nijkamp FP. Virus-induced airway hyperresponsiveness in guinea pigs is related to a deficiency in nitric oxide. *J Clin Invest* 1995; 95:26–30.

144. Lee Y, Cheon K, Lee H *et al*. Gene polymorphisms of endothelial nitric oxide synthase and angiotensin-converting enzyme in patients with asthma. *Allergy* 2000; 55:959–963.

145. Storm van's Gravensande K, Wechsler M, Grasemann H *et al*. Association of missense mutation in the NOS3 gene with exhaled nitric oxide levels. *Am J Respir Crit Care Med* 2003; 168:228–231.

146. Grasemann H, Yandava CN, Drazen JM. Neuronal NO synthase (NOS1) is a major candidate gene for asthma. *Clin Exp Allergy* 1999; 29(suppl 4):39–41.

147. Ali M, Khoo SK, Turner S *et al*. NOS1 polymorphism is associated with atopy but not exhaled nitric oxide levels in healthy children. *Pediatr Allergy Immunol* 2003; 14:261–265.

148. Holla LI, Schuller M, Buckova D *et al*. Neuronal nitric oxide synthase gene polymorphism and IgE-mediated allergy in the Central European population. *Allergy* 2004; 59:548–552.

149. Cockcroft D, Ruffin R, Dolovich J *et al*. Allergen-induced increase in non-allergic bronchial reactivity. *Clin Allergy* 1977; 7:503–513.

150. Folkerts G, Busse WW, Nijkamp FP *et al*. Virus-induced airway hyperresponsiveness and asthma. *Am J Respir Crit Care Med* 1998; 157:1708–1720.

151. Ricciardolo FLM, Timmers M, Geppetti P *et al*. Allergen-induced impairment of bronchoprotective nitric oxide synthesis in asthma. *J Allergy Clin Immunol* 2001; 108:198–204.

152. Ricciardolo FLM, Geppetti P, Mistretta A *et al*. Randomized double-blind placebo-controlled study of the effect of inhibition of nitric oxide synthesis in bradykin-induced asthma. *Lancet* 1996; 348:374–377.

153. Ricciardolo FLM, Di Maria GU, Mistretta A *et al*. Impairment of bronchoprotection by nitric oxide in severe asthma. *Lancet* 1997; 350:1297–1298.

154. Black P, Brodie S. Nitric oxide and response to inhaled bradykinin in severe asthma. *Lancet* 1998; 351:449–450.

155. Straub DA, Minocchieri S, Moeller A *et al*. The effect of montelukast on exhaled nitric oxide and lung function in asthmatic children 2 to 5 years old. *Chest* 2005; 127:509–514.

156. Redington AE, Meng Q-H, Springall DR *et al.* Increased expression of inducible nitric oxide synthase and cyclo-oxygenase-2 in the airway epithelium of asthmatic subjects and the regulation by corticosteroid treatment. *Thorax* 2001; 56:351–357.

157. De Gouw HWFM, Verbruggen MB, Twiss IM *et al.* Effect of oral L-arginine on airway hyperresponsiveness to histamine in asthma. *Thorax* 1999; 54:1033–1035.

158. Redington AE. Modulation of nitric oxide pathways: therapeutic potential in asthma and chronic obstructive pulmonary disease. *Eur J Pharmacol* 2006; 533:263–276.

159. Hamad A, Johnson S, Knox A. Antiproliferative effects of NO and ANP in cultured human airway smooth muscle. *Am J Physiol* 1999; 277:L910–L918.

160. Patel H, Belvisi M, Donnelly L *et al.* Constitutive expressions of type I NOS in human airway smooth muscle cells: evidence for an antiproliferative role. *FASEB J* 1999; 13:1810–1816.

161. Hamad A, Knox A. Mechanisms mediating the antiproliferative effects of nitric oxide in cultured human airway smooth muscle cells. *FEBS Lett* 2001; 506:91–96.

7

Metalloproteinases and asthma: untried potential for new therapeutic strategies

P. S. Thomas

INTRODUCTION

Metalloproteinases (MMPs) are becoming recognized as important modifiers of the extra cellular matrix. Now that asthma is recognized as a disease, which not only has an inflammatory component in addition to airway smooth muscle hyperresponsiveness, but which also leads to chronic, and possibly irreversible changes in the airway, it is important to consider the mediators which may be involved in the subepithelial fibrosis which characterizes chronic asthma. One of the important classes of enzymes that are becoming established as modulators of the extracellular matrix are the MMPs, and they are now becoming clearly associated with asthma. This review has focused upon human studies, rather than murine data, since there is incomplete congruity between man and mouse in terms of MMPs, and in addition, there is no naturally occurring form of asthma in the mouse.

STRUCTURE OF MMPS

MMPs form a subfamily of the metzincin superfamily of proteases, which constitute several metalloendopeptidase families. The metzincins are so named because they share a methionine or met-turn in their structure, which lies beneath the zinc ion associated with the enzymatic active site. The metzincins have conserved topology of their structure with three histidines within the catalytic domain which provides the zinc binding domain. The metzincins can be further subdivided into four groups: serralysins, adamalysins, astracins and matrixins or MMPs.

Initially, MMPs were classified on the basis of their known connective tissue substrates, with the main designated groups being collagenases, gelatinases, stromelysins and matrilysins. Unfortunately it became readily apparent that this classification was imprecise and the MMPs have largely been classified by numerical order in which they were identified, which has now nearly 30 in total (Table 7.1). Further subgrouping is now being attempted, but there are a number of features which typify the groups and subgroups. The MMPs are generated in a latent form or zymogen which contains a propeptide which needs to be cleaved for activation, and a secretary signal sequence (Figure 7.1). The propeptide sequence is followed by the catalytic domain which contains the common zinc binding motif. Some MMPs have

Paul S. Thomas, MD, FRCP, FRACP, Associate Professor and Consultant Physician, Faculty of Medicine, UNSW and Respiratory Medicine, Prince of Wales' Hospital, Sydney, Australia

Table 7.1 The matrix MMPs family* (adapted from reference [68])

Name	Substrates
Interstitial collagenases	
MMP-1 (Collagenase-1)	Collagen I, II, III, VII, VIII, X, aggrecan, gelatin, pro-MMP-2, pro-MMP-9
MMP-8 (Collagenase-2)	Collagen I, II, III, VII, VIII, X, aggrecan, gelatin
MMP-13 (Collagenase-3)	Collagen I, II, III, aggrecan, gelatin
MMP-18 (Collagenase-4)	
Gelatinases	
MMP-2 (Gelatinase-A)	Collagen I, II, III, IV, V, VII, X, XI, XIV, gelatin, elastin, fibronectin, aggrecan
MMP-9 (Gelatinase-B)	Collagen IV, V, VII, X, XIV, gelatin, pro-MMP-9, pro-MMP-13, elastin, aggrecan
Stomelysins	
MMP-3 (Stomelysin-1)	Collagen II, III, IV, IX, X, XI, elastin, pro-MMP-1, MMP-7, pro-MMP-7, pro-MMP-8, pro-MMP-9, pro-MMP-13
MMP-10 (Stomelysin-2)	Collagen III, IV, V, gelatin, fibronectin
MMP-11 (Stomelysin-3)	Fibronectin, laminin, gelatin, aggrecan
Membrane-type MMPs	
MMP-14 (MT1-MMP)	Pro-MMP-2, pro-MMP-13, collagen I, II, III, gelatin, aggrecan, fibronectin, laminin
MMP-15 (MT2-MMP)	Pro-MMP-2, gelatin, fibronectin, laminin
MMP-16 (MT3-MMP)	Pro-MMP-2
MMP-17 (MT4-MMP)	Unknown
MMP-24 (MT5-MMP)	Pro-MMP-2
MMP-25 (MT6-MMP)	Gelatin
Others	
MMP-7 (Matrilysin-2)	Collagen II, III, IV, IX, X, X1, elastin, pro-MMP-1, pro-MMP-7, pro-MMP-8, pro-MMP-9, pro-MMP-13, gelatin, aggrecan, fibronectin
MMP-26 (Matrilysin)	Collagen IV, gelatin, fibronectin
MMP-12 (Metalloelastase)	Elastin
MMP-19	Tenascin, gelatin, aggrecan
MMP-20 (Enamelysin)	Enamel, gelatin
MMP-21	Unknown
MMP-23	Unknown
MMP-27	Unknown
MMP-28 (Epilysin)	Unknown

*MMPs are shown grouped by their extracellular matrix substrate specificities. Many of the additional substrates that are able to be cleaved by the MMPs have yet to be determined in man, but include cytokines, chemokines and receptors.

only the signal peptide, propeptide and a catalytic domain (e.g. MMP-7 and MMP-26), others have a haemopexin-like domain that is thought to confer substrate specificity. Others may contain serine protease recognition motifs and fibronectin-like repeats. A few family members have a transmembrane domain. For detailed reviews see [1, 2].

REGULATION OF THE MMPs

There are numerous points for the regulation of MMPs, but the most clearly identified are those of gene transcription, activation of the enzyme and the interaction with naturally-occurring inhibitors.

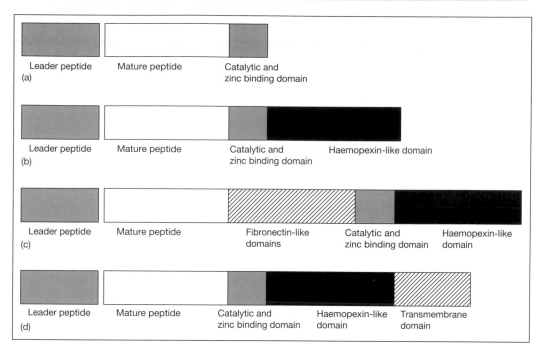

Figure 7.1 Schematic of the types of peptide domains found in the MMP family. The cysteine-containing leader sequence is cleaved from the propeptide to create the active enzyme, which is known as the 'cysteine switch'. The active site is connected to the COOH terminal by a flexible 'hinge' region of up to 75 amino acids. The haemopexin and fibronectin-like domains determine substrate specificity and the transmembrane domain will anchor cell surface MMPs (or MT-MMPs). Examples of the various types: (a) MMP-7; (b) MMP-1, -3,-8, -10 etc; (c) MMP-2, -9; (d) MMP-14 to -17. Adapted from reference [2].

Transcription

A number of cytokines have been identified as being able to upregulate gene transcription of MMPs, which include tumour necrosis factor alpha (TNFα) and interleukin (IL)-1β. Cytokines associated with downregulation include: IL-4, -10 and interferon-γ and involve intracellular signal transduction pathways which in turn interact with the gene. The 5' upstream region of inducible MMP genes contains an activator protein-1 (AP-1) *cis*-regulatory element, and other sites which cooperate to activate the promoters of MMP-1, -3 and -9. MMPs -7, -8 and -9 are also able to be constitutively stored in granules of secretory epithelial cells, but importantly in both neutrophils and eosinophils, which has implications for the inflammation associated with asthma. Glucocorticosteroids generally downregulate MMPs. In terms of MMP-9, this is indirect and not *via* a glucocorticoid response element in the 5' untranslated region of the gene, but probably *via* nuclear factor-κB (NF-κB) and Ets-1 interactions in this promoter region [3, 4].

Activation of MMPs

The majority of MMPs are secreted in a zymogen or latent precursor form. There is usually a cysteine residue within the propeptide which interacts with the catalytic zinc molecule, and this masks the active site. Cleavage and release of the propeptide is thought to abolish this interaction and expose the active site. This cleavage can be effected by other MMPs, but the *in vivo* mechanisms have yet to be defined. Another way in which MMPs can be regulated is by their association with the cell surface. If the MMP is not secreted, then intracellular trafficking and docking of the MMP protein on the cell surface is under the control of a variety of intracellular and extracellular messengers.

Inhibitors of MMPs

Tissue inhibitors of MMPs (TIMPs) are the best known of the naturally-occurring regulators of MMP activity, but other inhibitors also exist, e.g. α_2-macroglobulin, and thrombospondin, which can bind to and inactivate the MMPs. At least four TIMPs have been identified which bind on a 1:1 basis and irreversibly inactivate the activity of MMPs. The TIMPs differ in their expression characteristics and their binding affinities for the MMPs. In general terms, TIMPs-1 and -2 are able to inhibit a wide range of the MMPs while TIMP-3 can also inhibit ADAM-17, (ADAM family: a disintegrin and MMP) which is a distant cousin of the MMPs.

FUNCTIONAL CHARACTERISTICS OF MMPS

EXTRACELLULAR MATRIX DEGRADATION

The MMPs have long been recognized as being able to degrade all of the components of the extracellular matrix (ECM), and the potential substrates overlap between individual enzymes. In broad terms, they were traditionally grouped as collagenases (MMP-1, -8, -13); gelatinases (MMP-2, -9); stromelysins (MMP-3, -10, -11); elastases (MMP-7, -12), and membrane anchored MMPs such as MMP-14, -15, -16, -17. Such overlapping substrate targets indicate the importance of the homeostasis of the ECM. Initially, it was considered that MMPs were primarily concerned with the ECM, with cells such as fibroblasts generating collagen and other connective tissue matrices, while MMPs degraded these soft tissue components allowing remodelling to occur, but in addition, the MMPs are clearly involved in many other functions.

OTHER FUNCTIONS OF MMPS

It has since become apparent that these enzymes have more complex attributes and activities. At the very least, MMPs have been implicated in the release of ECM-sequestered mediators such as cytokines. In addition, some of the MMPs such as MMP-14 can activate latent transforming growth factor β (TGFβ). Other growth factors can be released from the cell surface by MMPs, such as members of the EGF family, which can be cleaved from their precursor form to be activated. Additional targets for MMP activity are thought to include growth factor receptors, adhesion molecules and proteoglycans. Examples are the EGF receptors, FGF receptor 1, integrins, such as integrin β_4, ICAM-1, syndecan-1 and this latter receptor in association with chemokines may regulate neutrophil influx.

To add to the complexity, a number of cytokines, chemokines and their receptors are now known to be potential targets of the MMP family. Some of those identified include Fas ligand, monocyte chemoattractant protein-3, and IL-8. Some are inactivated by MMPs, e.g. those of the chemokine family: CXCL-1, CXCL-4 and CXCL-12, which are inactivated by MMP-9. TNFα is released from its 26 kDa membrane bound form to the free, active 17 kDa cytokine by ADAM-17, MMP-1, -3 and -7.

The MMPs are expressed on cell membranes and their translocation to the cell surface is thought to indicate not just optimal positioning, but also suggests that they may play a role in the interaction between adhesion molecules and extracellular matrix products such as proteoglycan. Thus, MMP-7 has been shown to bind to heparan sulphate proteoglycans, this and MMP-9 can bind to the hyaluronan CD44 receptor, ICAM-1, and to integrins. This close association of the MMPs with connective tissue obviously may allow for remodelling to occur under tightly controlled circumstances in the vicinity of the host cell. It has important implications for cancer research in that expression of these enzymes by transformed cells may be one of the mechanisms by which neoplastic cells are able to invade local tissues and to migrate along tissue planes.

ROLE OF THE MMPS IN ASTHMA AND AIRWAY DISEASE

Airway inflammation, remodelling and the deposition of connective tissue leading to an increase in basement membrane thickness have been recognized as a feature of chronic asthma for many years. The exact mechanism by which these changes in the connective tissue occur are poorly understood. It has become clear that migration of inflammatory cells not only relies on appropriate cellular adhesion molecules, but also upon mediators which allow inflammatory cells to migrate through the basement membrane of vessels. It has been demonstrated that, *in vitro*, MMPs are important in eosinophilic migration through basement membrane components, and these findings have been demonstrated in other inflammatory cells such as neutrophils and lymphocytes as well [5]. In these eosinophil experiments, MMP-2 and -9 appeared to be crucial to this role and the latter has been shown to be over-expressed in eosinophils taken from the airways of asthmatic subjects. In a murine model of asthma, allergen challenge led to an increase in the expression of MMP-2 and -9 with detectable levels in the airway lavage fluid [6]. Antagonizing the effect of these MMPs with TIMP-2, showed reduced airway responsiveness and reduced the airway inflammation associated with eosinophils and lymphocytes. Similar results were seen in a MMP-9 murine knockout model. Inhibition of the inflammatory cellular infiltrate was also seen with TIMP-1 and a synthetic MMP inhibitor [7, 8]. Using data derived from murine knockout models undergoing inhalational challenge, it has been suggested that MMP-2 and -9 facilitate the ingress and control of inflammatory cells in the lung, but the applicability of these results to man remains unclear [9–11].

In human asthma, some of the observations seen in murine models have been confirmed, since MMP-9 and gelatinase activity have been shown to be more commonly isolated from sputum, lavage fluid and in bronchial biopsies of those with asthma, when compared with those subjects who are either normal or who have other lung diseases. When compared with normal subjects, increased sputum and bronchial lavage MMP-9 in those with asthma has been found both at baseline and during exacerbations [12–19] in biopsies [20], and in some studies elevated levels of circulating MMP-9 have also been found [21–23]. MMP-9 immunoreactivity has been co-localized to neutrophils and *ex vivo* in eosinophils after stimulation with TNFα [24, 25], and associated with diurnal variation in nocturnal asthma [19].

Further confirmatory studies have identified an increase in MMP-9 activity in sputum after allergen challenge [18, 26–29] and in lavage fluid from those asthmatic patients with severe exacerbations requiring mechanical ventilation [30, 31], but levels of MMP-9 may be higher in smokers and those with COPD also [32].

Some studies have established positive correlations between disease activity or severity with the expression of MMP-9: Han *et al.* found MMP-9 activity in the bronchial submucosa correlated with the degree of eosinophilia, while Wenzel *et al.* showed a link between MMP-9 expression and the severity of asthma [33–35], although not all have shown such a link [24, 36]. In addition, an inverse relationship between MMP-9 and airway wall thickness has been documented [37]. Some studies have demonstrated an effect of inhaled glucocorticosteroids (iGCS) with a fall in MMP-9 and an increase in the MMP-9/TIMP ratios after the administration of these drugs [38, 39]. This would appear logical, and MMP gene transcription is downregulated by GCS as well as TGFβ.

In summary, MMP-9 appears to be established as being upregulated in human asthma. Most of these studies have also looked for evidence of the other MMPs that were easily detectable by immunostaining or assays with reagents that were available at the time that the investigations were performed, such as MMP-2. There are a few reports of MMP-2 being elevated in asthma, and it may be involved in smooth muscle proliferation, but the findings are not as consistent as those of MMP-9 [15, 40–42]. Likewise MMP-1 may also play a role in smooth muscle hypertrophy [43].

The suggestion that MMP-9 is the sole important MMP in asthma is unlikely to be sustained as the molecular tools for the other members of the MMP family become available. In addition, interpretation of MMP levels has to be made in the context of active enzyme, the presence of inhibitors of these enzymes, including TIMPs, α-macroglobulin and thrombospondins.

The subset of asthma that is associated with neutrophilic inflammation may implicate MMP-8, which is stored within the neutrophilic granules of these inflammatory cells. There are data which suggest that MMP-8 expression is increased in bronchial biopsies and bronchoalveolar lavage to corroborate this view [44–46].

No review of the data relating to the MMPs would be complete without assessing the levels of the TIMPs. TIMPs are thought to act as one of the regulators of the MMP family and to maintain homeostasis. Accordingly, many of the reports relating to MMP-9 have studied markers of TIMP expression and have related these as the MMP-9/TIMP-1 ratio. Those that have reported such a relationship have shown an increase in both TIMP-1 expression and the ratio. The explanation may be that while MMP-9 is upregulated in exacerbations of asthma, TIMP expression may initially lag behind, allowing such an increase in the ratio, but as the asthmatic episode resolves, the ratio declines as TIMP-1 levels increase further and the MMP-9 levels decrease [15–19, 47–49]. It has also been suggested that the levels of TIMP-1 and the MMP-9/TIMP-1 ratio rise after the administration of inhaled glucocorticosteroids and later fall again, while other studies seem to indicate that TIMPs may be associated with pathological airway wall thickening [37, 47, 50, 51].

One study has identified a novel TIMP-1 polymorphism (536C > T, Ile158Ile), which was associated with asthma in women, but not in men. Other known polymorphisms in the MMP-9 and TIMP-1 genes were not detected [52]. This finding is difficult to interpret until other studies in other populations have confirmed this result [52–54]. The TIMP-1 polymorphism is not associated with an amino acid change, but could be associated with a splice variant, but until functional significance has been established, this association remains of uncertain importance.

THERAPEUTIC POTENTIAL OF MMP INHIBITION

While iGCS are the main therapeutic anti-inflammatory drugs in asthma, not all of the literature suggests that this class of agent is able to suppress the pro-inflammatory effect of the MMPs.

Doxycycline is a broad spectrum MMP inhibitor and in a murine model of occupational asthma, this drug has shown a decrease in the ability of toluene di-isocyanate to maintain inflammation in the airways. This was associated with a decline in airway inflammation, responsiveness, and MMP-9 expression [55]. Interestingly, this is the only licensed MMP inhibitor of use in man. As a commercial product called 'Periostat' (CollaGenex), doxycycline is marketed in sub-antimicrobial doses to reduce periodontal disease. At these doses it is believed to possess MMP inhibition and to reduce periodontal disease, not by antibacterial activity but by a reduction in the activity of the MMPs.

Synthetic inhibitors generally work on the principle of chelating the catalytic zinc atom at the MMP active site. Hydroxamates, phosphinyls, thiols, and carboxylates are examples. Therapeutic studies of MMP inhibitors have been carried out over the last decade, particularly in regard to the treatment of metastatic cancers. These trials have shown some beneficial effects, but few of the drugs studied in clinical trials have progressed to Phase II or III trials and none as yet have found general applicability. Many of the agents were synthetic compounds chosen for their effects upon the MMPs, such as hydroxamic acid derivatives.

Some examples were batimastat and marimastat, which are thought to work via the chelation or sequestration of zinc which is necessary for the MMPs to function [56, 57]. Marimastat showed some beneficial effects in terms of survival, initially in gastric cancer and later with some encouraging results in ovarian and pancreatic cancers [56, 57]. When larger trials were conducted, mainly in advanced disease, the response rate was less favourable and the drug has not been studied further. The discontinuation of these studies, and those of other MMP inhibitors was, in the majority of cases, mainly due to the modest effect of the drugs and to some of the musculoskeletal side-effects, usually tendonitis and a reversible fibrosis resembling Dupuytren's contractures affecting the flexor retinaculum. One of the possible problems of those studies that showed a lack of efficacy, was that the drugs were nearly always used in neoplasia with metastatic disease. While the concept of MMPs being over-expressed in cancers is well-founded, it is possible that the use of these drugs in early disease, prior to metastatic spread might be a valid option. The relevance to asthma is that MMPs, particularly MMP-9, are upregulated in asthma, it is feasible for them to be inhibited, and their inhibition may offer key insights into their role in asthma, not just at the level of ECM regulation, but also in terms of control of inflammation.

A number of these low molecular weight MMP inhibitors are also able to inhibit TNFα converting enzyme (TACE). For this reason, some effects may be due to TACE inhibition rather than MMP inhibition, and in addition, it is quite likely that additional classes of enzymes are also inhibited. This is a major problem in terms of non-specific MMP inhibitors as some MMPs are clearly involved in more 'protective' effects while others are involved in inflammatory changes. This effects means that blanket inhibition of MMPs can lead to undesirable imbalance of the MMPs, as well as inhibition of other zinc or metal-dependent enzymes. TACE is one such enzyme which is not closely related to the MMPs, which cleaves membrane-bound 26 kDa TNFα to the 17 kDa active form [58].

TNFα has been implicated in asthma and airway hyperresponsiveness, with data indicating that mast cells store this cytokine, i.e. it is released on allergen presentation both *in vitro* and *in vivo* and elevated levels have been found in the sputum and lavage of asthmatic subjects post-allergen challenge. In addition, exogenous inhalation of TNFα can mimic some of the classic airway changes seen in asthma, such as an inflammatory infiltrate and increased airway responsiveness [58–61]. Since marimastat is a potent inhibitor of TACE, as well as a broad spectrum inhibitor of MMPs including MMP-9, it was logical to study this drug in asthma [62]. Mild atopic, asthmatic subjects were studied in a double-blind, crossover design and challenged with dust mite antigen after 3 weeks of marimastat. After taking marimastat, there was a significant shift of the dose response to allergen to the right when compared to placebo, indicative of a fall in the airway responsiveness (Figure 7.2). The dose of marimastat used was sufficient to reduce peripheral blood mononuclear cell TNFα generation by more than half. There was a non-significant fall in airway inflammation as measured by sputum inflammatory cells. These data suggest that it is possible to inhibit MMPs and TACE, with a reduction in airway hyperresponsiveness, even in mild human asthma [62].

Other inhibitors have been shown to have effects in murine models with inhibition of TACE and MMP-1, -2, -3, -9, -13 [63, 64]. More recent confirmation of the concept of TNFα as playing a role in human asthma, has been the inhibition of this cytokine using humanized monoclonal antibodies directed against TNFα as being a way to reduce asthmatic reactivity and to improve lung function in those who are already on maximal therapy [65–67].

USE OF TIMPS OR OTHER MORE SPECIFIC INHIBITORS AS A THERAPEUTIC OPTION

The problem with our current modes of inhibiting MMPs, is that the inhibitors lack specificity. This is well-reviewed in at least two recent articles and as mentioned above, simple

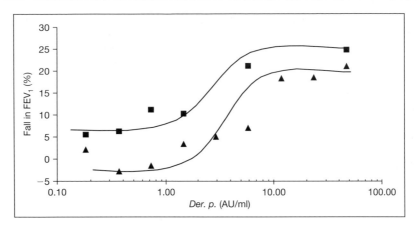

Figure 7.2 Effect of oral marimastat 5 mg twice daily for 21 days upon house dust mite (*Der. p.*) allergen challenge in *Der. p.* sensitive allergic asthmatic subjects. After marimastat (▲) there was a significant shift of the dose-response curve to the right, when compared to the placebo arm (■) of the protocol. The allergen-induced provocative concentration that induced a 20% fall in forced expiratory volume in the first second (FEV$_1$, allergen PC$_{20}$) after treatment with marimastat was significantly increased when compared with placebo, 22.2 AU/ml (95%CI = 11.7–32.6) compared with 17.0 AU/ml (95%CI = 7.6–26.4; *P* = 0.02). Thus, marimastat rendered the subjects less sensitive to the *Der. p.* allergen. Adapted from reference [62].

Zn chelation or sequestration will tend to confer blanket reduction in MMP activity [56, 57]. While MMPs have been described as having modulatory effects upon connective tissue, and many of the original classifications of these enzymes have been based upon their connective tissue substrates, it is clear that this is far too simplistic [56, 57]. If these enzymes do not just digest the 'gristle' that connects cells, but also modulate the release of cytokines, chemokines, angiostatic and angioblastic factors, then it is small wonder that inhibiting all of them may not lead to the desired effect, either in cancer treatment or in asthma therapy. We were fortunate in our studies of marimastat to show a response in mild asthmatic subjects in terms of allergen sensitivity. Reviewers, not surprisingly, could not decide whether this should be ascribed to inhibition of TNFα or MMPs, and such is the lack of specificity that it is difficult to determine in humans. Nonetheless, the fact that such changes, albeit modest, do occur should encourage us to try new therapies. Although the details of mechanisms and effects of MMPs are still being unravelled, the mode of action of many commonly used drugs, such as GCS, are also still incompletely understood.

Some of the problems of specificity could be overcome if it were possible to either over-express or find new ways to induce TIMPs. These inhibitors of MMPs should be more specific than current small molecular inhibitors of MMPs, substrate specificity would then be improved, and the shortcomings of the small molecular inhibitors might be overcome. In this post-modern human genome era, the translationalists are now emphasizing their importance. One of the major goals of therapy directed towards better inhibition of MMPs should be the identification of the 'substrate degradome', i.e. which MMP substrates are of importance in human asthma, or indeed whether we should be considering substrate or the modulation of known mediators such as the chemokines and cytokines by MMPs rather than the mere snipping of collagenous material.

Thus, these studies are able to show that additional therapeutic manoeuvres are possible, beyond the idea of inhaled GCS. Such drugs may fulfil several roles. They may be able to be used as an adjunct to inhaled GCS, particularly in difficult asthma, as shown in the studies by

Howarth *et al.* [66] and Berry *et al.* [67], or, they may be used as iGCS – sparing agents to assist in reducing the long-term side-effects of these inhaled agents which are known for long-term to be associated with cataracts, skin thinning, osteoporosis and glucose intolerance.

Few new classes of drugs of great consequence have been introduced into the daily management of asthma in the last few decades. Long-acting β_2 adrenergic agonists, anti IgE, leukotriene inhibitors and antagonists have shown some modest benefits, but there is no place for complacency and there is a real need for a continuing research until we have completely new classes of treatment for this common disease. Selective MMP inhibition may be one such approach.

REFERENCES

1. Stamenkovic I. Matrix metalloproteinases in tumor invasion and metastasis. *Cancer Biol* 2000; 10:415–433.
2. Stamenkovic I. Extracellular matrix remodelling: the role of matrix metalloproteinases. *J Pathol* 2003; 200:488–464.
3. Eberhardt W, Schulze M, Engels C, Klasmeier E, Pfeilschifter J. Glucocorticoid-mediated suppression of cytokine-induced matrix metalloproteinase-9 expression in rat mesangial cells: involvement of nuclear factor kB and Ets transcription factors. *Mol Endocrinol* 2002; 16:1752–1766.
4. Scneikert J, Peterziel H, Defossez PA, Klocker H, Launoit Y, Cato AC. Androgen receptor-Ets protein interaction is a novel mechanism for steroid hormone-mediated down-modulation of matrix metalloproteinase gene expression. *J Biol Chem* 1996; 271:23907–23913.
5. Okada S, Kita H, George TJ, Gleich GJ, Leiferman KM. Migration of eosinophil through basement membrane components in vitro: role of matrix metalloproteinase-9. *Am J Respir Cell Mol Biol* 1997; 17:519–528.
6. Lee KS, Jin SM, Lee H, Lee YC. Imbalance between matrix metalloproteinase-9 and tissue inhibitor of metalloproteinase-1 in toluene diisocyanate-induced asthma. *Clin Exp Allergy* 2004; 34:276–284.
7. Kumagai K, Ohno I, Okada S et al. Inhibition of matrix metalloproteinase prevents allergen-induced airway inflammation in a murine model of asthma. *J Immunol* 1999; 162:4212–4219.
8. Cataldo DD, Tournoy KG, Vermaelen K et al. Matrix metalloproteinase-9 deficiency impairs cellular infiltration and bronchial hyperresponsiveness during allergen-induced airway inflammation. *Am J Pathol* 2002; 161:491–498.
9. Corry DB, Rishi K, Kanellis J et al. Decreased allergic lung inflammatory cell egression and increased susceptibility to asphyxiation in MMP-2 deficiency. *Nat Immunol* 2002; 3:347–353.
10. McMillan SJ, Kearley J, Campbell JD et al. Matrix metalloproteinase-9 deficiency results in enhanced allergen-induced airway inflammation. *J Immunol* 2004; 172:2586–2594.
11. Corry DB, Kiss A, Song ALZ et al. Overlapping and independent contributions of MMP-2 and MMP-9 to lung allergic inflammatory cell egression through decreased CC chemokines. *FASEB J* 2004; 18:995–997.
12. Mautino G, Oliver N, Chanez P, Bousquet J, Capony F. Increased release of matrix metalloproteinase-9 in bronchoalveolar lavage fluid and by alveolar macrophages of asthmatics. *Am J Respir Cell Mol Biol* 1997; 17:583–591.
13. Warner JA, Julius P, Luttimann W, Kroegel C. Matrix metalloproteinases in bronchoalveolar lavage fluid following antigen challenge. *Int Arch Allergy Immunol* 1997; 113:318–320.
14. Vignola AM, Riccobono L, Mirabella A et al. Sputum metalloproteinase-9/tissue inhibitor of metalloproteinase-1 ratio correlates with airflow obstruction in asthma and chronic bronchitis. *Am J Respir Crit Care Med* 1998; 158:1945–1950.
15. Cataldo D, Munault C, Noel A et al. MMP-2 and MMP-9 linked gelatinolytic activity in the sputum from patients with asthma and chronic obstructive pulmonary disease. *Int Arch Allergy Immunol* 2000; 123:259–267.
16. Lee YC, Lee HB, Rhee YK, Song CH. The involvement of matrix metalloproteinase-9 in airway inflammation of patients with acute asthma. *Clin Exp Allergy* 2001; 31:1623–1630.
17. Suzuki R, Kato T, Miyazaki Y et al. Matrix metalloproteinases and tissue inhibitors of matrix metalloproteinases in sputum from patients with bronchial asthma. *J Asthma* 201; 38:477–484.
18. Mattos W, Lim S, Russell R, Jakatanon A, Chung KF, Barnes PJ. Matrix metalloproteinase-9 expression in asthma: effect of asthma severity, allergen challenge, and inhaled corticosteroids. *Chest* 2002; 122:1543–1552.

19. Pham DN, Chu HW, Martin RJ, Kraft M. Increased matrix metalloproteinase-9 with elastolysis in nocturnal asthma. *Ann Allergy Asthma Immunol* 2003; 90:72–78.

20. Hoshino M, Nakamura Y, Sim J, Shimojo J, Isogai S. Bronchial subepithelial fibrosis and expression of matrix metalloproteinase-9 in asthmatic airway inflammation. *J Allergy Clin Immunol* 1998; 102:783–788.

21. Bosse M, Chakir J, Rouabhia M, Boulet LP, Audette M, Laviolette M. Serum matrix metalloproteinase-9: tissue inhibitor of metalloproteinase-1 correlates with steroid responsiveness in moderate to severe asthma. *Am J Respir Crit Care Med* 1999; 159:562–602.

22. Belleguic C, Corbel M, Germain N *et al*. Increased release of matrix metalloproteinase-9 in the plasma of acute severe asthmatic patients. *Clin Exp Allergy* 2002; 32:217–223.

23. Oshita Y, Koga T, Kamimura T, Matsuo K, Rikimaru T, Aizawa H. Increased circulating 92 kDa matrix metalloproteinase (MMP-9) activity in exacerbations of asthma. *Thorax* 2003; 58:757–760.

24. Dahlen B, Shute J, Howarth P. Immunohistochemical localization of the matrix metalloproteinases MMP-3 and MMP-9 within the airways in asthma. *Thorax* 1999; 54:590–596.

25. Schwingsshackl A, Duszyk D, Brown N, Moqbel R. Human eosinophils release matrix metalloproteinase-9 on stimulation with TNF alpha. *J Allergy Clin Immunol* 1999; 104:983–989.

26. Kelly EA, Busse WW, Jarjour NN. Increased matrix metalloproteinase-9 in the airway after allergen challenge. *Am J Respir Crit Care Med* 2000; 162:1157–1161.

27. Boulay ME, Prince P, Deschesnes F, Chakir J, Boulet LP. Matrix metalloproteinase-9 in induced sputum correlates with the severity of the late allergen-induced asthmatic response. *Respiration* 2004; 71:216–224.

28. Cataldo DD, Bettiol J, Noel A, Bartsch P, Foidart JM, Louis R. Matrix metalloproteinase-9, but not tissue inhibitor of matrix metalloproteinase-1, increases in the sputum from allergic asthmatic patients after allergen challenge. *Chest* 2002; 122:1553–1559.

29. Park HS, Kim HA, Jung JW *et al*. Metalloproteinase-9 is increased after toluene diisocyanate exposure in the induced sputum from patients with toluene diisocyanate-induced asthma. *Clin Exp Allergy* 2003; 33:113–118.

30. Lemjabbar H, Gosset P, Lamblin C *et al*. Contribution of 92 kDa gelatinase type IV collagenase in bronchial inflammation during status asthmaticus. *Am J Respir Crit Care Med* 1999; 159:1298–1307.

31. Cundall M, Sun Y, Miranda C, Trudeau JB, Barnes S, Wenzel SE. Neutrophi-derived matrix metalloproteinase-9 is increased in severe asthma and poorly inhibited by glucocorticoids. *J Allergy Clin Immunol* 2003; 112:1064–1071.

32. Culpitt SV, Rogers DF, Travers SL, Barnes PJ, Donnelly LE. Sputum matrix metalloproteinases: comparison between chronic obstructive pulmonary disease and asthma. *Respir Med* 2005; 99:703–710.

33. Han Z, Junxu, Zhong N. Expression of matrix metalloproteinases MMP-9 within the airways in asthma. *Respir Med* 2003; 97:563–567.

34. Wenzel SE, Balzar S, Cundall M, Chu HW. Subepithelial basement membrane immunoreactivity for matrix metalloproteinase-9: association with asthma severity, neutrophil inflammation, and wound repair. *J Allergy Clin Immunol* 2003; 111:1345–1352.

35. Ko FWS, Diba C, Roth M *et al*. A comparison of airway and serum matrix metalloproteinase-9 activity among normal subjects, asthmatic patients and patients with asthmatic mucus hypersecretion. *Chest* 2005; 127:1919–1927.

36. Doherty GM, Kamath SV, de Courcey F *et al*. Children with stable asthma have reduced airway matrix metalloproteinase-9 and matrix metalloproteinase-9/tissue inhibitor of metalloproteinase-1 ratio. *Clin Exp Allergy* 2005; 35:1168–1174.

37. Matsumoto H, Niimi A, Takemura M *et al*. Relationship of airway wall thickening to an imbalance between matrix metalloproteinase-9 and its inhibitor in asthma. *Thorax* 2005; 60:277–281.

38. Hoshino M, Takahashi M, Takai Y, Sim J. Inhaled corticosteroids decrease subepithelial collagen deposition by modulation of the balance between matrix metalloproteinase-9 and tissue inhibitor of metalloproteinase-1 expression in asthma. *J Allergy Clin Immunol* 1999; 104:356–363.

39. Vignola AM, Riccobono L, Profita M *et al*. Effects of low doses of inhaled fluticasone propionate on inflammation and remodelling in persistent mild asthma. *Allergy* 2005; 60:1511–1517.

40. Johnson S, Knox A. Autocrine production of matrix metalloproteinase-2 is required for human airway smooth muscle proliferation. *Am J Physiol* 1999; 277:L1109–L1117.

41. Maisi P, Prikk K, Sepper R *et al*. Soluble membrane type-1 matrix metalloproteinase (MT1-MMP) and gelatinase A (MMP-2) in induced sputum and bronchoalveolar lavage fluid of human bronchial asthma and bronchiectasis. *APMIS* 2002; 110:771–782.

42. Elshaw SR, Henderson N, Knox AJ, Watson SA, Buttle DJ, Johnson SR. Matrix metalloproteinase expression and activity in human airway smooth muscle cells. *Br J Pharmacol* 2004; 142:1318–1324.

43. Rajah R, Nachajon RV, Collins MH, Hakonarson H, Grunstein MM, Cohen P. Elevated levels of the IGF-binding protein MMP-1 in asthmatic airway smooth muscle. *Am J Respir Cell Mol Biol* 1999; 20:199–208.

44. Cataldo D, Munault C, Noel A *et al*. Matrix metalloproteinases and TIMP-1 production by peripheral blood granulocytes from COPD patients and asthmatics. *Allergy* 2001; 56:145–151.

45. Prikk K, Maisi P, Pirila E *et al*. Airway obstruction correlates with collagenase-2 (MMP-8) expression and activation in bronchial asthma. *Lab Invest* 2002; 82:1535–1545.

46. Gueders MM, Balbin M, Rocks N *et al*. Matrix metalloproteinase-8 deficiency promotes granulocytic allergen induced airway inflammation. *J Immunol* 2005; 175:2589–2597.

47. Mautino G, Henriquet C, Jaffuel D, Bousquet J, Capony F. Tissue inhibitor of metalloproteinase-1 levels in bronchoalveolar lavage fluid from asthmatic subjects. *Am J Respir Crit Care Med* 1999; 160:324–330.

48. Tanaka H, Miyazaki N, Oashi K, Tanaka S, Ohmichi M, Abe S. Sputum matrix metalloproteinase-9: tissue inhibitor of metalloproteinase-1 ratio in acute asthma. *J Allergy Clin Immunol* 2000; 105:900–905.

49. Cataldo DD, Gueders M, Munaut C *et al*. Matrix metalloproteinases and tissue inhibitors of matrix metalloproteinase mRNA transcripts in the bronchial mucosa of asthmatics. *Lab Invest* 2004; 84:418–424.

50. Mautino G, Henriquet C, Gougat C *et al*. Increased expression of tissue inhibitor of metalloproteinase-1 and loss of correlation with matrix metalloproteinase-9 by macrophage in asthma. *Lab Invest* 1999; 79:39–47.

51. Profita M, Gagliardo R, Di Giorgi R *et al*. In vitro effects of flunisolide on MMP-9, TIMP-1, fibronectin, TGF beta1 release and apotosis in sputum cell freshly isolated from mild to moderate asthmatics. *Allergy* 2004; 59:927–932.

52. Lose F, Thompson PJ, Duffy D, Stewart GA, Kedda MA. A novel tissue inhibitor of metalloproteinase-1 (TIMP-1) polymorphism associated with asthma in Australian women. *Thorax* 2005; 60:617–618.

53. Holla LI, Vasku A, Stejskalova A, Znojil V. Functional polymorphism in the gelatinase B gene and asthma. *Allergy* 2000; 55:900–901.

54. Ganter K, Deichman KA, Heinzmann A. Association study of polymorphisms within matrix metalloproteinase 9 with bronchial asthma. *Int J Immunogenet* 2005; 32:233.

55. Lee KS, Jin SM, Kim SS, Lee YC. Doxycycline reduces airway inflammation and hyperresponsiveness in a murine model of toluene diisocyanate-induced asthma. *J Allergy Clin Immunol* 2004; 113:903–909.

56. Peterson JT. Matrix metalloproteinase inhibitor development and the remodeling of drug discovery. *Heart Fail Rev* 2004; 9:63–79.

57. Overall CM, Kleifeld O. Validating matrix metalloproteinases as drug targets and anti-targets for cancer therapy. *Nat Rev Cancer* 2006; 6:227–239.

58. Thomas PS. Tumor necrosis factor-alpha: the role of this multifunctional cytokine in asthma. *Immunol Cell Biol* 2001; 38:477–484.

59. Thomas PS, Yates DH, Barnes PJ. Tumor necrosis factor alpha increases airway responsiveness and sputum neutrophilia in normal human subjects. *Am J Respir Crit Care Med* 1995; 152:76–80.

60. Thomas PS, Pennington DW, Schreck RE, Levine T, Lazarus SC. Authentic 17 kD tumor necrosis factor alpha is synthesized and released from canine mast cells and up-regulated by stem cell factor. *Clin Exp Allergy* 1996; 26:710–718.

61. Thomas PS, Heywood G. Effects of inhaled tumor necrosis factor alpha in subjects with mild asthma. *Thorax* 2002; 57:774–778.

62. Bruce C, Thomas PS. The effect of marimastat, a metalloprotease inhibitor on allergen-induced asthmatic hyper-reactivity *Toxicol Appl Pharmacol* 2005; 205:126–132.

63. Lee YC, Song CH, Lee HB *et al*. A murine model of toluene diisocyanate-induced asthma can be treated with matrix metalloproteinase inhibitor. *J Allergy Clin Immunol* 2001; 108:1021–1026.

64. Trifilieff A, Walker C, Keller C, Kottirsch G, Neumann U. Pharmacological profile of PKF242-484 and PKF241-466, novel dual inhibitors of TNF alpha converting enzyme and matrix metalloproteinases, in models of airway inflammation. *Br J Pharmacol* 2002; 135:1655–1664.

65. Russo C, Polosa R. TNF-a as a promising therapeutic target in chronic asthma: a lesson from rheumatoid arthritis. *Clin Sci* 2005; 109:135–142.

66. Howarth PH, Babu KS, Arshad HS *et al*. Tumour necrosis factor alpha (TNFα) as a novel therapeutic target in symptomatic corticosteroid-dependent asthma. *Thorax* 2005; 60:1012–1018.

67. Berry MA, Hargadon B, Shelley M *et al*. Evidence of a role of tumor necrosis factor in refractory asthma. *N Engl J Med* 2006; 354:697–708.
68. Gueders MM, Foidart J-M, Noel A, Cataldo DD. Matrix metalloproteinases (MMPs) and tissue inhibitors of MMPs in the respiratory tract: potential implications in asthma and other lung diseases. *Eur J Pharmacol* 2006; 533:133–144.

Section III

Sensory nerves and sensory neuropeptides

8

Sensory neuropeptides as innovative targets in asthma

G. Joos

INTRODUCTION

Neural mechanisms have for a long time been regarded as factors contributing to the pathogenesis of asthma [1, 2]. The target organs involved in the pathogenesis of asthma, the airway epithelium, submucosal glands, airway smooth muscle, blood vessels and inflammatory cells are all under nervous control. Neurotransmitters may cause changes in airway calibre, affect bronchial responsiveness and airway inflammation. In the seventies and eighties of the past century, the classical view that cholinergic excitatory and adrenergic inhibitory nerves regulate airways, was considerably changed by the demonstration of a non-adrenergic, non-cholinergic (NANC) system. This NANC system can be either inhibitory (iNANC) or excitatory (eNANC). Various purines and peptides have been suggested as candidate neurotransmitters for the NANC. The sensory neuropeptides substance P and neurokinin A were found to be the main neurotransmitters responsible for the eNANC response [3].

The four major mammalian tachykinins are substance P, neurokinin A, neurokinin B, and haemokinin 1. They are derived from three pre-protachykinin genes, termed *TAC1*, *TAC3* and *TAC4*. Tachykinins are present in human airways, both in sensory nerves and in non-neuronal cells, including airway epithelium, airway smooth muscle, and immune cells such as eosinophils, monocytes, macrophages, lymphocytes and dendritic cells [4]. Tachykinins can be recovered from the airways after inhalation of ozone, cigarette smoke or allergen. They interact in the airways with tachykinin receptors to cause bronchoconstriction, plasma protein extravasation, and mucus secretion and to attract and activate immune cells. In preclinical studies substance P and neurokinin A have been implicated in the pathophysiology of asthma and chronic obstructive pulmonary disease (COPD), including the allergen- and cigarette smoke-induced airway inflammation and bronchial hyperresponsiveness. In this chapter, the therapeutic potential of tachykinin receptor antagonists in asthma will be discussed.

LOCALIZATION AND PRODUCTION OF TACHYKININS IN THE AIRWAYS

Tachykinins (substance P, neurokinin A and neurokinin B) have previously been considered as a group of neuropeptides because of their widespread distribution in the central and the peripheral nervous system. However, their presence in a variety of non-neuronal structures has been demonstrated repeatedly [5, 6]. Furthermore, mRNA expression studies suggest that the tachykinin haemokinin 1 has a unique distribution outside neuronal tissues [7].

Guy Joos, MD, PhD, Pulmonologist, Professor of Medicine, Director, Department of Respiratory Diseases, Ghent University Hospital, Ghent, Belgium

In the airways, substance P and neurokinin A positive nerves have been located beneath and within the epithelium, around blood vessels and submucosal glands and within the bronchial smooth muscle layer [8, 9]. In guinea pigs, airway sensory nerves containing tachykinins are easily demonstrated but in human airways, tachykinergic innervation is sparse. Additional, non-neuronal sources of tachykinins in the airways have been reported. Chu et al. [10] demonstrated staining for substance P in the airway epithelium and Maghni et al. [11] reported the presence of substance P in airway smooth muscle cells. There is also evidence for the production of substance P by eosinophils, monocytes and macrophages, lymphocytes and dendritic cells [12–15]. Immunoreactivity for neurokinin B has not been found in the airways yet. PCR-techniques demonstrated transcripts of the mouse and the human *TAC4* gene in lung tissue [16, 17], which may result in the formation of the haemokinin 1, representing another source of tachykinins in the airways.

AIRWAY TACHYKININ RECEPTORS

The biological activity of tachykinins depends on their interaction with three specific receptors, the tachykinin NK_1, NK_2 and NK_3 receptors [18, 19]. The tachykinin receptor displaying highest affinity for substance P was termed the tachykinin NK_1 receptor. The receptor showing highest affinity for neurokinin A was termed the tachykinin NK_2 receptor and the receptor with the highest affinity for neurokinin B was called the tachykinin NK_3 receptor [20]. Haemokinin 1 and its elongated forms act as tachykinin NK_1 receptor preferring agonists [21]. It should be emphasized, however that all tachykinins can act as full agonists on the three different receptors but with lower affinities than on the preferred receptor [22].

An overwhelming amount of functional data demonstrates indirectly the broad expression of tachykinin NK_1 and NK_2 receptors in the airways. Functional evidence for the presence of tachykinin NK_3 receptors also exists, including in human airways [23, 24]. mRNA for the tachykinin NK_1 and NK_3 receptors has been found in human pulmonary veins, arteries and bronchi. mRNA for the tachykinin NK_2 receptor was abundantly expressed in human bronchi, whereas a low expression of this receptor was found in human pulmonary veins and arteries [25]. In a study on surgical specimens, using specific antibodies, tachykinin NK_1 and NK_2 receptor protein was detected in human bronchial glands, bronchial vessels and bronchial smooth muscle. Tachykinin NK_1 receptors were occasionally found in nerves and tachykinin NK_2 receptors in inflammatory cells, such as T lymphocytes, macrophages and mast cells [26]. A study on endobronchial biopsies revealed immunoreactivity for the tachykinin NK_1 receptor in the epithelium and the submucosa. Goblet cells appeared to be the cells with the strongest staining. In the submucosa, staining was localized on the endothelial cells of the blood vessels, the surfaces of inflammatory cells, and some smooth muscle cells [10]. Immunohistochemistry on human pulmonary vessels from tissue obtained at lobectomy, revealed positive staining for tachykinin NK_1 receptors on the endothelium of both veins and arteries [27]. Inflammatory cells such as macrophages, lymphocytes, neutrophils, dendritic cells and mast cells, also express functional tachykinin NK_1 receptors [12, 14, 15, 28, 29]. Using confocal microscopy, the tachykinin NK_3 receptor was identified on human parasympathetic ganglion neurons. These neurons could be depolarized by activation of sensory nerve fibres [24].

AIRWAY EFFECTS OF TACHYKININS

EFFECTS ON AIRWAY SMOOTH MUSCLE TONE

Tachykinins are also potent contractors of human airways. Substance P contracts human bronchi and bronchioli, but is less potent than histamine or acetylcholine [30, 31]. Neurokinin A is a more potent constrictor and is, on a molar base, 2–3 orders of magnitude more potent than histamine or acetylcholine. Neurokinin B does not exert a contractile activity on human airways [32]. The tachykininergic contraction was demonstrated to become more important in more distal airways [33].

In human airways, tachykinins have both direct and indirect bronchoconstrictor effects [34]. It has long been thought that only tachykinin NK_2 receptors were involved in the direct contractile effect of tachykinins on isolated bronchi [35]. However, in small and medium-sized diameter bronchi, tachykinins also cause contraction *via* tachykinin NK_1 receptor stimulation [36, 37]. Part of the bronchoconstrictor effect of tachykinins in human airways is indirect and occurs by stimulation of cholinergic nerves and/or mast cells. Substance P facilitated release of acetylcholine from post-ganglionic cholinergic airway nerves [38–40, 41], probably through the tachykinin NK_1 receptor. In guinea pig trachea, tachykinin NK_2 receptors were also found to be involved in the facilitation of acetylcholine release [42]. Substance P is also known to induce degranulation of human and rat mast cells with subsequent release of histamine and serotonin, which in their turn could cause contraction [43, 44]. Leukotrienes have also been found to be involved in the indirect bronchoconstrictor effect of tachykinins [45].

COUGH

An afferent (sensory) and an efferent arm that synapses in the brainstem areas, including the nucleus tractus solitarius, make up the reflex arch that mediates the cough reflex [46]. Mediators and mechanisms of the sensory arm of the reflex pathway are not completely understood. Pharmacological evidence exists for the involvement of substance P [47, 48]. The role of tachykinins in the regulation of the cough response appears to be complex since antagonists for the three tachykinin receptors have antitussive activity in pre-clinical models [49–51]. In guinea pigs, substance P locally applied into the airways has been shown to produce [52] or potentiate cough produced by other stimuli [51]. These findings support a role for substance P at a peripheral site of action but also central sites of action have been reported [53].

SECRETION OF MUCUS, WATER AND ELECTROLYTES

Relatively strong evidence exists that tachykinins, released from sensory nerve fibres are physiological (and pathological) regulators of secretion in the upper and lower airways. A local release of tachykinins in the nasal mucosa could play a role in the defensive response to irritants. In the lower tracheobronchial tree, seromucous glands and goblet cells produce mucus. Both sources are under neural control. Depending upon species and airway level, innervation comprises parasympathetic, sympathetic and 'sensory-efferent' pathways [54]. The transmitters of the latter pathway are substance P and neurokinin A, which act *via* tachykinin NK_1 receptors [55, 56]. Recently, an involvement of tachykinin NK_3 receptors in porcine airways has been suggested [56]. Compared with cholinergic control, the eNANC neural control of human airway secretion appears to form a rather minor component [54].

Inflammatory cells may be an additional source of tachykinin-induced mucus secretion: indeed, in human tissue, obtained at thoracotomy, immunoreactivity for the NK_1 receptor was found in myoepithelial cells, which were in direct contact with pre-protachykinin mRNA and tachykinin-positive inflammatory cells [57]. Mucus secretion is closely coupled to liquid secretion to ensure optimal ciliary transport and presence of adequate concentrations of antibacterial substances on the airway surface. Substance P has also been shown to be involved in this process in porcine airways [58].

PLASMA PROTEIN EXTRAVASATION

Substance P, released from sensory nerves, mediates neurogenic inflammation in the airways [3, 59, 60]. Plasma extravasation, induced by cold air, hypertonic saline or isocapnic hyperpnoea also depends on stimulation of sensory fibres and is inhibited by tachykinin receptor antagonists [61, 62]. Once plasma extravasation occurs, leucocytes initiate a process that results in slowing down their velocity, rolling on and adhering to the venular endothelium. The involvement of the tachykinin NK_1 receptor in all these phenomena has been demonstrated by the use of specific antagonists [61, 63, 64]. It is not known how much of the effect is due to a tachykinin NK_1 receptor-mediated effect on leucocytes and endothelial cells or merely the consequence of inhibition of tachykinin NK_1 receptor-mediated plasma extravasation. Tachykinin NK_2 receptors also mediate part of the neurogenic plasma extravasation in the secondary bronchi and intraparenchymal airways of the guinea pig [65].

Direct evidence for neurogenic plasma extravasation in human airways could not be demonstrated for a long time due to difficulties in the assessment [66]. However, microvascular leakage can now be measured in human airways with a 'dual induction' model. First, substance P is inhaled and then sputum is induced by inhalation of hypertonic saline solution. With this method, it was demonstrated that inhalation of substance P induced significant increases in the levels of α_2-macroglobulin, ceruloplasmin and albumin in induced sputum [67].

CELL GROWTH AND PROLIFERATION OF MESENCHYMAL CELLS

Tachykinins stimulate the proliferation of a number of cell types, including fibroblasts [68], smooth muscle cells [69], epithelial [70] and endothelial cells [71]. This could have important implications in wound healing and tissue repair. The substance P-induced proliferation of human fibroblasts is mediated by interaction with tachykinin NK_1 receptors [72, 73]. The proliferation of rabbit airway smooth muscle also involves tachykinin NK_1 receptors [69]. The proliferation of smooth muscle cells in response to tachykinins is coupled to inositoltriphospate formation and DNA synthesis. In the tracheal epithelium of guinea pigs, it was shown that, besides tachykinin NK_1 and NK_2 receptors, CGRP-receptors are involved in the proliferative response [74]. Endothelial cell proliferation induced by tachykinins is a likely mechanism in the neovascularization observed *in vivo* in response to peptides of this family [75].

IMMUNOMODULATION

Tachykinins are known to have a wide variety of modulatory effects on inflammatory/ immune cell functions. This topic has been reviewed elsewhere [76–78].

ROLE OF TACHYKININS IN ANIMAL MODELS OF ASTHMA

In various animal models tachykinins have been found to be involved in *antigen-induced bronchoconstriction, airway inflammation* and *enhanced bronchial responsiveness*. A combination of a tachykinin NK_1 receptor antagonist, CP-96,345 [79], and a tachykinin NK_2 receptor antagonist, SR 48968 [80], inhibited bronchoconstriction produced by ovalbumin challenge in sensitized guinea pigs [81]. The NK_1 receptor antagonist, CP-96,345, was also able to limit antigen-induced plasma extravasation [82]. By using NK_1/NK_2 receptor blockade the involvement of endogenous tachykinins in antigen-induced bronchial hyperresponsiveness was demonstrated [83].

The relative contribution of the NK_1 and NK_2 receptors in antigen-induced airway changes has been studied in guinea pigs and rats. In conscious, unrestrained guinea pigs the NK_1 receptor is involved in both the development of antigen-induced airway hyperresponsiveness to histamine and the antigen-induced infiltration of eosinophils, neutrophils and lymphocytes [84]. On the other hand, the NK_2 receptor is involved in the development of the antigen-induced late reaction [85]. The effect of allergen challenge has also been studied in the Brown Norway rat model [86]. Substance P was found to increase 2.4-fold in bronchoalveolar lavage (BAL) after challenge with ovalbumin. The tachykinin NK_1 receptor antagonist CP-99,994 and the tachykinin NK_2 receptor antagonist SR 48968 were not able to reduce the early airway response to ovalbumin, but both antagonists reduced the ovalbumin-induced late airway responses. An interesting finding in this study was that the NK_2 tachykinin receptor antagonist decreased the number of eosinophils in BAL fluid and decreased the expression of both Th1 (IFNγ) and Th2 (IL-4 and -5) cytokines in BAL cells. In a mouse model of asthma, we observed no influence of the tachykinin NK_1 receptor on the development of acute allergic airway inflammation. However, allergen-induced goblet cell hyperplasia, one of the features of airway remodelling, was decreased in mice lacking the tachykinin NK_1 receptor [87].

So from animal studies, it seems that both the tachykinin NK_1 and the NK_2 receptor are involved in antigen-induced airway effects. In addition, it is possible that tachykinin NK_3 receptors are also involved in this process: administration of the tachykinin NK_3 receptor antagonist SR 142801 *via* aerosol caused a significant reduction in neutrophil and eosinophil influx in the airways of ovalbumin-sensitized and -challenged mice [88].

Tachykinins and their receptors have also been involved in *airway responses to non-specific stimuli*. Both the NK_1 and the NK_2 tachykinin receptors have been involved in airway contraction induced by cold air [89, 90], hyperventilation and cigarette smoke [91], in plasma extravasation induced by hypertonic saline [92, 93], and in airway hyperresponsiveness induced by viruses [94], IL-5 and nerve growth factor [95, 96]. In addition, the tachykinin NK_3 receptor was found to be involved in citric acid-induced cough and enhanced bronchial responsiveness [49]. From studies performed in tachykinin NK_1 receptor knockout mice, it is becoming apparent that the tachykinin NK_1 receptor plays a role in cigarette smoke-induced airway inflammation [97].

Neurogenic mucus secretion results from the contribution of different components and shows marked variation among species. Adrenergic and cholinergic agonists may stimulate mucus secretion in the ferret and human airways. Tachykinins also cause marked mucus secretion in the ferret, an effect exclusively mediated by NK_1 receptors. Endogenous tachykinins mediate mucus secretion induced by electrical stimuli and part of the response produced by exposure to antigen *via* NK_1 receptor activation [55].

SENSORY NEUROPEPTIDES AS TARGETS IN THE TREATMENT OF ASTHMA

Studies on rodents have demonstrated that a number of strategies are possible to interfere with the action of sensory neuropeptides in the airways: (1) depletion of neuropeptides within nerves (e.g. by the neurotoxin capsaicin); (2) inhibition of the release of sensory neuropeptides (e.g. by β_2-adrenoceptor agonist, theophylline, cromoglycate or phophodiesterase [PDE4] inhibitors) and (3) inhibition of tachykinin receptors by receptor antagonists [98].

Potent tachykinin receptor antagonists have only recently become available and some of them have not been considered for application in airways diseases, but for depression, emesis or inflammatory bowel disease [99]. From the data presented above, it is clear that substance P and neurokinin A may have a wide variety of effects on the airways. These effects occur by interaction with three tachykinin receptors. Several tachykinin receptor antagonists have been reported with activity in the airways. At the present time, clinical trials with at least seven tachykinin receptor antagonists have been performed and reported.

Reports studying the effects of FK224, a cyclic peptide tachykinin antagonist for NK_1 and NK_2 receptors, CP-99,994, a non-peptide NK_1 tachykinin receptor antagonist, FK888, a peptidic tachykinin NK_1 receptor antagonist, and SR 48968 (saredutant), a non-peptide NK_2 tachykinin receptor antagonist have been published (Table 8.1). In our centre, in the past few years, we completed three additional studies, one with the bicyclic peptidic tachykinin

Table 8.1 Tachykinin receptor antagonists in clinical developments for asthma

Drug name	Dose and route of administration	Molecular targets	Biological effects	References
FK224	4 mg by inhalation	NK_1 and NK_2 receptor	Inhibition of bradykinin-induced bronchoconstriction	[100]
			No effect on neurokinin A-induced bronchoconstriction	[102]
CP-99,994	250 μg/2 h by intravenous route	NK_1 receptor	No effect on bronchoconstriction and cough induced by hypertonic saline	[103]
FK888	2.5 mg by inhalation	NK_1 receptor	Reduction of the time of recovery from exercise-induced broncoconstriction	[104]
Saredutant	100 mg by oral route	NK_2 receptor	Significant inhibition of neurokinin A-induced bronchoconstriction	[105]
Nepadutant	2 and 8 mg by intravenous route	NK_2 receptor	Significant inhibition of neurokinin A-induced bronchoconstriction	[107]
DNK333A	100 mg *via* oral route	NK_1 and NK_2 receptor	Significant inhibition of neurokinin A-induced bronchoconstriction	[109]
CS003	200 mg *via* oral route	NK_1 NK_2 and NK_3 receptor	Significant inhibition of neurokinin A-induced bronchoconstriction	[110]

NK = Neurokinin.

NK_2 receptor antagonist MEN 11420 (nepadutant), one with the dual NK_1/NK_2 tachykinin receptor antagonist DNK333A, and one with the triple $NK_1/NK_2/NK_3$ receptor antagonist CS003.

FK244, 4 mg given by metred dose inhaler, was shown to inhibit bradykinin-induced bronchoconstriction and cough in nine asthmatics [100]. These findings suggested that bradykinin causes bronchoconstriction by release of tachykinins from sensory nerves. However, in a similar study, using a lower dose, FK224 had no effect on bradykinin-induced bronchoconstriction [101]. Moreover, inhaled FK224 had no effect on baseline lung function and offered no protection against neurokinin A (NKA)-induced bronchoconstriction in patients with asthma [102].

The non-peptide NK_1 tachykinin receptor antagonist CP-99,994 had no effect on the bronchoconstriction and cough induced by hypertonic saline [103]. However, it remains to be proven whether this compound at the dose given, was able to block the airway responses induced by inhaled SP or NKA.

The NK_1 tachykinin receptor antagonist FK888 had no effect on baseline lung function, and on the maximal decrease in lung function occurring after exercise, but reduced the time of recovery from exercise-induced bronchoconstriction [104].

The NK_2 tachykinin receptor antagonist SR 48968 (saredutant) (100 mg/os) caused a significant inhibition of neurokinin A-induced bronchoconstriction, with a mean 3–5-fold shift of the dose–response curve for NKA to the right [105]. Administration of saredutant during

Table 8.2 Airway effects of tachykinins and the receptors involved

Airway effects of tachykinins	Tachykinin receptor
Smooth muscle contraction	NK_1, NK_2
Submucosal gland secretion	NK_1
Vasodilatation	NK_1
Increase in vascular permeability	NK_1
Stimulation of cholinergic nerves	NK_1, NK_3
Stimulation of mast cells	NK_1, NK_2
Stimulation of B and T lymphocytes	NK_1
Stimulation of macrophages	NK_1, NK_2
Chemo-attraction of eosinophils and neutrophils	NK_1
Vascular adhesion of neutrophils	NK_1

9 days (100 mg/os, each day) did not however affect baseline airway calibre or bronchial responsiveness to adenosine [106]. Moreover, the NK_2 tachykinin receptor antagonist MEN 11420 (nepadutant) (2 and 8 mg i.v.) shifted the dose–response curve for NKA to the right, in a similar way to that observed in the study with SR 48968 [107]. These studies are the first to demonstrate activity of a tachykinin NK_2 receptor antagonist in human airways. It is, however, clear that although these agents are potent antagonists *in vitro* [35, 108], their potential to inhibit the bronchoconstrictor effect of neurokinin A in patients with asthma is rather limited. This can be explained by an additional involvement of tachykinin NK_1 receptors in the bronchoconstrictor effect of neurokinin [36, 37]. This idea is supported by our findings with a dual NK_1/NK_2 receptor antagonist: in a study on 19 patients with asthma, DNK333A, a newly developed NK_1/NK_2 receptor tachykinin receptor antagonist, was able to shift the dose–response curve to inhaled neurokinin A to a large extent (4.8 doubling doses) [109]. Similar findings were obtained using a triple $NK_1/NK_2/NK_3$ tachykinin receptor antagonist, CS003 [110] (Table 8.2).

SUMMARY AND FUTURE PERSPECTIVES

The tachykinins substance P and neurokinin A are present in human airways, in sensory nerves and immune cells. Tachykinins can be recovered from the airways after inhalation of ozone, cigarette smoke or allergen. They interact in the airways with tachykinin NK_1, NK_2 and NK_3 receptors to cause bronchoconstriction, plasma protein extravasation, and mucus secretion and to attract and activate immune cells. In pre-clinical studies, they have been implicated in the pathophysiology of asthma, including allergen- and cigarette smoke-induced airway inflammation and bronchial hyperresponsiveness.

Tachykinins are produced in human airways and mimic various features of asthma. So, tachykinin receptor antagonists have potential in the treatment of asthma [19, 23, 111]. However, the development of tachykinin receptor antagonists for airways diseases has been rather slow and up to now somehow disappointing. This is in contrast to the extensive and overwhelming pre-clinical data suggesting a role for tachykinins in asthma. There are several explanations for this apparent paradox [112]:

1. The lack of efficacy can be easily explained by the low potency or defective pharmacokinetics of the compounds tested so far.
2. Blocking either the NK_1 or the NK_2 receptor is probably an insufficient approach, as most of the effects of tachykinins in the airways are mediated by more than one tachykinin receptor.

3. In the application of a new tachykinin receptor antagonist to airways diseases, it is crucial that one first demonstrates that the antagonist is indeed able to block airway effects of an agonist (e.g. substance P or neurokinin A). This allows us to determine the *in vivo* activity of the antagonist under consideration and to determine dose and dosing frequency for further clinical study.

4. Once a potent drug that can be administered twice, or preferably once a day, is identified, clinical studies are to be conducted to define the potential therapeutic benefit in asthma. These clinical studies will need to last for at least 3, preferably 6 or 12 months, in order to demonstrate changes in relevant clinical outcomes. This is especially important to detect a possible effect on exacerbations of asthma, a situation where it is suggested a release of tachykinins from human airway tissue occurs [113, 114]. The arrival of more potent, dual or triple tachykinin recetor antagonists [115, 116] should allow us to obtain a final judgment on the role of tachykinins in asthma.

REFERENCES

1. Barnes PJ. Asthma as an axon reflex. *Lancet* 1986; i:242–244.
2. Joos GF, Geppetti P. Neural mechanisms in asthma. *Eur Respir Mon* 2003; 23:138–163.
3. Lundberg JM, Saria A. Capsaicin-induced desensitization of airway mucosa to cigarette smoke, mechanical and chemical irritants. *Nature* 1983; 302:215–253.
4. Joos G, De Swert K. Tachykinins. In: Laurent GJ, Shapiro SD (eds). *Encyclopedia of Respiratory Medicine*. Elsevier Ltd., 2006, vol. 2, pp 509–517.
5. Severini C, Improta G, Falconieri-Erspamer G, Salvadori S, Erspamer V. The tachykinin Peptide family. *Pharmacol Rev* 2002; 54:285–322.
6. Pennefather JN, Lecci A, Candenas ML, Patak E, Pinto FM, Maggi CA. Tachykinins and tachykinin receptors: a growing family. *Life Sci* 2004; 74:1445–1463.
7. Patacchini R, Lecci A, Holzer P, Maggi CA. Newly discovered tachykinins raise new questions about their peripheral roles and the tachykinin nomenclature. *Trends Pharmacol Sci* 2004; 25:1–3.
8. Lundberg JM, Hökfeldt T, Martling C-R, Saria A, Cuello C. Substance P-immunoreactive sensory nerves in the lower respiratory tract of various mammals including man. *Cell Tissue Res* 1984; 235:251–261.
9. Luts A, Uddman R, Alm P, Basterra J, Sundler F. Peptide-containing nerve fibers in human airways: distribution and coexistence pattern. *Int Arch Allergy Appl Immunol* 1993; 101:52–60.
10. Chu HW, Kraft M, Krause JE, Rex MD, Martin RJ. Substance P and its receptor neurokinin 1 expression in asthmatic airways. *J Allergy Clin Immunol* 2000; 106:713–722.
11. Maghni K, Michoud MC, Alles M *et al*. Airway smooth muscle cells express functional neurokinin-1 receptors and the nerve-derived preprotachykinin-a gene: regulation by passive sensitization. *Am J Respir Cell Mol Biol* 2003; 28:103–110.
12. Lai J-P, Douglas SD, Ho W-Z. Human lymphocytes express substance P and its receptor. *J Neuroimmunol* 1998; 86:80–86.
13. Aliakbar J, Sreedharan SP, Turck CW, Goetzl EJ. Selective localization of vasoactive intestinal peptide and substance P in human eosinophils. *Biochem Biophys Res Commun* 1987; 148:1440–1445.
14. Ho W-Z, Lai J-P, Zhu X-H, Uvaydova M, Douglas SD. Human monocytes and macrophages express substance P and neurokinin-1 receptor. *J Immunol* 1997; 159:5654–5660.
15. Lambrecht BN, Germonpre PR, Everaert EG *et al*. Endogenously produced substance P contributes to lymphocyte proliferation induced by dendritic cells and direct TCR ligation. *Eur J Immunol* 1999; 29:3815–3825.
16. Page NM, Bell NJ, Gardiner SM *et al*. Characterization of the endokinins: human tachykinins with cardiovascular activity. *Proc Natl Acad Sci USA* 2003; 100:6245–6250.
17. Duffy RA, Hedrick JA, Randolph G *et al*. Centrally administered hemokinin-1 (HK-1), a neurokinin NK1 receptor agonist, produces substance P-like behavioral effects in mice and gerbils. *Neuropharmacology* 2003; 45:242–250.
18. Maggi CA. Tachykinin receptors and airway pathophysiology. *Eur Respir J* 1993; 6:735–742.
19. Almeida TA, Rojo J, Nieto PM *et al*. Tachykinins and tachykinin receptors: structure and activity relationships. *Curr Med Chem* 2004; 11:2045–2081.
20. Maggi CA. The troubled story of tachykinins and neurokinins. *Trends Pharmacol Sci* 2000; 21:173–175.

21. Kurtz MM, Wang R, Clements MK et al. Identification, localization and receptor characterization of novel mammalian substance P-like peptides. *Gene* 2002; 296:205–212.

22. Maggi CA, Patacchini R, Rovero P, Giachetti A. Tachykinin receptors and tachykinin receptor antagonists. *J Auton Pharmacol* 1993; 13:23–93.

23. Joos GF, De Swert KO, Pauwels RA. Airway inflammation and tachykinins; prospects for the development of tachykinin receptor antagonists. *Eur J Pharmacol* 2001; 429:239–250.

24. Myers AC, Goldie RG, Hay DW. A novel role for tachykinin neurokinin-3 receptors in regulation of human bronchial ganglia neurons. *Am J Respir Crit Care Med* 2005; 171:212–216.

25. Pinto FM, Almeida TA, Hernandez M, Devillier P, Advenier C, Candenas ML. mRNA expression of tachykinins and tachykinin receptors in different human tissues. *Eur J Pharmacol* 2004; 494:233–239.

26. Mapp CE, Miotto D, Braccioni F et al. The distribution of neurokinin-1 and neurokinin-2 receptors in human central airways. *Am J Respir Crit Care Med* 2000; 161:207–215.

27. Mechiche H, Koroglu A, Candenas L et al. Neurokinins induce relaxation of human pulmonary vessels through stimulation of endothelial NK1 receptors. *J Cardiovasc Pharmacol* 2003; 41:343–355.

28. Wiedermann CJ, Wiedermann FJ, Apperl A, Kieselbach G, Konwalinka G, Braunsteiner H. In vitro human polymorphonuclear leukocyte chemokinesis and human monocyte chemotaxis are different activities of aminoterminal and carboxyterminal substance P. *N-S Arch Pharmacol* 1989; 340:185–190.

29. Cooke HJ, Fox P, Alferes L, Fox CC, Wolfe SA. Presence of NK1 receptors on a mucosal-like mast cell line, RBL-2H3 cells. *Can J Physiol Pharmacol* 1998; 76:188–193.

30. Finney MJB, Karlsson JA, Persson CGA. Effects of bronchoconstrictors and bronchodilators on a novel human small airway preparation. *Br J Pharmacol* 1985; 85:29–36.

31. Martling C-R, Theodorsson-Norheim E, Lundberg JM. Occurrence and effects of multiple tachykinins; substance P, neurokinin A and neuropeptide K in human lower airways. *Life Sci* 1987; 40:1633–1643.

32. Advenier C, Naline E, Drapeau G, Regoli D. Relative potencies of neurokinins in guinea-pig trachea and human bronchus. *Eur J Pharmacol* 1987; 139:133–137.

33. Frossard N, Barnes PJ. Effect of tachykinins in small human airways. *Neuropeptides* 1991; 19:157–161.

34. Van Schoor J, Joos GF, Pauwels RA. Indirect bronchial hyperresponsiveness in asthma: mechanisms, pharmacology and implications for clinical research. *Eur Respir J* 2000; 16:514–533.

35. Advenier C, Naline E, Toty L et al. Effects on the isolated human bronchus of SR 48968, a potent and selective nonpeptide antagonist of the neurokinin A (NK2) receptors. *Am Rev Respir Dis* 1992; 146:1177–1181.

36. Naline E, Molimard M, Regoli D, Emonds-Alt X, Bellamy JF, Advenier C. Evidence for functional tachykinin NK1 receptors on human isolated small bronchi. *Am J Physiol* 1996; 271:L763–L767.

37. Amadesi S, Moreau J, Tognetto M et al. NK1 receptor stimulation causes contraction and inositol phosphate increase in medium-size human isolated bronchi. *Am J Respir Crit Care Med* 2001; 163:1206–1211.

38. Hall AK, Barnes PJ, Meldrum LA, Maclayan J. Facilitation by tachykinins of neurotransmission in guinea-pig pulmonary parasympathetic nerves. *Br J Pharmacol* 1989; 97:274–280.

39. Colasurdo GN, Loader JE, Graves JP, Larsen GL. Modulation of acetylcholine release in rabbit airways in vitro. *Am J Physiol Lung Cell Molec Physiol* 1995; 268:L432–L437.

40. Joos GF, Pauwels RA, Van Der Straeten ME. The effect of oxitropiumbromide on neurokinin A-induced bronchoconstriction in asthmatics. *Pulm Pharmacol* 1988; 1:41–45.

41. Black JL, Johnson PRA, Alouan L, Armour CL. Neurokinin A with K+ channel blockade potentiates contraction to electrical stimulation in human bronchus. *Eur J Pharmacol* 1990; 180:311–317.

42. D'Agostino G, Erbelding D, Kilbinger H. Tachykinin NK(2) receptors facilitate acetylcholine release from guinea-pig isolated trachea. *Eur J Pharmacol* 2000; 396:29–32.

43. Cross LJM, Heaney LG, Ennis M. Further characterization of substance P induced histamine release from human bronchoalveolar lavage mast cells. *Inflamm Res* 1996; 45:S11–S12.

44. Joos GF, Pauwels RA. The in vivo effect of tachykinins on airway mast cells in the rat. *Am Rev Respir Dis* 1993; 148:922–926.

45. Crimi N, Pagano C, Palermo F et al. Inhibitory effect of a leukotriene receptor antagonist (montelukast) on neurokinin A-induced bronchoconstriction. *J Allergy Clin Immunol* 2003; 111:833–839.

46. Higenbottam T. Chronic cough and the cough reflex in common lung diseases. *Pulm Pharmacol Ther* 2002; 15:241–247.

47. Mutoh T, Bonham AC, Joad JP. Substance P in the nucleus of the solitary tract augments bronchopulmonary C fiber reflex output. *Am J Physiol Regul Integr Comp Physiol* 2000; 279:R1215–R1223.

48. Advenier C, Lagente V, Boichot E. The role of tachykinin receptor antagonists in the prevention of bronchial hyperresponsiveness, airway inflammation and cough. *Eur Respir J* 1997; 10:1892–1906.

49. Daoui S, Cognon C, Naline E, Emonds-Alt X. Involvement of tachykinin NK3 receptors in citric acid-induced cough and bronchial responses in guinea pigs. *Am J Respir Crit Care Med* 1998; 158:42–48.

50. Girard V, Naline E, Vilain P, Emonds-Alt X, Advenier C. Effect of the two tachykinin antagonists, SR 48968 and SR 140333, on cough induced by citric acid in the unanaesthetized guinea pig. *Eur Respir J* 1995; 8:1110–1114.

51. Moreaux B, Nemmar A, Vincke G *et al*. Role of substance P and tachykinin receptor antagonists in citric acid-induced cough in pigs. *Eur J Pharmacol* 2000; 408:305–312.

52. Kohrogi H, Graf PD, Sekizawa K, Borson DB, Nadel JA. Neutral endopeptidase inhibitors potentiate substance P- and capsaicin-induced cough in awake guinea pigs. *J Clin Invest* 1988; 82:2063–2068.

53. Bolser DC, DeGennaro FC, O'Reilly S, McLeod RL, Hey JA. Central antitussive activity of the NK1 and NK2 tachykinin receptor antagonists, CP-99,994 and SR 48968, in the guinea-pig and cat. *Br J Pharmacol* 1997; 121:165–170.

54. Rogers DF. Motor control of airway goblet cells and glands. *Respir Physiol* 2001; 125:129–144.

55. Khan S, Liu Y-C, Khawaja AM, Manzini S, Rogers DF. Effect of the long-acting tachykinin NK1 receptor antagonist MEN 11467 on tracheal mucus secretion in allergic ferrets. *Br J Pharmacol* 2001; 132:189–196.

56. Phillips JE, Hey JA, Corboz MR. Tachykinin NK(3) and NK(1) receptor activation elicits secretion from porcine airway submucosal glands. *Br J Pharmacol* 2003; 138:254–260.

57. Springer J, Groneberg DA, Pregla R, Fischer A. Inflammatory cells as source of tachykinin-induced mucus secretion in chronic bronchitis. *Regul Pept* 2005; 124:195–201.

58. Trout L, Corboz MR, Ballard ST. Mechanism of substance P-induced liquid secretion across bronchial epithelium. *Am J Physiol Lung Cell Mol Physiol* 2001; 281:L639–L645.

59. Lundberg JM, Saria A. Capsaicin-sensitive vagal neurons involved in control of vascular permeability in rat trachea. *Acta Physiol Scand* 1982; 115:521–523.

60. Lundberg JM, Saria A, Brodin E, Rossel S, Folkers K. A substance P antagonist inhibits vagally induced increase in vascular permeability and bronchial smooth muscle contraction in the guinea-pig. *Proc Natl Acad Sci USA* 1983; 83:1120–1124.

61. Yoshihara S, Chan B, Yamawaki I *et al*. Plasma extravasation in the rat trachea induced by cold air is mediated by tachykinin release from sensory nerves. *Am J Respir Crit Care Med* 1995; 151:1011–1017.

62. Umeno E, McDonald DM, Nadel JA. Hypertonic saline increases vascular permeability in the rat by producing neurogenic inflammation. *J Clin Invest* 1990; 85:1905–1908.

63. Piedimonte G, Bertrand C, Geppetti P, Snider RM, Desai MC, Nadel JA. A new NK1 receptor antagonist (CP-99,994) prevents the increase in tracheal vascular permeability produced by hypertonic saline. *J Pharmacol Exp Ther* 1993; 266:270–273.

64. Baluk P, Bertrand C, Geppetti P, McDonald DM, Nadel JA. NK1 receptor antagonist CP-99,994 inhibits cigarette smoke-induced neutrophil and eosinophil adhesion in rat tracheal venules. *Exp Lung Res* 1996; 22:409–418.

65. Tousignant C, Chan CC, Guevremont D *et al*. NK2 receptors mediate plasma extravasation in guinea-pig lower airways. *Br J Pharmacol* 1993; 108:383–386.

66. Barnes PJ. Neurogenic inflammation in the airways. *Respir Physiol* 2001; 125:145–154.

67. Van Rensen EL, Hiemstra PS, Rabe KF, Sterk PJ. Assessment of microvascular leakage via sputum induction: the role of substance P and neurokinin A in patients with asthma. *Am J Respir Crit Care Med* 2002; 165:1275–1279.

68. Harrison NK, Dawes KE, Kwon OJ, Barnes PJ, Laurent GJ, Chung KF. Effects of neuropeptides on human lung fibroblast proliferation and chemotaxis. *Am J Physiol* 1995; 12:L278–L283.

69. Noveral JP, Grunstein MM. Tachykinin regulation of airway smooth muscle cell proliferation. *Am J Physiol* 1995; 269:L339–L343.

70. Kim JS, Rabe KF, Magnussen H, Green JM, White SR. Migration and proliferation of guinea pig and human airway epithelial cells in response to tachykinins. *Am J Physiol* 1995; 269:L119–L126.

71. Ziche M, Morbidelli L, Geppetti P, Maggi CA, Dolara P. Substance P induces migration of capillary endothelial cells: a novel NK-1 selective receptor mediated activity. *Life Sci* 1991; 48:L7–L11.

72. Ziche M, Morbidelli L, Pacini M, Dolara P, Maggi CA. NK1-receptors mediate the proliferative response of human fibroblasts to tachykinins. *Br J Pharmacol* 1990; 100:11–14.

73. Ziche M, Parenti A, Amerini S, Zawieja D, Maggi CA, Ledda F. Effect of the non-peptide blocker (±) CP 96,345 on the cellular mechanism involved in the response to NK1 receptor stimulation in human skin fibroblasts. *Neuropeptides* 1996; 30:345–354.

74. White SR, Garland A, Gitter B *et al*. Proliferation of guinea pig tracheal epithelial cells in coculture with rat dorsal root ganglion neural cells. *Am J Physiol* 1995; 268(pt 1):L957–L965.

75. Wiedermann CJ, Auer B, Sitte B, Reinisch N, Schratzberger P, Kahler CM. Induction of endothelial cell differentiation into capillary-like structures by substance P. *Eur J Pharmacol* 1996; 298:335–338.

76. Joos GF, Germonpre PR, Pauwels RA. Role of tachykinine in asthma. *Allergy* 2000; 55:321–337.

77. Joos GF, Pauwels RA. Pro-inflammatory effects of substance P: new perspectives for the treatment of airway diseases? *Trends Pharmacol Sci* 2000; 21:131–133.

78. O'Connor TM, O'Connell J, O'Brien DI, Goode T, Bredin CP, Shanahan F. The role of substance P in inflammatory disease. *J Cell Physiol* 2004; 201:167–180.

79. Snider RM, Constantine JW, Lowe III JA *et al*. A potent nonpeptide antagonist of the substance P (NK1) receptor. *Science* 1991; 251:435–437.

80. Emonds-Alt X, Vilain P, Goulaouic P *et al*. A potent and selective non-peptide antagonist of the neurokinin A (NK2) receptor. *Life Sci* 1992; 50:L101–L106.

81. Bertrand C, Geppetti P, Graf PD, Foresi A, Nadel JA. Involvement of neurogenic inflammation in antigen-induced bronchoconstriction in guinea pigs. *Am J Physiol* 1993; 265:L507–L511.

82. Bertrand C, Geppetti P, Baker J, Yamawaki I, Nadel JA. Role of neurogenic inflammation in antigen-induced vascular extravasation in guinea pig trachea. *J Immunol* 1993; 150:1479–1485.

83. Kudlacz EM, Knippenberg RW, Logan DE, Burkholder TP. Effect of MDL 105,212, a nonpeptide NK-1/NK-2 receptor antagonist in an allergic guinea pig model. *J Pharmacol Exp Ther* 1996; 279:732–739.

84. Schuiling M, Zuidhof A, Zaagsma J, Meurs H. Involvement of tachykinin NK1 receptor in the development of allergen-induced airway hyperreactivity and airway inflammation in conscious, unrestrained guinea-pigs. *Am J Respir Crit Care Med* 1999; 159:423–430.

85. Schuiling M, Zuidhof A, Meurs H, Zaagsma J. Role of tachykinin NK2-receptor activation in the allergen-induced late asthmatic reaction, airway hyperreactivity and airway inflammation cell influx in conscious, unrestrained guinea-pigs. *Br J Pharmacol* 1999; 127:1030–1038.

86. Maghni K, Taha R, Afif W, Hamid Q, Martin JG. Dichotomy between neurokinin receptor actions in modulating allergic airway responses in an animal model of helper T cell type 2 cytokine-associated inflammation. *Am J Respir Crit Care Med* 2000; 162:1068–1074.

87. De Swert KO, Tournoy KG, Joos GF, Pauwels RA. The role of the tachykinin NK1 receptor in airway changes in a mouse model of allergic asthma. *J Allergy Clin Immunol* 2004; 113:1093–1099.

88. Nénan S, Germain N, Lagente V, Emonds-Alt X, Advenier C, Boichot E. Inhibition of inflammatory cell recruitment by the tachykinin NK3-receptor antagonist, SR 14280, in a murine model of asthma. *Eur J Pharmacol* 2001; 421:210–205.

89. Yang XX, Powell WS, Hojo M, Martin JG. Hyperpnea-induced bronchoconstriction is dependent on tachykinin-induced cysteinyl leukotriene synthesis. *J Appl Physiol* 1997; 82:538–544.

90. Yoshihara S, Geppetti P, Hara M *et al*. Cold air-induced bronchoconstriction is mediated by tachykinin and kinin release in guinea pigs. *Eur J Pharmacol* 1996; 296:291–296.

91. Wu ZX, Lee LY. Airway hyperresponsiveness induced by chronic exposure to cigarette smoke in guinea pigs: role of tachykinins. *J Appl Physiol* 1999; 87:1621–1628.

92. Pedersen KE, Meeker SN, Riccio MM, Undem BJ. Selective stimulation of jugular ganglion afferent neurons in guinea pig airways by hypertonic saline. *J Appl Physiol* 1998; 84:499–506.

93. Piedimonte G, Hoffman JI, Husseini WK, Snider RM, Desai MC, Nadel JA. NK1 receptors mediate neurogenic inflammatory increase in blood flow in rat airways. *J Appl Physiol* 1993; 74:2462–2468.

94. Piedimonte G, Rodriguez MM, King KA, McLean S, Jiang X. Respiratory syncytial virus upregulates expression of the substance P receptor in rat lungs. *Am J Physiol* 1999; 277(pt 1):L831–L840.

95. Kraneveld AD, Nijkamp FP, Van Oosterhout AJM. Role for neurokinin-2 receptor in interleukin-5-induced airway hyperresponsiveness but not eosinophilia in guinea pigs. *Am J Respir Crit Care Med* 1997; 156:367–374.

96. De Vries A, Dessing MC, Engels F, Henricks PAJ, Nijkamp FP. Nerve growth factor induces a neurokinin-1 receptor-mediated airway hyperresponsiveness in guinea pigs. *Am J Respir Crit Care Med* 1999; 159:1541–1544.

97. De Swert KO, Pauwels RA, Joos GF. Influence of the tachykinin NK1 receptor on long term smoke-induced pulmonary changes in mice. *Am J Respir Crit Care Med* 2004; 169:A273 (abstract).

98. Lundberg JM. Pharmacology of cotransmission in the autonomic nervous system: integrative aspects on amines, neuropeptides, adenosine triphosphate, amino acids and nitric oxide. *Pharmacol Rev* 1996; 48:113–178.

99. Diemunsch P, Grelot L. Potential of substance P antagonists as antiemetics. *Drugs* 2000; 60:533–546.

100. Ichinose M, Nakajima N, Takahashi T, Yamauchi H, Inoue H, Takishima T. Protection against bradykinin-induced bronchoconstriction in asthmatic patients by neurokinin receptor antagonist. *Lancet* 1992; 340:1248–1251.

101. Schmidt D, Jorres RA, Rabe KF, Magnussen H. Reproducibility of airway response to inhaled bradykinin and effect of the neurokinin receptor antagonist FK-224 in asthmatic subjects. *Eur J Clin Pharmacol* 1996; 50:269–273.

102. Joos GF, Van Schoor J, Kips JC, Pauwels RA. The effect of inhaled FK244, a tachykinin NK-1 and NK-2 receptor antagonist, on neurokinin A-induced bronchoconstriction in asthmatics. *Am J Respir Crit Care Med* 1996; 153:1781–1784.

103. Fahy JV, Wong HH, Geppetti P *et al*. Effect of an NK1 receptor antagonist (CP-99,994) on hypertonic saline-induced bronchoconstriction and cough in male asthmatic subjects. *Am J Respir Crit Care Med* 1995; 152:879–884.

104. Ichinose M, Miura M, Yamauchi H *et al*. A neurokinin 1-receptor antagonist improves exercise-induced airway narrowing in asthmatic patients. *Am J Respir Crit Care Med* 1996; 153:936–941.

105. Van Schoor J, Joos G, Chasson B, Brouard R, Pauwels R. The effect of the NK2 receptor antagonist SR48968 (saredutant) on neurokinin A-induced bronchoconstrction in asthmatics. *Eur Respir J* 1998; 12:17–23.

106. Kraan J, Vink-Klooster H, Postma DS. The NK-2 receptor antagonist SR 48968C does not improve adenosine hyperresponsiveness and airway obstruction in allergic asthma. *Clin Exp Allergy* 2001; 31:274–278.

107. Joos G, Schelfhout V, Van De Velde V, Pauwels R. The effect of the tachykinin NK2 receptor antagonist MEN11420 (nepadutant) on neurokinin A-induced bronchoconstriction in patients with asthma. *Am J Respir Crit Care Med* 2001; 163:A628.

108. Catalioto R-M, Criscuoli M, Cucchi P *et al*. MEN 11420 (Nepadutant), a novel glycosylated bicyclic peptide tachykinin NK2 receptor antagonist. *Br J Pharmacol* 1998; 123:81–91.

109. Joos GF, Vincken W, Louis RE *et al*. Dual NK1/NK2 tachykinin receptor antagonist DNK333 inhibits neurokinin A-induced bronchoconstriction in asthma patients. *Eur Respir J* 2004; 23:76–81.

110. Schelfhout V, Louis R, Lenz W, Heyrman R, Pauwels R, Joos G. The triple neurokinin-receptor antagonist CS-003 inhibits neurokinin A (NKA)-induced bronchoconstriction in patients with asthma. *Pulm Pharmacol Ther* 2005, ePub ahead of print.

111. Groneberg DA, Quarcoo D, Frossard N, Fischer A. Neurogenic mechanisms in bronchial inflammatory diseases. *Allergy* 2004; 59:1139–1152.

112. Joos GF, Pauwels RA. Tachykinin receptor antagonists: potential in airways disease. *Curr Opin Pharmacol* 2001; 1:235–241.

113. Lilly CM, Bai TR, Shore SA, Hall AE, Drazen JM. Neuropeptide content of lungs from asthmatic and nonasthmatic patients. *Am J Respir Crit Care Med* 1995; 151:548–553.

114. Boschetto P, Miotto D, Bononi I *et al*. Sputum substance P and neurokinin A are reduced during exacerbations of chronic obstructive pulmonary disease. *Pulm Pharmacol Ther* 2005; 18:199–205.

115. Rumsey WL, Aharony D, Bialecki RA *et al*. Pharmacological characterization of zd6021: a novel, orally active antagonist of the tachykinin receptors. *J Pharmacol Exp Ther* 2001; 298:307–315.

116. Anthes JC, Chapman RW, Richard C *et al*. SCH 206272: a potent, orally active tachykinin NK(1), NK(2), and NK(3) receptor antagonist. *Eur J Pharmacol* 2002; 450:191–202.

9

Rationale for vanilloid receptor 1 antagonist-based therapies in asthma

P. Geppetti, R. Nassini, M. Trevisani

INTRODUCTION

A subpopulation of primary sensory neurons, also present in the airways, is characterized for the expression of the transient receptor potential (TRP) vanilloid 1 (TRPV1) and of proinflammatory neuropeptides. TRPV1 is a cation channel sensitive to pungent xenobiotics (capsaicin and resiniferatoxin), low extracellular pH, noxious heat, a variety of lipids (anandamide, n-arachidonoyl dopamine, leukotrienes and other eicosanoids) and various irritants of diverse chemical nature. Opening of the TRPV1 channel causes the excitation of the nerve terminal, which results in both activation of protective reflex responses and the local release of neuropeptides (neurogenic inflammation). TRPV1 activity is markedly regulated by the activation of G protein-coupled (bradykinin and protease-activated receptor-2 [PAR-2] receptors) and tyrosine kinase (nerve growth factor [NGF] receptor) receptors. A variety of stimulants of, and receptors that sensitize, TRPV1 have been proposed to play a role in the mechanism of chronic respiratory diseases. Here, we discuss the physiological and pathophysiological functions of TRPV1 in the airway with a particular focus on asthma. Localization of TRPV1 in non-neuronal cells and its relevance for airway inflammation and damage is also considered. Finally, special attention is paid to the role of TRPV1 in triggering and modulating the cough response.

THE TRANSIENT RECEPTOR POTENTIAL FAMILY OF CHANNELS

The TRP proteins are widely represented in the phylogenesis and currently a large family of TRPs has been cloned in mammals, including man. Three main subclasses, namely TRPC, TRPM and TRPV (V stands for vanilloid) of TRP channels have been described [1, 2]. All TRPs have six putative transmembrane domains and they are assembled as tetramers to form cation-permeable pores. Newly proposed subtypes of TRPs are the TRPP, TRPML and TRPN [1, 2]. Finally, a novel TRP-like channel, that responds to cold temperature ($<15°C$), has been cloned and termed ANKTM1 or TRPA1 [3, 4].

The precise role(s) of TRPs has not been completely defined. For instance, intracellular localization in the endoplasmic reticulum [5] and the contribution to cellular regulation of ion flux has suggested a role as modulators of Ca^{2+} homeostasis [1, 6]. TRPs could act downstream to G protein-coupled receptors, most probably *via* the phospholipase C pathway as phosphatidylinositol-4,5-bisphosphate (PIP_2) binding and PIP_2 hydrolysis inhibits and

Pierangelo Geppetti, MD, Professor of Clinical Pharmacology, Department of Critical Care Medicine and Surgery, Florence, Italy
Romina Nassini, BSc, Assistant Pharmacologist, Department of Critical Care Medicine and Surgery, Florence, Italy
Marcello Trevisani, PhD, Assistant Pharmacologist, Department of Critical Care Medicine and Surgery, Florence, Italy

activates, respectively, TRPL in the *Drosophila* [7] and the mammalian TRPV1 [8, 9]. However, this does not seem to be a general feature of TRPs as constitutive activity of TRPM7 is increased by PIP_2 binding and reduced by PIP_2 hydrolysis [10]. TRPs have been also proposed to regulate the so-called capacitance Ca^{2+} entry or store-operated Ca^{2+} entry (SOCE). However, conclusive evidence that one or more TRPs are the exclusive and select-ive mechanism that mediate SOCE is still lacking [1].

Although there is no evidence for one or more specific and high-affinity endogenous lig-ands for TRPs, a series of lipid derivatives, including arachidonic acid metabolites, have been claimed to gate TRPs. For example, the endocannabinoid anandamide activates directly TRPV1 [11] and arachodonic acid, *via* a cytochrome P-450 (CYP-450) epoxygenase-dependent formation of epoxyeicosatrienoic acids, TRPV4 [12]. TRPs have been proposed as sensors of thermal stimuli or of other sensory modalities, including osmolarity or pressure sweet and bitter tastes. Localization of TRPs in the plasma membranes of neurons or other cells and a large body of evidence collected using a plethora of stimuli support this proposal.

THE TRANSIENT RECEPTOR POTENTIAL VANILLOID 1

It is now evident that the unique sensitivity of a subset of primary sensory neurons to cap-saicin and other vanilloid molecules is conferred by the expression of the TRPV1, a 426 (in the rat) amino acid protein [13] activated also by low extracellular pH (pH 6–5) [14–16], and µM concentrations of anandamide [11], the lipoxygenase metabolites of arachidonic acid, leukotriene B_4 or 12-hydroperoxyeicosatetraenoic acids [17] and N-arachidonoyl-dopamine [18]. Noxious temperatures between 42–53°C [13] may also activate TRPV1 which, together with TRPA1, TRPM8, TRPV3, TRPV4, TRPV1 and TRPV2, enables mammals and humans to discriminate cold, warmth and heat [1, 2, 6]. TRPV1-expressing primary sensory neurons of the trigeminal, vagal and dorsal root ganglia (DRG) with C- and A-δ fibres are polymodal nociceptors, because they detect noxious chemical, thermal and high threshold mechanical stimuli. Expression of TRPV1 mRNA has been also found in the central nervous system [19], and in non-neuronal cells including epithelial cells of the urothelium [20], keratinocytes [21], epithelial cells of the palatal rugae [22] or human peripheral lymphocytes [23]. However, with a few exceptions, there is no conclusive evidence that, at these non-neuronal sites, mRNA expression is associated with a functional channel.

Activation of TRPV1 results in excitation of peripheral terminals of primary sensory neu-rons, with an ortodromic propagated action potential that initiates reflex responses (cough, urinary bladder voiding, peristalsis in the gut, etc.). Antidromic invasion of collateral fibres by the propagated action potential and direct, TRPV1-mediated, Ca^{2+} influx contribute to the release of pro-inflammatory neuropeptides. Localization of TRPV1 at the peripheral terminal of sensory neurons is justified by its putative role as sensor of noxious agents. Less clear is the role of TRPV1 localized to the central terminals of nociceptive fibres. The recent observations that a selective TRPV1 antagonist, SB-366791, had no effect on spontaneous or evoked excita-tory post-synaptic currents (sEPSC) in normal animals, but reduced sEPSC from animals inflamed with complete Freund adjuvant (CFA) as well as miniature glutamatergic EPSCs suggest that TRPV1 may contribute to the excitatory glutammatergic transmission at spinal cord synapses [24]. Central TRPV1 channels may also be activated by lipidic endovanilloids [25].

Genetic ablation of TRPV1 in mice demonstrated that TRPV1 is not required for appro-priate temperature sensing, but it is essential for the development of thermal hyperalgesia [26]. In addition, pharmacological studies in the guinea pig [27] and more recent studies in the rat [28, 29] have shown by using first and second generation TRPV1 antagonists that TRPV1 also contributes to mechanical hyperalgesia. A very recent observation that TRPV1 knockout mice developed reduced joint inflammation and associated mechanical hypersen-sitivity in CFA-induced arthritis indicated an important role of this channel in a relevant model of inflammatory pain [30].

TRPV1 STIMULATES NEUROGENIC INFLAMMATORY RESPONSES

Stimulation of peripheral terminals of primary sensory neurons by a variety of mechanisms, including TRPV1 induces a Ca^{2+}-dependent release of calcitonin gene-related peptide (CGRP) and the tachykinins, substance P (SP) and neurokinin A (NKA). Activation of CGRP receptors and tachykinin (NK_1, NK_2 and NK_3) receptors on effector cells causes a sequence of inflammatory responses, collectively referred to as neurogenic inflammation [31]. Neurogenic inflammation encompasses a series of vascular and extravascular responses. Arteriolar vasodilatation, plasma protein extravasation and leucocyte adhesion to the vascular endothelium of post-capillary venules are main vascular neurogenic inflammatory responses [31]. In the airways, neurogenic inflammation consists also of constriction/dilatation of the bronchial smooth muscle, secretion from seromucous glands and excitation of post-ganglionic cholinergic nerve terminals in the human bronchus [32–34]. There is no final evidence that SP- and tachykinin receptor-mediated neurogenic inflammation has a major role in man. In contrast, BIBN4096BS, a peptoid with high affinity for the CGRP receptor [35], was reported to reduce the pain and other symptoms associated with migraine attacks [36]. Thus, neurogenic inflammatory vasodilatation produced by CGRP stimulation of its vascular receptors seems to be important in migraine mechanism and perhaps in other diseases. However, the function and the impact in diseases of specific neurogenic inflammation responses in the human airways has not been completely elucidated.

PLASTICITY OF TRPV1 EXPRESSION AND FUNCTION

Expression of TRPV1 mRNA/protein undergoes marked plasticity by a series of regulatory and inflammatory mediators. Survival of newborn rat DRG neurons and expression of the TRPV1-fenotype in adult rat DRG neurons depend on NGF [37]. Increase in heat hypersensitivity associated with increased TRPV1 protein transport to peripheral endings of sensory neurons also depends on NGF *via* a p38 mitogen-activated protein kinase [38]. TRPV1 function is also regulated by protein kinases (PK) A and C, through diverse pathways. Thus, a major pro-inflammatory peptide, bradykinin *via* activation of the B_2 receptor, sensitizes TRPV1 PK C-ε [39, 40], displacement of PIP_2 from TRPV1 binding [9], and 12- and 5-lipoxygenase metabolite production [41, 42]. Bradykinin evokes membrane depolarization and action potential discharge through the additive effects of TRPV1 activation in vagal afferent C-fibres [43]. Sensitization of TRPV1 by PKC and cAMP-dependent protein kinase (PKA) pathways seems to be promiscuously used by different stimuli, including capsaicin, anandamide, heat and proton [39, 44–46].

In addition to the their recognized extracellular role, trypsin and tryptase are signalling molecules because they cleave their and activate PAR-2. PAR-2 is expressed in a large variety of cells, including TRPV1-positive sensory neurons, and PAR-2 stimulation promotes neurogenic inflammation and hyperalgesia [47, 48]. PAR-2 is largely diffused in the lung and its activation is associated with inflammatory responses, including exaggeration of allergic reaction [49] bronchoconstriction, plasma protein extravasation [50]. Neurogenic mechanisms play a significant role in the effects of PAR-2 activation. Previous and more recent findings show that PAR-2 stimulation upregulates the function of TRPV1 through PKC and PKA-dependent mechanisms [51, 52]. The interesting hypothesis that PKC-and PKA mediate TRPV1 sensitization that results in a lowered threshold to tussive stimuli is currently under intense scrutiny.

LOCALIZATION AND FUNCTION AND TRPV1 IN THE AIRWAYS

Localization of TRPV1 on airway sensory nerve has been reported [53]. TRPV1 positive axons seem to represent only a small proportion of the total number of PGP9.5 staining nerves within guinea pig tracheal epithelium and only half the number of TRPV1 axons is immunopositive for SP [54]. In contrast, in intrapulmonary airways most TRPV1-positive neurones colocalized with SP/CGRP. However, there is also report by RT-PCR that TRPV1, together with acid sensing ion channel 1a (ASIC1a), and ASIC3 subunits of proton-gated ion channels, are expressed in non-neuronal cells, namely immortalized human bronchial epithelial cells, normal human bronchial/tracheal epithelial cells, and normal human small airway epithelial cells from the distal airways [55]. In these cells, TRPV1 appeared to mediate apoptosis induced by particulate matter (PM), as the response was inhibited by capsazepine and because PM exposure induced apoptosis in mouse sensory neurons, but not in those neurons pre-treated with capsazepine, or taken from TRPV1 null mice [56]. Additional findings showed that both capsaicin- and acid-sensitive irritant receptors, located on somatosensory cell bodies and their nerve fibre terminals, contribute to PM-induced airway inflammation [57].

The distribution of TRPV1 has also been studied in human airways. Immuno-histochemistry and RT-PCR analysis showed TRPV1 on epithelial cells, vascular endothelial cells, submucosal glands and nerves in the human nasal mucosa [58]. A five-fold increase in TRPV1-positive nerve profiles was found in the airway epithelium of patients with chronic cough, whereas PGP-9.5-positive nerve fibres were not increased. A significant correlation between capsaicin tussive response and the number of TRPV1-positive nerves was also found in patients with chronic cough [59]. Expression of TRPV1, colocalized with a thapsi-gargin insensitive compartment, has also been found to be increased in the airway smooth muscle of patients with chronic cough [60].

A report of non-neuronal localization of TRPV1 is somehow linked to the hypothesis that the channel, like tachykinins and CGRP, contributes to the immune response [61]. The recent report that mouse dendritic cells (DC) express TRPV1, and its activation by capsaicin or heat leads to DC maturation and draining lymph nodes [62], has been rapidly followed by a study that failed to detect the occurrence of a factional TRPV1 in mouse DC [63]. TRPV1 expression has been recently detected in many other non-neuronal human cells in the skin (human mast cells, epidermal keratinocytes) [64], liver (HepG2 cells) [65], prostate (epithelial cell lines PC-3 and LNCaP) [66], stomach (parietal cells) [67], and in human peripheral lymphocytes [23]. However, it should be underlined that conclusive evidence that non-neuronal TRPV1 in different tissues, including the airways, is functional and exerts defined biological roles is still absent.

TRPV1 AND ASTHMA

A role for TRPV1-expressing neurons and neurogenic inflammation has been proposed in a large variety of diseases, including migraine, osteoarthrtitis, cystitis and detrusor hyper-reflexia, faecal urgency and inflammatory bowel diseases, post-herpetic neuralgia and post-mastectomy pain and asthma and chronic obstructive pulmonary disease (COPD) [31, 68–71]. Both old and recent work supports a role for TRPV1 and neurogenic mechanisms in models of asthma and COPD. It has been known for a long time that early inflammatory responses following exposure to cigarette smoke are entirely mediated by sensory neu-ropeptides [72, 73]. Very recent evidence shows that the TRPV1 antagonist, capsazepine, inhibited ovalbumin-induced tracheal contractile response in sensitized animals [74]. Apart from this most relevant allergic model of asthma, additional examples in experimental animals strengthen the role of TRPV1 in asthma as follows.

Gastro-oesophageal reflux disease (GERD) is not infrequently associated with symptoms outside the gastrointestinal tract. GERD-induced asthma is now a recognized clinical condition, most likely caused either by direct reflux of acid material into the airways or by activation of reflex responses from the oesophagus that involve the airways [75]. It has also been proposed that asthma exacerbations are characterized by a fall in the pH of the exhaled air, a phenomenon that should mirror acid production in the lining fluid of the airway

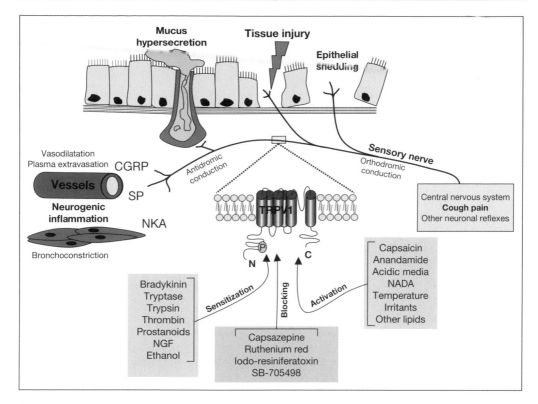

Figure 9.1 Schematic representation of putative functions exerted by neuronal TRPV1 in the airways and relevant for asthma.

epithelium [76, 77]. Neuronal and non-neuronal mechanisms may contribute to airway inflammation produced by acidic media. Whereas the non-neuronal effects of protons are poorly understood, neuronal mechanisms have attracted much attention. Extracellular pH may stimulate neurons by activating specified channels such as the ASIC1/2/3 or the TRPV1. There is evidence that the TRPV1+/ASIC3+ expressing spinal afferent neurons are between 44% (lung) and 48% (pleura) of total neurons in the rat, and half of them presumably conduct in the A-fibre range [78]. In rat vagal afferents, the response to low pH is in part mediated by an ASIC component (inhibited by amiloride), whereas a sustained component (significantly attenuated by capsazepine) is due to TRPV1 activation. All these mechanisms may contribute to the activation of neural reflex responses (including bronchoconstriction, hypersecretion an cough) and neurogenic inflammatory responses.

Several endogenous molecules seem to act through TRPV1 in the airways (Figure 9.1). H_2S is a malodorous gas with toxic effects in the lung. However, H_2S has been recognized as a signalling molecule in different cells and tissues [79]. More recently, H_2S has been found to activate sensory nerves [80]. In anaesthetized guinea pigs, intratracheal instillation of NaHS, which generates H_2S, was found to increase the lung resistance and airway plasma protein extravasation. These two effects were reduced by TRPV1 antagonism (capsazepine) and by tachykinin receptor (SR140333 and SR48968) blockade [81]. The bronchoconstrictive eicosanoid, 20-hydroxy-eicosatetraenoic acid (20-HETE), a product of CYP-450 ω-hydroxylase, causes a capsazepine-sensitive contraction of airway smooth muscle cells [82]. Thus, 20-HETE with several other eicosanoids may contribute to airway narrowing by stimulation of TRPV1 channels. Reactive oxygen species (ROS) are major contributors of tissue damage in

COPD, but they also participate in tissue injury in asthma. In rat vagal afferents, fibre responses to H_2O_2 were attenuated by capsazepine or the purinergic P_2X receptor antagonist, iso-pyridoxalphosphate-6-azophenyl-2',5'-disulphonate. These results suggest that capsaicin-sensitive vagal lung afferent fibres mediate the sensory transduction of ROS, especially H_2O_2 and $OH^\bullet$ by both the TRPV1 and P_2X receptors [83].

Ingestion of alcoholic beverages has been associated with the occurrence of asthma attacks in susceptible individuals [84]. Ethanol-induced asthma is still a poorly understood condition, where a primary role for acetaldehyde has been proposed [85]. The finding that TRPV1, usually stimulated at 42°C, is activated by lower temperatures in the presence of ethanol, is the mechanistic basis that explains the ability of ethanol to stimulate TRPV1 at the physiological temperature of 37°C [86]. By stimulating TRPV1 ethanol most likely causes the burning pain experienced after its application to wounds or mucosal surfaces. TRPV1 stimulation is also the mechanism by which ethanol contracts guinea pig bronchi *in vivo* and *in vitro* [87]. Thus, in a manner independent from the non-neuronal effects of acetaldehyde, ethanol may *per se* contribute to the symptoms of alcohol-induced asthma.

COUGH AND TRPV1

Participation of TRPV1 to the cough response is indisputable as in experimental animals and in man the channel selective agonist, capsaicin, is one of the most used tussive agents. Citric acid is another commonly used stimulus in cough challenge. Although ASICs contribute to the sensing of low extracellular pH [88], pharmacological evidence with two different TRPV1 antagonists, capsazepine [89] and iodo-resiniferatoxin (I-RTX) [90] supports the role of TRPV1 in citric acid-induced cough. The current understanding of the precise contribution of TRPV1 of C and A-δ fibres and of sensory neuropeptides to the cough response is far from complete. For instance, there is evidence that capsaicin and bradykinin substantially reduce the electrical threshold for initiating the cough reflex, and capsazepine prevents the increased cough sensitivity induced by capsaicin [91, 92]. However, it is known that C-fibre activation may also inhibit cough. Participation of SP/NKA to the cough response seems to be more relevant at the central synapses than at the periphery [92]. Despite these uncertainties, studies in man give further support to a key role for TRPV1 in chronic cough. A five-fold increase in TRPV1-positive nerve profiles was found in the airway epithelium of patients with chronic cough, whereas PGP-9.5-positive nerve fibres were not increased. A significant correlation between capsaicin tussive response and the number of TRPV1-positive nerves was also found in patients with chronic cough [59]. The lower threshold to capsaicin-induced cough in patients with asthma, cough variant asthma, and COPD supports the role of TRPV1 in the modulation of the exaggerated cough response in chronic airway inflammatory diseases [93–96]. Thus, novel therapeutic strategies in treating cough should consider selective TRPV1 antagonists.

THE THERAPEUTIC POTENTIAL OF TRPV1 ANTAGONISTS IN ASTHMA

A large series of molecules with high affinity and selectivity for the TRPV1 is currently available for pre-clinical investigation. Major focus on this research has been directed towards inflammatory and neuropathic pain and urinary bladder dysfunction. However, previous paragraphs of this chapter indicate clearly that attention should also be paid to the scrutiny of TRPV1 antagonists for the treatment of airway diseases, including asthma and COPD. We already described a variety of putative endogenous agonists of TRPV1 (endovanilloids). Anandamide [97] and N-arachidonoyl-dopamine [98] are powerful bronchoconstricors *via* TRPV1 activation. Exposure to endogenous and exogenous acids in the airways (acidopnoea) evokes cough, bronchoconstriction, airway hyper-reactivity, microvascular leakage, and heightened production of mucus. The role of acidity in the mechanism of asthma is being increasingly appreciated [75], and now the contribution of inhalation of acidic media in GERD patients and following exposure to acid fog, pollution or workplace exposure in asthma seem widely confirmed [75]. Citric acid produces a sensory nerve-mediated bronchoconstriction [99], and protons seem to play a major role as putative ligands of TRPV1 in the airways [14, 16]. The pro-inflammatory action of all these putative endovanilloids might be inhibited by TRPV1 antagonists.

As reported before, old generation TRPV1 antagonists, capsazepine and I-RTX, successfully inhibited pro-inflammatory and reflex (including cough) responses in the airways. New generation TRPV1 antagonists of diverse chemical structures have been used in the search for novel analgesics [28, 100–102]. However, one or more of these drugs could soon be investigated to prove or disprove the role of TRPV1 in models of asthma or other respiratory diseases in experimental animals and perhaps also in man. In this respect it is worth mentioning that the first study of a TRPV1 antagonist, SB705498, in man has been presented recently (Chizh B, *et al. Am Pain Soc Meeting, San Antonio, TX, May 3–6*, 2006). The findings that SB705498 reduced both capsaicin and ultraviolet irradiation-induced hyperalgesia in healthy volunteers open new avenues for clinical investigations in human diseases, including respiratory diseases.

ACKNOWLEDGMENTS

This work is supported in part by a grant from MURST, Rome, ARCA, Padua and Fondazione-DEI, Florence, Italy.

REFERENCES

1. Clapham DE. TRP channels as cellular sensors. *Nature* 2003; 426:517–524.
2. Montell C, Birnbaumer L, Flockerzi V *et al*. A unified nomenclature for the superfamily of TRP cation channels. *Mol Cell* 2002; 9:229–231.
3. Peier AM, Moqrich A, Hergarden AC *et al*. A TRP channel that senses cold stimuli and menthol. *Cell* 2002; 108:705–715.
4. McKemy DD, Neuhausser WM, Julius D. Identification of a cold receptor reveals a general role for TRP channels in thermosensation. *Nature* 2002; 416:52–58.
5. Karai LJ, Russell JT, Iadarola MJ, Olah Z. Vanilloid receptor 1 regulates multiple calcium compartments and contributes to Ca^{2+}-induced Ca^{2+} release in sensory neurons. *J Biol Chem* 2004; 279:16377–16387.
6. Montell C. New light on TRP and TRPL. *Mol Pharmacol* 1997; 52:755–763.
7. Hardie RC. Regulation of TRP channels via lipid second messengers. *Annu Rev Physiol* 2003; 65:735–759.
8. Prescott ED, Julius D. A modular PIP2 binding site as a determinant of capsaicin receptor sensitivity. *Science* 2003; 300:1284–1288.
9. Chuang HH, Prescott ED, Kong H *et al*. Bradykinin and nerve growth factor release the capsaicin receptor from PtdIns(4,5)P2-mediated inhibition. *Nature* 2001; 411:957–962.
10. Runnels LW, Yue L, Clapham DE. The TRPM7 channel is inactivated by PIP(2) hydrolysis. *Nat Cell Biol* 2002; 4:329–336.
11. Zygmunt PM, Petersson J, Andersson DA *et al*. Vanilloid receptors on sensory nerves mediate the vasodilator action of anandamide. *Nature* 1999; 400:452–457.
12. Watanabe H, Vriens J, Prenen J, Droogmans G, Voets T, Nilius B. Anandamide and arachidonic acid use epoxyeicosatrienoic acids to activate TRPV4 channels. *Nature* 2003; 424:434–438.
13. Caterina MJ, Schumacher MA, Tominaga M, Rosen TA, Levine JD, Julius D. The capsaicin receptor: a heat-activated ion channel in the pain pathway. *Nature* 1997; 389:816–824.
14. Tominaga M, Caterina MJ, Malmberg AB *et al*. The cloned capsaicin receptor integrates multiple pain-producing stimuli. *Neuron* 1998; 21:531–543.
15. Geppetti P, Del Bianco E, Patacchini R, Santicioli P, Maggi CA, Tramontana M. Low pH-induced release of calcitonin gene-related peptide from capsaicin-sensitive sensory nerves: mechanism of action and biological response. *Neuroscience* 1991; 41:295–301.

16. Bevan S, Geppetti P. Protons: small stimulants of capsaicin-sensitive sensory nerves. *Trends Neurosci* 1994; 17:509–512.

17. Hwang SW, Cho H, Kwak J *et al*. Direct activation of capsaicin receptors by products of lipoxygenases: endogenous capsaicin-like substances. *Proc Natl Acad Sci USA* 2000; 97:6155–6160.

18. Huang SM, Bisogno T, Trevisani M *et al*. An endogenous capsaicin-like substance with high potency at recombinant and native vanilloid VR1 receptors. *Proc Natl Acad Sci USA* 2002; 99:8400–8405.

19. Mezey E, Toth ZE, Cortright DN *et al*. Distribution of mRNA for vanilloid receptor subtype 1 (VR1), and VR1-like immunoreactivity, in the central nervous system of the rat and human. *Proc Natl Acad Sci USA* 2000; 97:3655–3660.

20. Birder LA, Kanai AJ, de Groat WC *et al*. Vanilloid receptor expression suggests a sensory role for urinary bladder epithelial cells. *Proc Natl Acad Sci USA* 2001; 98:13396–13401.

21. Inoue K, Koizumi S, Fuziwara S, Denda S, Denda M. Functional vanilloid receptors in cultured normal human epidermal keratinocytes. *Biochem Biophys Res Commun* 2002; 291:124–129.

22. Kido MA, Muroya H, Yamaza T, Terada Y, Tanaka T. Vanilloid receptor expression in the rat tongue and palate. *J Dent Res* 2003; 82:393–397.

23. Saunders CI, Kunde DA, Crawford A, Geraghty DP. Expression of transient receptor potential vanilloid 1 (TRPV1) and 2 (TRPV2) in human peripheral blood. *Mol Immunol* 2006; 13:13.

24. Lappin SC, Randall AD, Gunthorpe MJ, Morisset V. TRPV1 antagonist, SB-366791, inhibits glutamatergic synaptic transmission in rat spinal dorsal horn following peripheral inflammation. *Eur J Pharmacol* 2006; 540:73–81.

25. Tognetto M, Amadesi S, Harrison S *et al*. Anandamide excites central terminals of dorsal root ganglion neurons via vanilloid receptor-1 (VR-1) activation. *J Neurosci* 2000; 21:1104–1109.

26. Davis JB, Gray J, Gunthorpe MJ *et al*. Vanilloid receptor-1 is essential for inflammatory thermal hyperalgesia. *Nature* 2000; 405:183–187.

27. Walker KM, Urban L, Medhurst SJ *et al*. The VR1 antagonist capsazepine reverses mechanical hyperalgesia in models of inflammatory and neuropathic pain. *J Pharmacol Exp Ther* 2003; 304:56–62.

28. Pomonis JD, Harrison JE, Mark L, Bristol DR, Valenzano KJ, Walker K. N-(4-Tertiarybutylphenyl)-4-(3-cholorphyridin-2-yl)tetrahydropyrazine-1(2H)-carbox-amide (BCTC), a novel, orally effective vanilloid receptor 1 antagonist with analgesic properties: II. In vivo characterization in rat models of inflammatory and neuropathic pain. *J Pharmacol Exp Ther* 2003; 306:387–393.

29. Lee J, Kang M, Shin M *et al*. N-(3-acyloxy-2-benzylpropyl)-N'-[4-(methylsulfonylamino)benzyl]thiourea analogues: novel potent and high affinity antagonists and partial antagonists of the vanilloid receptor. *J Med Chem* 2003; 46:3116–3126.

30. Barton N, McQueen D, Thomson D *et al*. Attenuation of experimental arthritis in TRPV1R knockout mice. *Exp Mol Pathol* 2006; in press.

31. Geppetti P, Holzer P. *Neurogenic inflammation*. CRC Press, Boca Raton 1996.

32. Amadesi S, Moreau J, Tognetto M *et al*. NK1 receptor stimulation causes contraction and inositol phosphate increase in medium-size human isolated bronchi. *Am J Respir Crit Care Med* 2001; 163:1206–1211.

33. Myers AC, Goldie RG, Hay DW. A novel role for tachykinin neurokinin-3 receptors in regulation of human bronchial Ganglia neurons. *Am J Respir Crit Care Med* 2005; 171:212–216.

34. Geppetti P, Bertrand C, Bacci E, Huber O, Nadel JA. Characterization of tachykinin receptors in ferret trachea by peptide agonists and nonpeptide antagonists. *Am J Physiol* 1993; 265(pt 1):L164–L169.

35. Doods H, Hallermayer G, Wu D *et al*. Pharmacological profile of BIBN4096BS, the first selective small molecule CGRP antagonist. *Br J Pharmacol* 2000; 129:420–423.

36. Olesen J, Diener HC, Husstedt IW *et al*. Calcitonin gene-related peptide receptor antagonist BIBN 4096 BS for the acute treatment of migraine. *N Engl J Med* 2004; 350:1104–1110.

37. Bevan S, Winter J. Nerve growth factor (NGF) differentially regulates the chemosensitivity of adult rat cultured sensory neurons. *J Neurosci* 1995; 15(pt 1):4918–4926.

38. Ji RR, Samad TA, Jin SX, Schmoll R, Woolf CJ. p38 MAPK activation by NGF in primary sensory neurons after inflammation increases TRPV1 levels and maintains heat hyperalgesia. *Neuron* 2002; 36:57–68.

39. Premkumar LS, Ahern GP. Induction of vanilloid receptor channel activity by protein kinase C. *Nature* 2000; 408:985–990.

40. Sugiura T, Tominaga M, Katsuya H, Mizumura K. Bradykinin lowers the threshold temperature for heat activation of vanilloid receptor 1. *J Neurophysiol* 2002; 88:544–548.

41. Carr MJ, Kollarik M, Meeker SN, Undem BJ. A role for TRPV1 in bradykinin-induced excitation of vagal airway afferent nerve terminals. *J Pharmacol Exp Ther* 2003; 304:1275–1279.

42. Shin J, Cho H, Hwang SW et al. Bradykinin-12-lipoxygenase-VR1 signaling pathway for inflammatory hyperalgesia. *Proc Natl Acad Sci USA* 2002; 99:10150–10155.

43. Lee MG, Macglashan DW Jr, Undem BJ. Role of chloride channels in bradykinin-induced guinea pig airway vagal C-fibre activation. *J Physiol* 2005; 566(pt 1):205–212.

44. Vellani V, Mapplebeck S, Moriondo A, Davis JB, McNaughton PA. Protein kinase C activation potentiates gating of the vanilloid receptor VR1 by capsaicin, protons, heat and anandamide. *J Physiol* 2001; 534(pt 3):813–825.

45. De Petrocellis L, Harrison S, Bisogno T et al. The vanilloid receptor (VR1)-mediated effects of anandamide are potently enhanced by the cAMP-dependent protein kinase. *J Neurochem* 2001; 77:1660–1663.

46. Bhave G, Zhu W, Wang H, Brasier DJ, Oxford GS, Gereau RWT. cAMP-dependent protein kinase regulates desensitization of the capsaicin receptor (VR1) by direct phosphorylation. *Neuron* 2002; 35:721–731.

47. Steinhoff M, Vergnolle N, Young SH et al. Agonists of proteinase-activated receptor 2 induce inflammation by a neurogenic mechanism. *Nat Med* 2000; 6:151–158.

48. Vergnolle N, Bunnett NW, Sharkey KA et al. Proteinase-activated receptor-2 and hyperalgesia: a novel pain pathway. *Nat Med* 2001; 7:821–826.

49. Schmidlin F, Amadesi S, Dabbagh K et al. Protease-activated receptor 2 mediates eosinophil infiltration and hyperreactivity in allergic inflammation of the airway. *J Immunol* 2002; 169:5315–5321.

50. Su X, Camerer E, Hamilton JR, Coughlin SR, Matthay MA. Protease-activated receptor-2 activation induces acute lung inflammation by neuropeptide-dependent mechanisms. *J Immunol* 2005; 175:2598–2605.

51. Amadesi S, Nie J, Vergnolle N et al. Protease-activated receptor 2 sensitizes the capsaicin receptor transient receptor potential vanilloid receptor 1 to induce hyperalgesia. *J Neurosci* 2004; 24:4300–4312.

52. Amadesi S, Cottrell GS, Divino L et al. Protease-activated receptor 2 sensitizes TRPV1 by protein kinase c{epsilon}- and a-dependent mechanisms in rats and mice. *J Physiol* 2006; 22:22.

53. Watanabe N, Horie S, Michael GJ, Spina D, Page CP, Priestley JV. Immunohistochemical localization of vanilloid receptor subtype 1 (TRPV1) in the guinea pig respiratory system. *Pulm Pharmacol Ther* 2005; 18:187–197.

54. Watanabe N, Horie S, Michael GJ et al. Immunohistochemical co-localization of transient receptor potential vanilloid (TRPV)1 and sensory neuropeptides in the guinea-pig respiratory system. *Neuroscience* 2006; 8:8.

55. Agopyan N, Bhatti T, Yu S, Simon SA. Vanilloid receptor activation by 2- and 10-microm particles induces responses leading to apoptosis in human airway epithelial cells. *Toxicol Appl Pharmacol* 2003; 192:21–35.

56. Agopyan N, Head J, Yu S, Simon SA. TRPV1 receptors mediate particulate matter-induced apoptosis. *Am J Physiol Lung Cell Mol Physiol* 2004; 286:L563–L572.

57. Veronesi B, Oortgiesen M, Roy J, Carter JD, Simon SA, Gavett SH. Vanilloid (capsaicin) receptors influence inflammatory sensitivity in response to particulate matter. *Toxicol Appl Pharmacol* 2000; 169:66–76.

58. Seki N, Shirasaki H, Kikuchi M, Sakamoto T, Watanabe N, Himi T. Expression and localization of TRPV1 in human nasal mucosa. *Rhinology* 2006; 44:128–134.

59. Groneberg DA, Niimi A, Dinh QT et al. Increased expression of transient receptor potential vanilloid-1 in airway nerves of chronic cough. *Am J Respir Crit Care Med* 2004; 170:1276–1280.

60. Mitchell JE, Campbell AP, New NE et al. Expression and characterization of the intracellular vanilloid receptor (TRPV1) in bronchi from patients with chronic cough. *Exp Lung Res* 2005; 31:295–306.

61. van Hagen PM, Hofland LJ, ten Bokum AM et al. Neuropeptides and their receptors in the immune system. *Ann Med* 1999; 2:15–22.

62. Basu S, Srivastava P. Immunological role of neuronal receptor vanilloid receptor 1 expressed on dendritic cells. *Proc Natl Acad Sci USA* 2005; 102:5120–5125.

63. O'Connell PJ, Pingle SC, Ahern GP. Dendritic cells do not transduce inflammatory stimuli via the capsaicin receptor TRPV1. *FEBS Lett* 2005; 2:2.

64. Stander S, Moormann C, Schumacher M et al. Expression of vanilloid receptor subtype 1 in cutaneous sensory nerve fibers, mast cells, and epithelial cells of appendage structures. *Exp Dermatol* 2004; 13:129–139.

65. Vriens J, Janssens A, Prenen J, Nilius B, Wondergem R. TRPV channels and modulation by hepatocyte growth factor/scatter factor in human hepatoblastoma (HepG2) cells. *Cell Calcium* 2004; 36:19–28.

66. Sanchez MG, Sanchez AM, Collado B *et al*. Expression of the transient receptor potential vanilloid 1 (TRPV1) in LNCaP and PC-3 prostate cancer cells and in human prostate tissue. *Eur J Pharmacol* 2005; 515:20–27.

67. Faussone-Pellegrini MS, Taddei A, Bizzoco E, Lazzeri M, Vannucchi MG, Bechi P. Distribution of the vanilloid (capsaicin) receptor type 1 in the human stomach. *Histochem Cell Biol* 2005; 124:61–68.

68. Geppetti P, Trevisani M. Activation and sensitization of the vanilloid receptor: role in gastrointestinal inflammation and function. *Br J Pharmacol* 2004; 141:1313–1320.

69. Joos GF, Pauwels RA. Tachykinin receptor antagonists: potential in airways diseases. *Curr Opin Pharmacol* 2001; 1:235–241.

70. Barnes PJ. Asthma as an axon reflex. *Lancet* 1986; 1:242–245.

71. Bertrand C, Geppetti P. Tachykinin and kinin receptor antagonists: therapeutic perspectives in allergic disease. *Trends Pharmacol Sci* 1996; 17:255–259.

72. Baluk P, Bertrand C, Geppetti P, McDonald DM, Nadel JA. NK1 receptor antagonist CP-99,994 inhibits cigarette smoke-induced neutrophil and eosinophil adhesion in rat tracheal venules. *Exp Lung Res* 1996; 22:409–418.

73. Lundberg J, Saria A. Capsaicin induced desensitization of the airway mucosa to cigarette smoke, mechanical and chemical irritants. *Nature* 1983; 302:251–253.

74. van den Worm E, de Vries A, Nijkamp FP, Engels F. Capsazepine, a vanilloid receptor antagonist, inhibits allergen-induced tracheal contraction. *Eur J Pharmacol* 2005; 518:77–78.

75. Harding SM. Recent clinical investigations examining the association of asthma and gastroesophageal reflux. *Am J Med* 2003; 18:39S–44S.

76. Hunt JF, Fang K, Malik R *et al*. Endogenous airway acidification. Implications for asthma pathophysiology. *Am J Respir Crit Care Med* 2000; 161(pt 1):694–699.

77. Ricciardolo FL, Gaston B, Hunt J. Acid stress in the pathology of asthma. *J Allergy Clin Immunol* 2004; 113:610–619.

78. Groth M, Helbig T, Grau V, Kummer W, Haberberger RV. Spinal afferent neurons projecting to the rat lung and pleura express acid sensitive channels. *Respir Res* 2006; 7:96.

79. Li L, Bhatia M, Zhu YZ *et al*. Hydrogen sulfide is a novel mediator of lipopolysaccharide-induced inflammation in the mouse. *FASEB J* 2005; 19:1196–1198.

80. Patacchini R, Santicioli P, Giuliani S, Maggi CA. Hydrogen sulfide (H2S) stimulates capsaicin-sensitive primary afferent neurons in the rat urinary bladder. *Br J Pharmacol* 2004; 142:31–34.

81. Trevisani M, Patacchini R, Nicoletti P *et al*. Hydrogen sulfide causes vanilloid receptor 1-mediated neurogenic inflammation in the airways. *Br J Pharmacol* 2005; 6:6.

82. Rousseau E, Cloutier M, Morin C, Proteau S. Capsazepine, a vanilloid antagonist, abolishes tonic responses induced by 20-HETE on guinea pig airway smooth muscle. *Am J Physiol Lung Cell Mol Physiol* 2005; 288:L460–L470.

83. Ruan T, Lin YS, Lin KS, Kou YR. Sensory transduction of pulmonary reactive oxygen species by capsaicin-sensitive vagal lung afferent fibres in rats. *J Physiol* 2005; 565(pt 2):563–578.

84. Myou S, Fujimura M, Nishi K *et al*. Effect of ethanol on airway caliber and nonspecific bronchial responsiveness in patients with alcohol-induced asthma. *Allergy* 1996; 51:52–55.

85. Vally H, Thompson PJ. Allergic and asthmatic reactions to alcoholic drinks. *Addict Biol* 2003; 8:3–11.

86. Trevisani M, Smart D, Gunthorpe MJ *et al*. Ethanol elicits and potentiates nociceptor responses via the vanilloid receptor-1. *Nat Neurosci* 2002; 5:546–551.

87. Trevisani M, Gazzieri D, Benvenuti F *et al*. Ethanol causes inflammation in the airways by a neurogenic and TRPV1-dependent mechanism. *J Pharmacol Exp Ther* 2004; 309:1167–1173.

88. Kollarik M, Undem BJ. Mechanisms of acid-induced activation of airway afferent nerve fibres in guinea-pig. *J Physiol* 2002; 543(pt 2):591–600.

89. Lalloo UG, Fox AJ, Belvisi MG, Chung KF, Barnes PJ. Capsazepine inhibits cough induced by capsaicin and citric acid but not by hypertonic saline in guinea pigs. *J Appl Physiol* 1995; 79:1082–1087.

90. Trevisani M, Milan A, Gatti R *et al*. Antitussive activity of iodo-resiniferatoxin in guinea pigs. *Thorax* 2004; 59:769–772.

91. Undem BJ, Carr MJ, Kollarik M. Physiology and plasticity of putative cough fibres in the Guinea pig. *Pulm Pharmacol Ther* 2002; 15:193–198.

92. Mazzone SB, Mori N, Canning BJ. Synergistic interactions between airway afferent nerve subtypes regulating the cough reflex in guinea pigs. *J Physiol* 2005; 4:4.

93. Millqvist E. Cough provocation with capsaicin is an objective way to test sensory hyperreactivity in patients with asthma-like symptoms. *Allergy* 2000; 55:546–550.

94. Doherty MJ, Mister R, Pearson MG, Calverley PM. Capsaicin responsiveness and cough in asthma and chronic obstructive pulmonary disease. *Thorax* 2000; 55:643–649.
95. Fujimura M, Kamio Y, Hashimoto T, Matsuda T. Cough receptor sensitivity and bronchial responsiveness in patients with only chronic nonproductive cough: in view of effect of bronchodilator therapy. *J Asthma* 1994; 31:463–472.
96. Wong CH, Morice AH. Cough threshold in patients with chronic obstructive pulmonary disease. *Thorax* 1999; 54:62–64.
97. Tucker RC, Kagaya M, Page CP, Spina D. The endogenous cannabinoid agonist, anandamide stimulates sensory nerves in guinea-pig airways. *Br J Pharmacol* 2001; 132:1127–1135.
98. Harrison S, De Petrocellis L, Trevisani M *et al*. Capsaicin-like effects of N-arachidonoyl-dopamine in the isolated guinea pig bronchi and urinary bladder. *Eur J Pharmacol* 2003; 475:107–114.
99. Ricciardolo FL, Rado V, Fabbri LM, Sterk PJ, Di Maria GU, Geppetti P. Bronchoconstriction induced by citric acid inhalation in guinea pigs: role of tachykinins, bradykinin, and nitric oxide. *Am J Respir Crit Care Med* 1999; 159:557–562.
100. Honore P, Wismer CT, Mikusa J *et al*. A-425619 [1-isoquinolin-5-yl-3-(4-trifluoromethyl-benzyl)-urea], a novel transient receptor potential type V1 receptor antagonist, relieves pathophysiological pain associated with inflammation and tissue injury in rats. *J Pharmacol Exp Ther* 2005; 314:410–421.
101. Gavva NR, Tamir R, Qu Y *et al*. AMG 9810 [(E)-3-(4-t-butylphenyl)-N-(2,3-dihydrobenzo[b][1,4] dioxin-6-yl)acrylamide], a novel vanilloid receptor 1 (TRPV1) antagonist with antihyperalgesic properties. *J Pharmacol Exp Ther* 2005; 313:474–484.
102. Culshaw AJ, Bevan S, Christiansen M *et al*. Identification and biological characterization of 6-aryl-7-isopropylquinazolinones as novel TRPV1 antagonists that are effective in models of chronic pain. *J Med Chem* 2006; 49:471–474.

Section IV

Receptors in immunology

10

Anticytokines and cytokines as asthma therapy

K. F. Chung

INTRODUCTION

Asthma is a complex disorder of the airways that has increased in severity and prevalence over the last 30 years in many industrialized countries, and poses a significant burden to health. Effective treatments, including anti-inflammatories such as inhaled corticosteroids and bronchodilators such as β-adrenergic agonists, are available to control the disease. Many patients are reluctant to use inhaled corticosteroids regularly, due to the risks of side-effects. In addition, despite their use, there is continuing significant morbidity and mortality from asthma [1], and a sizeable proportion of asthmatics, particularly at the more severe end, remains uncontrolled from currently-available drugs [2]. There is therefore a need for better therapies, particularly those targeted towards the inflammatory process [3].

Because cytokines are important in the genesis of chronic inflammation, they are potentially therapeutic targets. Cytokines are extracellular signalling proteins usually of <80 kDa in size produced by different cell types and having an effect on closely adjacent cells. The effects of cytokines are mediated by binding to cell surface high-affinity receptors usually present in low numbers, but which may be upregulated with cell activation, thereby changing the responsiveness of both source and target cells. Cytokines are involved in multiple aspects of the inflammatory process of asthma [4], and therefore may be considered to work in a network, with overlapping properties. In asthma, there has already been some experience of the therapeutic effects of targeting specific cytokines, which will be summarized in this chapter.

T CELL-DERIVED CYTOKINES

Lymphokines, which are soluble factors generated by activated lymphocytes (particularly CD4+ T cells) in response to specific or polyclonal antigens were the first class of cytokines described. Subclasses of T helper (Th) cells can be identified on the basis of their expression of cytokines [5]. Allergens are taken up and processed by specialized cells, such as dendritic cells (antigen-presenting cells [APCs]), followed by presentation of peptide fragments to naïve T cells. The activation of naïve T cells occurs *via* the CD4+ T cell receptor through the APC-bound antigen to major histocompatibility complex (MHC)-II and then *via* the co-stimulatory pathway linked by the B7 family and T cell-bound CD28 [6]. CD28 itself has two major ligands, B7.1, which inhibits Th2 cell activation and development, and B7.2, which induces T cell activation and Th2 cell proliferation.

Kian Fan Chung, MD, DSc, FRCP, Professor of Respiratory Medicine and Honorary Consultant Physician, Section of Experimental Medicine, National Heart and Lung Institute, Imperial College, London, UK

Naïve Th0 cells produce mainly interleukin (IL)-2, but may also contribute cytokines of the Th1 and Th2 repertoire. Th1 cells produce interferon (IFN)γ and tumor necrosis factor (TNF)β, but not IL-4 or IL-5, while Th2 cells produce IL-4, IL-5, IL-9 and IL-25, but not IFNγ or transforming growth factor (TGF)β [7]. In addition to Th1 and Th2 cells, CD4+ T cells can produce immunosuppressive cytokines, TGFβ and IL-10 *in vitro* and are designated regulatory CD4+ T cells (Tr) mediating T cell-mediated natural self-tolerance [8]. These cells are naturally derived from the thymus and can also be locally induced, such as during immunotherapy or peptide-induced tolerance.

Lung T cells express and release high levels of Th2 type cytokines. Increased proportions of T cells in bronchial biopsies and in bronchoalveolar lavage (BAL) cells from atopic asthmatics express mRNA for IL-3, IL-4, IL-5, IL-13 and granulocyte-macrophage colony-stimulating factor (GM-CSF), the Th2 gene cluster, when compared with those of non-atopic control individuals [9–11]. However, these cytokines are not only restricted to T cells, as mast cells and eosinophils also express the cytokines IL-4 and IL-5 [12–14]. Alveolar macrophages from patients with asthma release more pro-inflammatory cytokines, specifically IL-1β, TNFα, GM-CSF and macrophage inflammatory protein (MIP)-1α [15, 16]. IFNγ expression in asthmatic tissues has been reported, but its expression and release are impaired [17].

MACROPHAGE-DERIVED CYTOKINES

Airway macrophages may be an important source of cytokines, such as IL-1, TNFα and IL-6, which may be released on exposure to inhaled allergens *via* FcεRI receptors. Indeed, this could also occur through the stimulation of the innate immune system using pattern recognition receptors to release TNF, IL-1, IL-6, IL-8, IL-12, IL-15, IL-18 and IL-23 [18]. These receptors could modulate Th2 responses to allergens [19]. The cytokines might then act on epithelial cells to cause release of another wave of cytokines, including GM-CSF, eotaxin and RANTES (regulated on activation normal T cell expressed and secreted), which then leads to influx of secondary cells, such as eosinophils, which themselves may release multiple cytokines. In addition, other cytokines IL-12, IL-18 and IL-23 can maintain Th1 cell differentiation, while IL-12 and IL-18 are particularly potent inducers of IFNγ [20].

THE IgE RESPONSE

IL-4 and IL-13 mediate immunoglobulin (Ig)E synthesis *via* isotype switching by B cells [21]. IL-4 also activates B cells through increasing the expression of class II MHC molecules and enhancing the expression of CD23, the low-affinity IgE (FcεRII) receptor. CD40 antigen is expressed on B cells after antigen recognition. IL-4 together with the engagement of CD40 antigen with its ligand, CD40-L on activated T cells, promotes IgE class switching and B cell growth. As IL-4 has surface CD40-L and can also be produced by basophils, mast cells and eosinophils, these cells may contribute to the amplification of IgE responses.

IgE produced in asthmatic airways binds to FcεRI receptors ('high-affinity' IgE receptors) on mast cells and basophils, priming them for activation by antigen. Cross-linking of FcεRI receptors causes upregulation of their own expression and leads to mast cell degranulation with the release of mediators such as histamine and cysteinyl-leukotrienes [22]. The low-affinity IgE receptor, FcεRII or CD23, is present on B cells, macrophages and eosinophils; it may serve principally as a negative regulator of IgE synthesis.

MAST CELLS

The maturation and expansion of mast cells from bone marrow cells involve growth factors and cytokines such as stem cell factor (SCF) or c-kit ligand and IL-3. Increased numbers of mast cells are present within airway smooth muscle bundles, implying direct interaction between these cells to induce bronchoconstriction [23]. Mast cells in mucosal biopsies from atopic asthmatics are positive for IL-3, IL-4, IL-5, IL-6 and TNFα by immunohistochemistry [12]. IL-4 also increases the expression of an inducible form of FcεRII on B lymphocytes and macrophages [24]. IL-4 drives the differentiation of CD4+ T cell precursors into Th2-like cells.

EOSINOPHIL-ASSOCIATED CYTOKINES

The differentiation, migration and pathobiological effects of eosinophils may occur through the actions of GM-CSF, IL-3, IL-5 and certain chemokines such as eotaxin [25, 26]. IL-5 influences the production, maturation and activation of eosinophils, acting predominantly at the later stages of eosinophil maturation and activation, and can prolong the survival of eosinophils. IL-5 causes the release of eosinophils from the bone marrow, while the local release of an eosinophil chemoattractant such as eotaxin may be necessary for the tissue localization of eosinophils [27]. Mature eosinophils may demonstrate increased survival in bronchial tissue, secondary to the effects of GM-CSF, IL-3 and IL-5 [28]. Eosinophils themselves may also generate other cytokines, such as IL-3, IL-5 and GM-CSF [14]. Cytokines such as IL-4 may also exert an important regulatory effect on the expression of adhesion molecules such as vascular cell adhesion molecule-1 on endothelial cells of bronchial blood vessels and on airway epithelial cells. IL-1 and TNFα increase the expression of intracellular adhesion molecule-1 in vascular endothelium and airway epithelium [29].

Eotaxin is a chemoattractant cytokine (chemokine) selective for eosinophils and acts through the chemokine receptor CCR3 present on eosinophils, basophils and T cells. Increased expression of eotaxin and CCR3 has been demonstrated in asthmatic airways [30, 31]. Cooperation between IL-5 and eotaxin appears necessary for the mobilization of eosinophils from the bone marrow during allergic reactions and for the local release of chemokines to induce homing and migration into tissues [27, 32]. When administered to mild asthmatic individuals, human recombinant IL-5 induces an increase in blood mature and immature eosinophils without lung eosinophilia or bronchial hyperresponsiveness, but increased CCR3 expression on mature eosinophils [33, 34]. Inhaled eotaxin had no effect on lung eosinophilia, but paradoxically caused lung neutrophilia [35].

ANTI-INFLAMMATORY CYTOKINES

TGFβ is constitutively produced in the healthy lung and may reduce allergic inflammation by inhibiting IgE synthesis and mast cell proliferation. IL-10 produced by Tr cells, B cells and monocytes inhibits IFNγ and IL-2 release by Th1 cells, IL-4 and IL-5 by Th2 cells, and IL-1β, IL-6, IL-8, IL-12 and TNFα by monocytes/macrophages. In addition, IL-10 inhibits eosinophil survival and IL-4-induced IgE synthesis, however, it stimulates B cell proliferation and is a cofactor for the growth of cytotoxic T cells. Other members of the IL-10 family include IL-19, IL-20, IL-22 and IL-24, but these do not inhibit cytokine release by mononuclear cells [36]. These anti-inflammatory cytokines may be selectively enhanced during specific immunotherapy and during innate immune stimulation such as with CpG DNA [37, 38].

AIRWAY WALL REMODELLING CYTOKINES

Overexpression of various Th2-associated cytokines in the airway epithelium of mice mimics features of asthma and airway wall remodelling. Overexpression of IL-13 causes eosinophilic and mononuclear inflammation with goblet cell hyperplasia, subepithelial fibrosis, airway obstruction and airway hyperresponsiveness [39]. IL-4, IL-5 and IL-9 overexpression lead to substantial mucus metaplasia, while IL-9 and IL-5 overexpression caused subepithelial fibrosis and airways hyperresponsiveness [40–42]. Proliferation of myofibroblasts and the hyperplasia of airway smooth muscle may also occur through the action of growth factors, such as platelet-derived growth factor (PDGF) and TGFβ, released by macrophages and eosinophils, airway epithelium, endothelial cells and fibroblasts [43]. These growth factors may stimulate fibrogenesis by recruiting and activating fibroblasts or transforming myofibroblasts. Epithelial cells may release growth factors, as collagen deposition occurs underneath the basement membrane of the airway epithelium [44]. Growth factors such as PDGF and epidermal growth factor (EGF) may also stimulate the proliferation and growth of airway smooth muscle cells. Airway smooth muscle cells have the capacity to elaborate a range of cytokines, including IL-4, IL-5, GM-CSF, IL-8, eotaxin and MCP-1, and therefore, may play a role in the induction of local inflammatory responses [45].

SPECIFIC CYTOKINE-BASED THERAPIES FOR ASTHMA

Although there is a wide pleiotropy and element of redundancy in the cytokine family, in that each cytokine has many overlapping functions, with each function potentially mediated by more than one cytokine, therapies based on single specific cytokines continue to be considered for the treatment of asthma. Blocking antibodies, soluble receptors or receptor antagonists have been used to block the effects of a particular cytokine. In cases of anti-inflammatory cytokines, the cytokine itself may be used. The results of such approaches would need to be compared to other therapies, such as corticosteroids, which have more general inhibitory effects on many cytokines and which can also promote certain anti-inflammatory cytokines. More recent general inhibitory approaches include the inhibition of specific signal transduction pathways that are either involved in the generation of many types of cytokines or in the downstream action of many cytokines, such as signalling through kinases.

INHIBITION OF IL-5 USING ANTI-IL-5 ANTIBODY

Two humanized anti-human IL-5 monoclonal antibodies, Sch-55700 and mepolizumab (SB-240563), have been developed and studies have been conducted in patients with asthma (Table 10.1). The effect of mepolizumab was examined against allergen challenge in a double-blind, randomized, placebo-controlled trial, in which a single intravenous infusion of SB-240563 was given at doses of 2.5 mg/kg ($n = 8$) or 10.0 mg/kg ($n = 8$) [46]. Following one single dose of mepolizumab, there was an immediate fall in circulating eosinophil counts, which was maximal at the dose of 10 mg/kg, an effect that persisted for up to 3 months (Figure 10.1). After inhaled allergen challenge, 9 days after treatment with mepolizumab, the percentage sputum eosinophils were 12.2% in the placebo group and lowered to 0.9% (-1.2 to 3.0; $P = 0.0076$) in the 10 mg/kg group; this effect persisted at day 30 after the dose. There was no significant effect of monoclonal antibody to IL-5 on the late asthmatic response or on airway hyperresponsiveness to histamine (Figure 10.2).

In a study of twenty-four patients with mild asthma receiving three intravenous doses of either 750 mg of mepolizumab or placebo in a randomized, double-blind, parallel-group fashion over 20 weeks, fiberoptic bronchoscopy was performed in order to sample airway tissue. A persistent suppression of blood eosinophils and a greater than 90% reduction in bronchoalveolar lavage eosinophilia was observed after mepolizumab, but it was less efficient at decreasing mucosal eosinophils in the airways (by only 55%) [47]. There were no effects on bronchial hyperresponsiveness or forced expiratory volume in 1s (FEV_1), although the groups studied were small. In another study, mepolizumab has been shown to decrease mature eosinophil numbers in the bone marrow by 70% in comparison with placebo and decrease numbers of eosinophil myelocytes and metamyelocytes by 37% and 44%, respectively [48]. However, mepolizumab had no effect on numbers of blood or bone marrow CD34+, CD34 /IL-5Rα+ cells, or eosinophil/basophil colony-forming units. There was a significant decrease in bronchial mucosal CD34+ /IL-5Rα+ mRNA-positive cell numbers in the

Table 10.1 Published studies of anticytokine therapies in asthma

Cytokine	Cytokine blocking	Compound	Study	Effect	Reference
IL-4	rhuIL-4R	Nuvance	Inhaled steroid withdrawal in mild–moderate asthma	Maintain asthma while inhaled steroids are reduced	[51, 52]
IL-5	Humanized monoclonal antibody	SB-240563 (Mepolizumab)	Allergen challenge late-phase response	No effect on late-phase response	[46]
	Humanized monoclonal antibody	SB-240563	Treatment of mild asthma	Reduction in extracellular matrix deposition	[50]
	Humanized monoclonal antibody	Sch-55700	Treatment of severe persistent asthma	Trend for an improvement in FEV_1	[49]
TNFα	Soluble TNF receptor	Etanercept	Steroid-dependent asthma	Improvement in FEV_1 and PC_{20}	[74]
		Etanercept	Severe refractory asthma	Improvement in quality of life, post-bronchodilator FEV_1 and PC_{20}	[75]

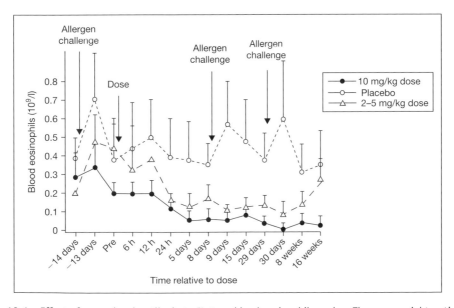

Figure 10.1 Effect of monoclonal antibody to IL-5 on blood eosinophil number. There were eight patients per group up to day 30, after which sample sizes were smaller. Raw data is expressed as arithmetic mean with 95% CI. Reproduced by permission from reference [46].

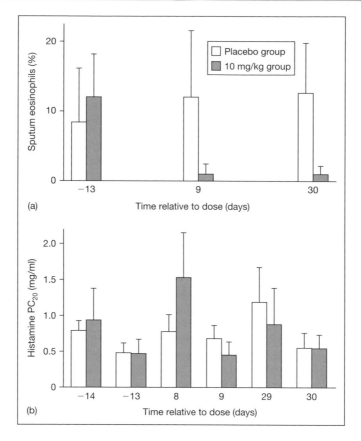

Figure 10.2 Effect of monoclonal antibody to IL-5 on sputum eosinophils and histamine PC_{20}. (a) Mean percentage of total leukocytes. (b) Histamine PC_{20} was done before inhaled allergen challenge on day -14, 8 and 29 and repeated 24 days later. Raw data are expressed as arithmetic mean with 95% CI for sputum eosinophils and geometric mean with geometric SE for histamine PC_{20}. Reproduced by permission from reference [46].

anti-IL-5 treated group. These studies indicated that at the doses of mepolizumab used, there was only partial depletion of eosinophils in the airway tissues and of eosinophil progenitors in the bone marrow and in the airway tissues. This raised the possibility that the dose administered was not sufficient, or else IL-5 may not be the only cytokine important in eosinophil recruitment or in eosinophil maturation. Cooperation between IL-5 and eotaxin in these aspects has been previously demonstrated in murine models, and therefore the possibility that a combined approach to blocking the effects of IL-5 and eotaxin simultaneously may be important.

The lack of clinical response observed in the initial studies with mepolizumab were reflected also in clinical studies with anti-IL5 antibody. In a phase II, double-blind, placebo-controlled study of 378 moderately severe symptomatic patients, mepolizumab (250 or 750 mg iv) was administered monthly for 3 months [C Compton, unpublished data]. There was a significant reduction in blood eosinophil counts and sputum eosinophil counts at the 750 mg dose; however, no significant changes in FEV_1 were observed but there was a trend towards a reduction in exacerbations in the mepolizumab-treated group. Perhaps a study to look specifically at exacerbations in a more severe group of asthmatic patients with evidence of eosinophilia should be performed.

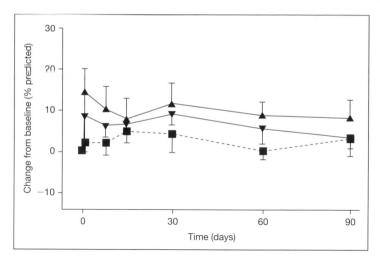

Figure 10.3 Change in baseline FEV$_1$, expressed as a percentage ($\pm$SEM) of the predicted value, after intravenous administration of placebo ($n = 8$) (■), or a single dose of anti-IL-5 antibody, Sch-55700 at 0.3 mg/kg ($n = 6$) (▲) or 1 mg/kg ($n = 12$) (▼). $P = 0.019$, placebo vs. Sch-55700 (0.3 mg/kg) at 24 h (analysis of variance). Reproduced by permission from reference [49].

In a group of patients with severe persistent asthma on oral or high doses of inhaled corticosteroids, the humanized anti-IL5 antibody, Sch-55700, administered as a single dose (0.03, 0.1, 0.3 or 1.0 mg/kg subcutaneously) dose-dependently reduced blood eosinophil counts. A trend towards improvement in baseline FEV$_1$ was noted and reached significance 24 h after the 0.3 mg/kg dose, but no changes in other parameters of asthma activity were achieved [49]. A phase II study in symptomatic asthma with Sch-55700 has been completed, but the data have not been presented and development of this compound has been discontinued (Figure 10.3).

Finally, one study with mepozulimab indicated that this compound may have beneficial effects in reversing some of the features of airway wall remodelling [50]. In this randomized, double-blind, placebo-controlled study, bronchial biopsies were obtained before and after three infusions of mepolizumab in 24 atopic asthmatics. The anti-IL-5 antibody specifically decreased airway eosinophil numbers, and significantly reduced the expression of tenascin, lumican and procollagen III in the bronchial mucosal reticular basement membrane when compared with placebo. Anti-IL-5 treatment was associated with a significant reduction in the numbers and percentage of airway eosinophils expressing mRNA for TGFβ1 and the concentration of TGFβ1 in BAL fluid. This study indicated that eosinophils may be important effectors of extracellular matrix deposition, perhaps through the production of TGFβ.

In these studies in asthma patients with either Sch-55700 or mepolizumab, no serious adverse events were observed, in particular the potential problems of antibody generation or anaphylaxis.

INHIBITION OF IL-4 USING SOLUBLE IL-4 RECEPTOR

IL-4 and IL-13 share the α chain of the IL-4 receptor (IL-4Rα). The IL-4R is a cell surface heterodimeric complex consisting of a specific, high-affinity chain and a second chain that could be either the common γ chain or the α chain of the IL-13 receptor. IL-4 binds to IL-4Rα alone, but both chains are necessary for cellular activation. On engagement of the ligand with IL4Rα, signal transducer and activator of transcription 6 (STAT6) translocates to the nucleus and germline ε mRNA transcription is initiated together with ε class switching of immunoglobulin genes. Secreted forms of IL-4Rα occur naturally, and soluble IL-4R can bind to IL-4, without leading to cellular activation. Therefore, soluble IL-4R can bind and sequester IL-4, and therefore acts as an antagonist for IL-4. Soluble recombinant human IL-4 receptor (Nuvance) is the extracellular portion of human IL-4Rα and is non-immunogenic.

In the first study of Nuvance, mild or moderate asthmatics were withdrawn from inhaled corticosteroid therapy and received either placebo or rhuIL-4R (0.5 or 1.5 mg by nebulizer) [51]. No adverse events were observed and no patients developed any antibodies. The serum half-life was approximately 5 days. Following discontinuation of inhaled steroids, two out of eight patients in the placebo group and three out of eight in the rhuIL-4R 0.5 mg group had exacerbations, while none of the patients in the rhuIL-4R 1.5 mg group experienced exacerbations. The latter group also demonstrated an improvement in FEV_1 at 2 h, and on days 2, 4 and 15 after treatment, with improved symptom scores and reduction in β_2-agonist use. Improvement was also reflected in the improved scores on the asthma quality of life questionnaire in the rhuIL-4R 1.5 mg group, while these scores worsened in the placebo-treated group. An anti-inflammatory effect was supported by the reduction in exhaled nitric oxide levels in the patients receiving rhuIL-4R.

In the second phase I/II double-blind, placebo-controlled study, 62 moderate persistent asthmatics were randomized to receive 12 weekly nebulizations of 0.75, 1.5 or 3.0 mg of rhuIL-4R or placebo [52]; inhaled steroids were discontinued. A significant decline in FEV_1 and an increase in symptom score was observed in the placebo group, but this was not seen in the 3.0 mg treatment group. Although these results were promising, further development of Nuvance as a therapy for asthma was suspended. It is likely that the clinical response observed was not deemed to have been of sufficient impact compared with the clinical benefits obtained from inhaled corticosteroids.

INHIBITION OF IL-13

The extensive properties of IL-13 in regulating IgE production, eosinophilic inflammation, airway smooth muscle hyperplasia and induction of goblet cell hyperplasia with mucus production make it an interesting mediator in asthma [53], and it is currently a target for the treatment of asthma. Acute administration of IL-13 into naïve mice reproduces many of the features of asthma such as airway hyperresponsiveness (AHR), eosinophilic inflammation and mucus cell hyperplasia [54, 55]. Targeted overexpression of IL-13 in murine lung also reproduces these features, in addition to subepithelial fibrosis and the presence of Charcot-Leyden particles [39]. Specific blockade of IL-13 was achieved in the mouse by using a soluble form of the IL-13Rα2 chain which binds only to IL-13 but not to IL-4, and this led to reversal of airway hyperresponsiveness and mucus production in the allergen-exposed sensitized mouse [54]. IL-13 can facilitate the recruitment of eosinophils, monocytes/macrophages and T cells into the airway spaces through the induction of vascular cell adhesion molecule 1 [56], and can also cause the upregulation of many chemokines such as MCP-1, MCP-3, eotaxin, and MIP-1α [57]. IL-13 can also induce and activate TGFβ, thus contributing to subepithelial fibrosis [58]. IL-13 may induce proliferation of airway smooth muscle cells indirectly *via* LTD4 receptors [59] and can directly induce increased intracellular calcium fluxes in isolated smooth muscle strips induced by histamine, bradykinin and acetylcholine, and increased contractile responses to carbachol [60].

IL-13 binds to a low-affinity binding chain, IL-13Rα1, and a high-affinity complex made up of IL-13Rα1 and IL-4R. Binding to the latter complex leads to phosphorylation dependent activation of JAK1 and JAK2 and STAT 6 proteins. IL-13 and not IL-4 binds also to another receptor IL-13Rα2, which may function top and inhibits the activity of IL-13, therefore not contributing to IL-13 signalling. A soluble form of IL-13Rα2 that binds IL-13 at a 100-fold greater affinity than IL-13Rα1 has been observed in murine serum. Antagonizing IL-13 may be achieved by administering soluble IL-13 receptors (as for IL-4 targeting), anti-IL-13 monoclonal antibodies and anti-receptor antibodies. sIL-13R has an extended half-life and high-affinity binding to IL-13 using a fully humanized peptide, and may be administered by inhalation to patients, but there has been no reports of any clinical trial yet.

INHIBITION OF EOTAXIN

The importance of eotaxin in allergic eosinophilic inflammation has been underlined in murine models through the studies of CCR3 knockout mice [61, 62]. Eotaxin selectively mediates its effects through the CCR3 receptor and allergen-sensitized CCR3 knockout mice were protected against allergen challenge-induced AHR. This was accompanied by a reduction in CCR3 positive cells in the lungs, usually eosinophils and epithelial mast cells. Therefore, one of the therapeutic ways of blocking the effects of eotaxin has been to block the CCR3 receptor, which is a member of the G protein-coupled receptor super-family. Both peptide-derived and small molecule CCR3 antagonists have been developed [63]. Many potent small molecule CCR3 receptor antagonists have been described, and a novel way of measuring the activity of these antagonists in whole blood using white blood cell shape change and chemokine receptor internalization will help to assess the activity of these molecules *in vivo* [64]. Although some of these compounds are known to have entered clinical trials, there are no results that have been published yet [65, 66].

INHIBITION OF IgE USING HUMANIZED MONOCLONAL ANTI-IgE ANTIBODY

Omalizumab is a humanized murine anti-IgE antibody that binds to the FcεRI binding site of human IgE, such that IgE can no longer bind to cells such as basophils and mast cells. Free serum IgE levels fall to very low levels and a reduction in high-affinity IgE receptors is observed on basophils. Omalizumab can be considered as an anti-inflammatory agent for asthma, as it caused inhibition of sputum eosinophils and submucosal eosnophils and T cells in patients with mild asthma [67]. Omalizumab reduced the early- and late-phase bronchoconstrictor response to allergen, together with a reduction in the percentage of induced sputum eosinophils, and in the number of circulating eosinophils. In two studies of 1071 moderate-to-severe patients, omalizumab was added to standard inhaled steroid therapy and then the steroid was gradually reduced over a 12-week period [68, 69]. The percentage of patients having at least one exacerbation of asthma was nearly twice as high in the placebo group as in the omalizumab group. In an analysis of patients at high risk of serious asthma-related morbidity and mortality, treatment with omalizumab halved the rate of asthma exacerbations and improved disease control in this particularly severe group [70]. In a study of 419 patients, inadequately controlled despite treatment with high doses of inhaled corticosteroids and long-acting β-agonists with reduced lung function, treatment with omalizumab reduced exacerbation rates by 26%, together with an improvement in quality of life, morning peak expiratory flows and asthma symptom scores [71].

Omalizumab is now available for treating patients with severe asthma particularly those experiencing frequent exacerbations of asthma despite being on high-dose inhaled corticosteroids and on long-acting β-agonists. The costs of this treatment are high and issues about cost-effectiveness have yet to be resolved.

INHIBITION OF TNFα

Inhibition of TNFα in rheumatoid arthritis either by using monoclonal antibodies, anti-TNFα or recombinant soluble TNF receptors has been successful in modifying the activity of the disease. There are good indications that TNFα may be involved in asthma [72], and particularly so in patients with severe asthma. First, TNFα stored in granules of mast cells can be released through IgE-mediated mechanisms [12]. Other cell types that may release

TNFα in asthma include epithelial cells, eosinophils, macrophages and neutrophils. T cells from asthmatic airways also express and release TNFα. An excess expression of TNFα mRNA in asthmatic airways has been demonstrated [73], and following allergen challenge TNFα levels in BAL fluid of asthmatic subjects is increased. In severe asthma, TNFα levels in bronchoalveolar lavage fluid were increased compared to mild asthmatics, together with an increase in TNFα positive cells in the airway submucosa [74]. Patients with refractory asthma have been shown to have an increased expression of membrane-bound TNFα, TNFα receptor 1, and TNF α-converting enzyme by peripheral-blood monocytes [75].

TNFα has been implicated in facilitating the migration of eosinophils and neutrophils since it can upregulate the expression of adhesion molecules and can induce the release of chemotactic factors such as chemokines from a variety of cells including airway epithelium, macrophages, vascular endothelium and muscle cells. In addition, TNFα can modulate the levels of various proteolytic enzymes such as MMP-9, and extracellular matrix proteins such as tenascin and collagen; TNFα may also induce the proliferation and activation of subepithelial myofibroblasts and fibroblasts. These properties place TNFα in the thick of airway wall remodelling. TNFα can also induce goblet cell hyperplasia in the mouse through the expression of gob-5 and MUC-5AC [76], in addition to its direct mucus secretagogue role. TNFα has direct effects on airway smooth muscle cells such as enhancing calcium signalling pathways leading to hypercontractility [77]. TNFα increases maximal isotonic contraction to methacholine in guinea pig tracheal preparations [78]. In an allergen exposure model, a TNF receptor fusion protein that blocked the effects of TNFα prevented allergen-induced bronchial hyperresponsiveness (BHR) in sensitized guinea pigs [79]. Direct administration of TNFα induces BHR in sensitized rats [80]. Similarly, healthy volunteers or asthmatics develop BHR when inhaling rh-TNFα [81].

Therapeutic blockade of TNFα has been successful in the treatment of severe refractory rheumatoid arthritis, and there are several clinically-available TNFα blockers. These are infliximab, a chimeric mouse/human monoclonal anti-TNFα antibody, etanercept, a soluble fusion protein made of two p65 TNF receptors with an Fc fragment of human IgG1, and adalimumab, a human monoclonal anti-TNFα antibody. These have been safe in patients with rheumatoid arthritis, and the major side-effects have been tuberculosis reactivation, demyelination, and possibly increased risk of lymphoma.

In an open uncontrolled study, 17 patients with corticosteroid-dependent asthma were treated with etanercept 25 mg twice daily for 12 weeks. At the end of 12 weeks, there was a significant improvement in symptom scores, a 12% improvement in FEV_1 and bronchial responsiveness improved by 2.5 doubling doses [74]. In a clinical trial of 10 patients with refractory asthma, 10 patients with mild-to-moderate asthma, and 10 control subjects, treatment with a soluble TNF receptor, etanercept, for 10 weeks was associated with a significant increase in the concentration of methacholine required to provoke a 20% decrease in the FEV_1 (PC_{20}; mean difference in doubling concentration changes between etanercept and placebo 3.5; 95% confidence interval [CI] 0.07–7.0; $P = 0.05$), an improvement in the asthma-related quality-of-life score (by 0.85-point; 95% CI 0.16–1.54 on a 7-point scale; $P = 0.02$), and a 0.32 l increase in post-bronchodilator FEV_1 (95% CI 0.08–0.55; $P = 0.01$) [75]. Larger studies of etanercept in severe asthma are now being performed.

IL-12 INJECTIONS

In a small study, IL-12 subcutaneous injections in patients with mild asthma inhibited circulating blood eosinophils following allergen challenge but not sputum eosinophilia, but with no effect on late phase response or bronchial hyperresponsiveness [82]. The most notable feature of this study was the incidence of side-effects with flu-like symptoms, abnormal liver function tests and cardiac arrhythmias. This study illustrates the limitations of using anti-inflammatory cytokines as a form of therapy in asthma. Such therapies will require systemic administration as aerosol administration may not allow for sufficient tissue penetration with tight epithelial airway and alveolar barriers to large molecules. In addition, systemic administration is associated with significant systemic side-effects, as each specific cytokine usually possesses a plethora of effects.

IL-10 INJECTIONS

Administration of IL-10 to normal volunteers induced a fall in circulating CD2, CD3, CD4 and CD8 lymphocytes with a suppression of mitogen-induced T cell proliferation and reduction of TNFα and IL-1β production from whole blood stimulated with endotoxin *ex vivo* [83]. There have been no reports of IL-10 administration in asthma, although IL-10 therapy has been studied in rheumatoid arthritis, inflammatory bowel disease and psoriasis [84].

IFNγ ADMINISTRATION

IFNγ, a Th1 cytokine, may inhibit Th2-mediated allergic inflammation [85], but studies of administration of IFNγ to asthmatics have been disappointing [86, 87]. Daily subcutaneous injections of $0.05 \, mg/M^2$ of r-IFNγ in nine patients with steroid-dependent asthma for 90 days did not lead to any changes in the maintenance dose of prednisone or in lung function. There was a greater fall in blood eosinophil count after IFNγ compared to the effect of placebo in a parallel group of patients, but this did not achieve statistical significance [87]. In a later study, incremental doses of nebulized r-IFNγ was administered in five mild atopic asthmatics. No changes in symptoms or lung function or bronchial responsiveness were noted. In four of the five patients there was a fall in eosinophil count measured in bronchoalveolar lavage fluid, but overall statistical significance was not achieved [86].

SUMMARY

Targeting individual cytokines in asthma may represent a valid approach to develop new therapies in asthma, despite the redundancy and pleiotropic nature of the cytokine network. Asthma is a heterogeneous disease in its clinical presentation, and there is increasing evidence that this is also reflected in the mucosal inflammation. There may be subgroups of asthmatics that could particularly benefit from these specific therapies and these subgroups may need to be identified. At present, the greatest unmet need is that of patients with severe asthma who are relatively less responsive to existing therapies, and these patients are likely to be the recipients of many of the novel therapies based on inhibition of specific cytokines or administration of anti-asthmatic cytokines. Recent studies of the therapeutic inhibition of cytokines using recombinant antibodies or receptors have been encouraging from the safety aspect, and these treatments may conceivably equal inhaled steroids in efficacy; however, the main issue is which cytokine target or combination of cytokine targets this will be. Of the Th2 cytokine targets, much more work is needed, and we are awaiting studies of IL-13 inhibitors with great interest since targeting IL-4 and IL-5 has now been virtually abandoned. Although not classified as a cytokine target, IgE inhibition with an anti-IgE monoclonal antibody has now been successfully launched for the treatment of severe asthma. Single cytokine targeting of TNFα in rheumatoid arthritis, a disease with similarities to asthma, has been successful. These successes indicate that there will be cytokine targets for human asthma that may well work, but one needs to keep in mind that there may be subcategories of patients that may respond particularly well. The issue may not be identifying the target, but with greater difficulty, the suitable patient that will respond to these very specific therapies. These can only be discovered from doing focused clinical trials in asthma patients.

REFERENCES

1. Rabe KF, Vermeire PA, Soriano JB, Maier WC. Clinical management of asthma in 1999: the Asthma Insights and Reality in Europe (AIRE) study. *Eur Respir J* 2000; 16:802–807.
2. Chung KF, Godard P, Adelroth E *et al*. Difficult/therapy-resistant asthma: the need for an integrated approach to define clinical phenotypes, evaluate risk factors, understand pathophysiology and find novel therapies. ERS Task Force on Difficult/Therapy-Resistant Asthma. European Respiratory Society [In Process Citation]. *Eur Respir J* 1999; 13:1198–1208.
3. Chung KF. Individual cytokines contributing to asthma pathophysiology: valid targets for asthma therapy? *Curr Opin Investig Drugs* 2003; 4:1320–1326.
4. Chung KF, Barnes PJ. Cytokines in asthma. *Thorax* 1999; 54:825–857.
5. Mossman TR, Coffman RL. TH1 and TH2 cells: different patterns of lymphokine secretion lead to different functional properties. *Ann Rev Immunol* 1989; 7:145–173.
6. Green JM. The B7/CD28/CTLA4 T cell activation pathway. Implications for inflammatory lung disease. *Am J Respir Cell Mol Biol* 2000; 22:261–264.
7. Umetsu DT, DeKruyff RH. TH1 and TH2 CD4+ cells in human allergic diseases. *J Allergy Clin Immunol* 1997; 100:1–6.
8. Akdis M, Blaser K, Akdis CA. T regulatory cells in allergy: novel concepts in the pathogenesis, prevention, and treatment of allergic diseases. *J Allergy Clin Immunol* 2005; 116:961–968.
9. Hamid Q, Azzawi M, Ying S *et al*. Expression of mRNA for interleukins in mucosal bronchial biopsies from asthma. *J Clin Invest* 1991; 87:1541–1546.
10. Broide DH, Lotz M, Cuomo AJ. Cytokines in symptomatic asthma. *J Allergy Clin Immunol* 1992; 89:958–967.
11. Humbert M, Durham SR, Kimmitt P *et al*. Elevated expression of messenger ribonucleic acid encoding IL-13 in the bronchial mucosa of atopic and nonatopic subjects with asthma. *J Allergy Clin Immunol* 1997; 99:657–665.
12. Bradding P, Roberts JA, Britten KM, Montefort S, Djukanovic R, Mueller R *et al*. Interleukin-4, -5 and -6 and tumor necrosis factor-α in normal and asthmatic airways: evidence for the human mast cell as a source of these cytokines. *Am J Respir Cell Mol Biol* 1994; 10:471–480.
13. Broide D, Paine MM, Firestein GS. Eosinophils express interleukin S and granulocyte-macrophage colony-stimulating factor mRNA at sites of allergic inflammation in asthmatics. *J Clin Invest* 1992; 90:1414–1424.
14. Moqbel R, Hamid Q, Ying S *et al*. Expression of mRNA and immunoreactivity for the granulocyte/macrophage colony-stimulating factor (GM-CSF) in activated human eosinophils. *J Exp Med* 1991; 174:749–752.
15. John M, Lim S, Seybold J *et al*. Inhaled corticosteroids increase interleukin-10 but reduce macrophage inflammatory protein-1a, granulocyte-macrophage colony-stimulating factor and interferon-y release from alveolar macrophages in asthma. *Am J Respir Crit Care Med* 1998; 157:256–262.
16. Hallsworth MP, Soh CPC, Lane SJ, Arm JP, Lee TH. Selective enhancement of GM-CSF, TNF-α, IL-1β and IL-8 production by monocytes and macrophages of asthmatic subjects. *Eur Respir J* 1994; 7:1096–1102.
17. Smart JM, Horak E, Kemp AS, Robertson CF, Tang ML. Polyclonal and allergen-induced cytokine responses in adults with asthma: resolution of asthma is associated with normalization of IFN-gamma responses. *J Allergy Clin Immunol* 2002; 110:450–456.
18. Barton GM, Medzhitov R. Toll-like receptors and their ligands. *Curr Top Microbiol Immunol* 2002; 270:81–92.
19. Eisenbarth SC, Piggott DA, Huleatt JW, Visintin I, Herrick CA, Bottomly K. Lipopolysaccharide-enhanced, toll-like receptor 4-dependent T helper cell type 2 responses to inhaled antigen. *J Exp Med* 2002; 196:1645–1651.
20. Langrish CL, McKenzie BS, Wilson NJ, de Waal MR, Kastelein RA, Cua DJ. IL-12 and IL-23: master regulators of innate and adaptive immunity. *Immunol Rev* 2004; 202:96–105.
21. Minty A, Chalon P, Derocq J-M *et al*. Interleukin-13 is a new human lymphokine regulating inflammatory and immune responses. *Nature* 1993; 362:248–250.
22. Gould HJ, Sutton BJ, Beavil AJ *et al*. The biology of IgE and the basis of allergic disease. *Annu Rev Immunol* 2003; 21:579–628.
23. Brightling CE, Bradding P, Symon FA, Holgate ST, Wardlaw AJ, Pavord ID. Mast-cell infiltration of airway smooth muscle in asthma. *N Engl J Med* 2002; 346:1699–1705.

24. Vercelli D, Jabara HH, Lee BW, Woodland N, Geha RS, Leung DY. Human recombinant interleukin-4 induces FC4RII/CD23 on normal human monocytes. *J Exp Med* 1988; 167:1406–1416.

25. Jose PJ, Griffiths-Johnson DA, Collins PD *et al.* Eotaxin: a potent eosinophil chemoattractant cytokine detected in a guinea pig model of allergic airways inflammation. *J Exp Med* 1994; 179:881–887.

26. Sanderson CJ, Warren DJ, Strath M. Identification of a lymphokine that stimulates eosinophil differentiation in vitro. Its relationship to interleukin 3, and functional properties of eosinophils produced in cultures. *J Exp Med* 1985; 162:60–74.

27. Collins PD, Griffiths-Johnson DA, Jose PJ, Williams TJ, Marleau S. Co-operation between interleukin-5 and the chemokine, eotaxin, to induce eosinophil accumulation in vivo. *J Exp Med* 1995; 182: 1169–1174.

28. Rothenberg ME, Owen WFJ, Siberstein DS. Human eosinophils have prolonged survival, enhanced functional properties and become hypodense when exposed to human interleukin. *J Clin Invest* 1988; 81:1986–1992.

29. Tosi MF, Stark JM, Smith WC, Hamedani A, Gruenert DC, Infeld MD. Induction of ICAM-1 expression on human airway epithelial cells by inflammatory cytokines: effects on neutrophil-epithelial cell adhesion. *Am J Respir Cell Mol Biol* 1992; 7:214–221.

30. Ying S, Robinson DS, Meng Q *et al.* Enhanced expression of eotaxin and CCR3 mRNA and protein in atopic asthma. Association with airway hyperresponsiveness and predominant co-localization of eotaxin mRNA to bronchial epithelial and endothelial cells. *Eur J Immunol* 1997; 27:3507–3516.

31. Ying S, Meng Q, Zeibecoglou K *et al.* Eosinophil chemotactic chemokines (eotaxin, eotaxin-2, RANTES, monocyte chemoattractant protein-3 (MCP-3), and MCP-4), and C-C chemokine receptor 3 expression in bronchial biopsies from atopic and nonatopic (Intrinsic) asthmatics. *J Immunol* 1999; 163:6321–6329.

32. Hisada T, Hellewell PG, Teixeira MM *et al.* Alpha4 integrin-dependent eotaxin induction of bronchial hyperresponsiveness and eosinophil migration in interleukin-5 transgenic mice. *Am J Respir Cell Mol Biol* 1999; 20:992–1000.

33. Stirling RJ, van Rensen ELJ, Barnes PJ, Chung KF. Interleukin-5 induces CD34+ eosinophil progenitor mobilization and eosinophil CCR3 expression in asthma. *Am J Respir Crit Care Med* 2001; 164:1403–1409.

34. van Rensen EL, Stirling RG, Scheerens J *et al.* Evidence for systemic rather than pulmonary effects of interleukin-5 administration in asthma. *Thorax* 2001; 56:935–940.

35. Bumbacea D, Scheerens J, Mann BS, Stirling RG, Chung KF. Failure of sputum eosinophilia after eotaxin inhalation in asthma. *Thorax* 2004; 59:372–375.

36. Conti P, Kempuraj D, Frydas S *et al.* IL-10 subfamily members: IL-19, IL-20, IL-22, IL-24 and IL-26. *Immunol Lett* 2003; 88:171–174.

37. Jutel M, Akdis M, Budak F *et al.* IL-10 and TGF-beta cooperate in the regulatory T cell response to mucosal allergens in normal immunity and specific immunotherapy. *Eur J Immunol* 2003; 33:1205–1214.

38. Yi AK, Yoon JG, Yeo SJ, Hong SC, English BK, Krieg AM. Role of mitogen-activated protein kinases in CpG DNA-mediated IL-10 and IL-12 production: central role of extracellular signal-regulated kinase in the negative feedback loop of the CpG DNA-mediated Th1 response. *J Immunol* 2002; 168:4711–4720.

39. Zhu Z, Homer RJ, Wang Z *et al.* Pulmonary expression of interleukin-13 causes inflammation, mucus hypersecretion, subepithelial fibrosis, physiologic abnormalities, and eotaxin production. *J Clin Invest* 1999; 103:779–788.

40. Rankin JA, Picarella DE, Geba GP *et al.* Phenotypic and physiologic characterization of transgenic mice expressing interleukin 4 in the lung: lymphocytic and eosinophilic inflammation without airway hyperreactivity. *Proc Natl Acad Sci USA* 1996; 93:7821–7825.

41. Temann UA, Geba GP, Rankin JA, Flavell RA. Expression of interleukin 9 in the lungs of transgenic mice causes airway inflammation, mast cell hyperplasia, and bronchial hyperresponsiveness. *J Exp Med* 1998; 188:1307–1320.

42. Lee NA, McGarry MP, Larson KA, Horton MA, Kristensen AB, Lee JJ. Expression of IL-5 in thymocytes/T cells leads to the development of a massive eosinophilia, extramedullary eosinophilopoiesis, and unique histopathologies. *J Immunol* 1997; 158:1332–1344.

43. Davies DE, Wicks J, Powell RM, Puddicombe SM, Holgate ST. Airway remodelling in asthma: new insights. *J Allergy Clin Immunol* 2003; 111:215–225.

44. Brewster CEP, Howarth PH, Djukanovic R, Wilson J, Holgate ST, Roche WR. Myofibroblasts and subepithelial fibrosis in bronchial 'asthma'. *Am J Resp Cell Mol Biol* 1990; 3:507–511.

45. Chung KF. Airway smooth muscle cells: contributing to and regulating airway mucosal inflammation? *Eur Respir J* 2000; 15:961–968.

46. Leckie MJ, ten Brinke A, Khan J *et al.* Effects of an interleukin-5 blocking monoclonal antibody on eosinophils, airway hyper-responsiveness, and the late asthmatic response. *Lancet* 2000; 356:2144–2148.

47. Flood-Page PT, Menzies-Gow AN, Kay AB, Robinson DS. Eosinophil's role remains uncertain as anti-interleukin-5 only partially depletes numbers in asthmatic airway. *Am J Respir Crit Care Med* 2003; 167:199–204.

48. Menzies-Gow A, Flood-Page P, Sehmi R *et al.* Anti-IL-5 (mepolizumab) therapy induces bone marrow eosinophil maturational arrest and decreases eosinophil progenitors in the bronchial mucosa of atopic asthmatics. *J Allergy Clin Immunol* 2003; 111:714–719.

49. Kips JC, O'Connor BJ, Langley SJ *et al.* Effect of SCH55700, a humanized anti-human interleukin-5 antibody, in severe persistent asthma: a pilot study. *Am J Respir Crit Care Med* 2003; 167:1655–1659.

50. Flood-Page P, Menzies-Gow A, Phipps S, Ying S *et al.* Anti-IL-5 treatment reduces deposition of ECM proteins in the bronchial subepithelial basement membrane of mild atopic asthmatics. *J Clin Invest* 2003; 112:1029–1036.

51. Borish LC, Nelson HS, Lanz MJ *et al.* Interleukin-4 receptor in moderate atopic asthma. A phase I/II randomized, placebo-controlled trial. *Am J Respir Crit Care Med* 1999; 160:1816–1823.

52. Borish LC, Nelson HS, Corren J *et al.* Efficacy of soluble IL-4 receptor for the treatment of adults with asthma. *J Allergy Clin Immunol* 2001; 107:963–970.

53. Wills-Karp M. Interleukin-13 in asthma pathogenesis. *Immunol Rev* 2004; 202:175–190.

54. Wills-Karp M, Luyimbazi J, Xu X *et al.* Interleukin-13: central mediator of allergic asthma [In Process Citation]. *Science* 1998; 282:2258–2261.

55. Grunig G, Warnock M, Wakil AE *et al.* Requirement for IL-13 independently of IL-4 in experimental asthma [In Process Citation]. *Science* 1998; 282:2261–2263.

56. Bochner BS, Klunk DA, Sterbinsky SA, Coffman RL, Schleimer RP. IL-13 selectively induces vascular cell adhesion molecule-1 expression in human endothelial cells. *J Immunol* 1995; 154:799–803.

57. Zhu Z, Ma B, Zheng T *et al.* IL-13-induced chemokine responses in the lung: role of CCR2 in the pathogenesis of IL-13-induced inflammation and remodelling. *J Immunol* 2002; 168:2953–2962.

58. Lee CG, Homer RJ, Zhu Z *et al.* Interleukin-13 induces tissue fibrosis by selectively stimulating and activating transforming growth factor beta(1). *J Exp Med* 2001; 194:809–821.

59. Espinosa K, Bosse Y, Stankova J, Rola-Pleszczynski M. CysLT1 receptor upregulation by TGF-beta and IL-13 is associated with bronchial smooth muscle cell proliferation in response to LTD4. *J Allergy Clin Immunol* 2003; 111:1032–1040.

60. Tliba O, Deshpande D, Chen H *et al.* IL-13 enhances agonist-evoked calcium signals and contractile responses in airway smooth muscle. *Br J Pharmacol* 2003; 140:1159–1162.

61. Humbles AA, Lu B, Friend DS *et al.* The murine CCR3 receptor regulates both the role of eosinophils and mast cells in allergen-induced airway inflammation and hyperresponsiveness. *Proc Natl Acad Sci USA* 2002; 99:1479–1484.

62. Ma W, Bryce PJ, Humbles AA *et al.* CCR3 is essential for skin eosinophilia and airway hyperresponsiveness in a murine model of allergic skin inflammation. *J Clin Invest* 2002; 109:621–628.

63. Elsner J, Escher SE, Forssmann U. Chemokine receptor antagonists: a novel therapeutic approach in allergic diseases. *Allergy* 2004; 59:1243–1258.

64. Bryan SA, Jose PJ, Topping JR *et al.* Responses of leukocytes to chemokines in whole blood and their antagonism by novel CC-chemokine receptor 3 antagonists. *Am J Respir Crit Care Med* 2002; 165:1602–1609.

65. Wacker DA, Santella JB III, Gardner DS *et al.* CCR3 antagonists: a potential new therapy for the treatment of asthma. Discovery and structure-activity relationships. *Bioorg Med Chem Lett* 2002; 12:1785–1789.

66. De Lucca GV, Kim UT, Vargo BJ *et al.* Discovery of CC chemokine receptor-3 (CCR3) antagonists with picomolar potency. *J Med Chem* 2005; 48:2194–2211.

67. Djukanovic R, Wilson SJ, Kraft M *et al.* Effects of treatment with anti-immunoglobulin E antibody omalizumab on airway inflammation in allergic asthma. *Am J Respir Crit Care Med* 2004; 170:583–593.

68. Soler M, Matz J, Townley R, Buhl R *et al.* The anti-IgE antibody omalizumab reduces exacerbations and steroid requirement in allergic asthmatics. *Eur Respir J* 2001; 18:254–261.

69. Busse W, Corren J, Lanier BQ *et al.* Omalizumab, anti-IgE recombinant humanized monoclonal antibody, for the treatment of severe allergic asthma. *J Allergy Clin Immunol* 2001; 108:184–190.

70. Holgate S, Bousquet J, Wenzel S, Fox H, Liu J, Castellsague J. Efficacy of omalizumab, an anti-immunoglobulin E antibody, in patients with allergic asthma at high risk of serious asthma-related morbidity and mortality. *Curr Med Res Opin* 2001; 17:239–240.

71. Humbert M, Beasley R, Ayres J *et al.* Benefits of omalizumab as add-on therapy in patients with severe persistent asthma who are inadequately controlled despite best available therapy (GINA 2002 step 4 treatment): INNOVATE. *Allergy* 2005; 60:309–316.

72. Russo C, Polosa R. TNF-alpha as a promising therapeutic target in chronic asthma: a lesson from rheumatoid arthritis. *Clin Sci (Lond)* 2005; 109.135–142.

73. Ying S, Robinson DS, Varney V *et al.* TNF-α mRNA expression in allergic inflammation. *Clin Exp Allergy* 1991; 21:745–750.

74. Howarth PH, Babu KS, Arshad HS *et al.* Tumour necrosis factor (TNF alpha) as a novel therapeutic target in symptomatic corticosteroid dependent asthma. *Thorax* 2005; 60:1012–1018.

75. Berry MA, Hargadon B, Shelley M *et al.* Evidence of a role of tumor necrosis factor alpha in refractory asthma. *N Engl J Med* 2006; 354:697–708.

76. Busse PJ, Zhang TF, Srivastava K *et al.* Chronic exposure to TNF-alpha increases airway mucus gene expression in vivo. *J Allergy Clin Immunol* 2005; 116:1256–1263.

77. Amrani Y, Krymskaya V, Maki C, Panettieri RA Jr. Mechanisms underlying TNF-alpha effects on agonist-mediated calcium homeostasis in human airway smooth muscle cells. *Am J Physiol* 1997; 273:L1020–L1028.

78. Pennings HJ, Kramer K, Bast A, Buurman WA, Wouters EF. Tumour necrosis factor-alpha induces hyperreactivity in tracheal smooth muscle of the guinea-pig in vitro. *Eur Respir J* 1998; 12:45–49.

79. Renzetti LM, Paciorek PM, Tannu SA *et al.* Pharmacological evidence for tumor necrosis factor as a mediator of allergic inflammation in the airways. *J Pharmacol Exp Ther* 1996; 278:847–853.

80. Kips JC, Tavernier J, Pauwels RA. Tumor necrosis factor causes bronchial hyperresponsiveness in rats. *Am Rev Respir Dis* 1992; 145:332–336.

81. Thomas PS, Yates DH, Barnes PJ. Tumor necrosis factor-alpha increases airway responsiveness and sputum neutrophilia in normal human subjects. *Am J Respir Crit Care Med* 1995; 152:76–80.

82. Bryan SA, O'Connor BJ, Matti S *et al.* Effects of recombinant human interleukin-12 on eosinophils, airway hyper-responsiveness, and the late asthmatic response. *Lancet* 2000; 356:2149–2153.

83. Chernoff AE, Granowitz EV, Shapiro L *et al.* A randomized, controlled trial of IL-10 in humans. Inhibition of inflammatory cytokine production and immune responses. *J Immunol* 1995; 154:5492–5499.

84. Asadullah K, Sterry W, Volk HD. Interleukin-10 therapy – review of a new approach. *Pharmacol Rev* 2003; 55:241–269.

85. Huang TJ, Macary PA, Eynott P *et al.* Allergen-specific Th1 cells counteract efferent Th2 cell-dependent bronchial hyperresponsiveness and eosinophilic inflammation partly via IFN-gamma. *J Immunol* 2001; 166:207–217.

86. Boguniewicz M, Martin RJ, Martin D *et al.* The effects of nebulized recombinant interferon-gamma in asthmatic airways. *J Allergy Clin Immunol* 1995; 95:133–135.

87. Boguniewicz M, Schneider LC, Milgrom HN *et al.* Treatment of steroid-dependent asthma with recombinant interferon-gamma. *J Allergy Clin Immunol* 1992; 89:288.

11

Tumour necrosis factor alpha and asthma

M. A. Berry, I. D. Pavord

INTRODUCTION

A link between exposure to infectious organisms and necrosis of tumours has been established since the late 19th century [1] and the presence of a serum factor responsible for this observation was postulated following experiments in the 1960s in which serum from mice inoculated with bacterial lipopolysaccharide was demonstrated to have the ability to damage cultured sarcoma cell lines [2]. In the 1970s the convergence of investigations into septic shock syndrome, cachexia and tumour necrosis led to the characterization of a protein named cachectin/tumour necrosis factor (TNF) which later was determined to be two highly homologous proteins which were named TNFα, produced by macrophages and monocytes and TNFβ or lymphotoxin which is produced by lymphocytes [3]. There followed an intense period of investigation into the biological actions of TNF and, although a role as a chemotherapeutic agent in cancer medicine has been prevented by side-effects, much of great biological importance has been learnt about this pleiotropic, pro-inflammatory cytokine which plays a key role in the innate immune response and diseases associated with dysregulated innate immunity.

INNATE IMMUNITY

Innate immunity provides immediate host defence against invading organisms prior to activation of the adaptive immune system [4]. A key element of the innate immune system is the activation of membrane-bound pattern recognition molecules, which detect common bacterial cell surface products such as polysaccharide, carbohydrates and lipopolysaccharides, which leads to increased cellular production of pro-inflammatory cytokines including IL-1, -6 and -12 and TNFα, primarily by macrophages. These cytokines orchestrate an immediate immune response and are involved in activation of the adaptive immune response.

BIOLOGY OF TNFα

TNFα is initially produced as a 26 kDa membrane-anchored precursor protein [5] which is subsequently cleaved, principally by TNFα converting enzyme (TACE) [6], to release the 17 kDa free protein [7]. These proteins form into biologically active homotrimers [8], which act on the ubiquitously expressed TNFα receptors 1 and 2 (p55 and p75 or TNFRi and

Mike A. Berry, MRCP, Research Fellow, Institute for Lung Health, Department of Respiratory Medicine, Thoracic Surgery and Allergy, University Hospitals of Leicester NHS Trust, Glenfield Hospital, Leicester, UK

Ian D. Pavord, DM, FRCP, Consultant Physician and Honorary Professor of Medicine, Institute for Lung Health, Department of Respiratory Medicine, Thoracic Surgery and Alllergy, University Hospitals of Leicester NHS Trust, Glenfield Hospital, Leicester, UK

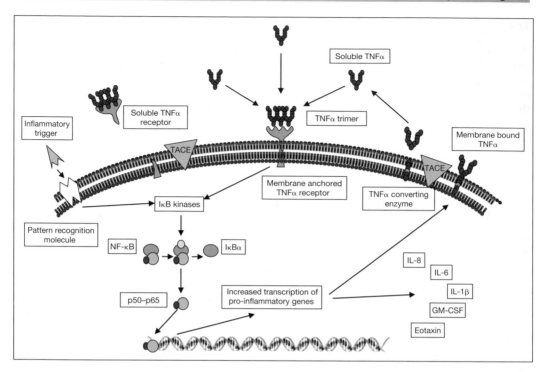

Figure 11.1   Biology of TNFα. Recognition of conserved molecules associated with inflammatory triggers by pattern recognition molecules leads to increased transcription of various pro-inflammatory cytokines including the 26 kDa transmembrane precursor protein (membrane TNFα). Membrane TNFα is cleaved by TACE to form the 17 kDa free TNFα which subsequently forms highly active homotrimers. These interact with two distinct TNFα receptors on the cell surface. The effect of TNFα activation is reduced by cleavage of the receptor from the cell surface to become soluble TNFα receptors.

TNFRii) [9]. The receptor–ligand interaction causes intracellular signalling without internalization of the complex which leads to phosphorylation of nuclear factor-κB (NF-κB) to activate the p50–p65 subunit which interacts with the DNA chromatin structure to increase transcription of pro-inflammatory genes, such as IL-8, IL-6 and TNFα itself [10], which leads to inflammatory responses such as neutrophil activation and recruitment (Figure 11.1).

As well as causing increased secretion of inflammatory cytokines, TNFα has direct systemic effects which are highly dose-dependent: chronic low-dose exposure causes anorexia, protein catabolism, insulin resistance and subendocardial inflammation, whereas acute exposure to high doses causes fever, shock, adult respiratory distress syndrome and acute tubular necrosis [11]. Response to TNFα activation is balanced by shedding of the extracellular domain of the TNFα receptors which occurs in response to stimulation by TNFα [12], lipopolysaccharides [13], mitogens and IL-10 [14]. Humans with a mutation of the TNFα receptor 1 gene express a non-sheddable TNFα receptor 1 and suffer from and auto-inflammatory periodic syndrome known as TNFα receptor 1 associated periodic syndromes (TRAPS); this condition is characterized by fever and severe localized inflammation [15]. Mice 'knocked in' to express the non-sheddable TNFα receptor 1 have enhanced macrophage activation and increased release of effector molecules in response to Toll-like receptor stimulation [16]. In addition, these mice suffered from an auto-inflammatory condition with evidence of inflammatory arthritis.

TNFα IN INFLAMMATORY CONDITIONS

An autoimmune inflammatory arthritis mediated by TNFα is known to occur in humans: rheumatoid arthritis is a common destructive arthropathy in which TNFα is produced by macrophages and monocytes in response to activation by CD4+ T cells. TNFα is measurable in increased concentration in the synovial fluid and in the serum [17]. Antagonism of the TNFα either by treatment with recombinant soluble receptors or neutralizing antibodies in patients with rheumatoid disease leads to improvement in disease activity scores [18]. Similarly positive results are seen in treatment of other conditions mediated by TNFα, including Crohn's disease and Beçhet's disease.

A POTENTIAL ROLE FOR TNFα IN ASTHMA

The possibility that TNFα contributes to the dysregulated inflammatory response seen in the asthmatic airway is raised by the findings of increased TNFα mRNA [19] and protein [20] in the airway of patients with asthma. Moreover, the administration of inhaled recombinant TNFα to normal subjects leads to the development of airway hyperresponsiveness and an airway neutrophilia [21] and administration of TNFα to patients with asthma leads to an increase in airway hyperresponsiveness as reflected by a reduction in methacholine PC_{20} [22]. The mechanism behind this observation has not been fully elucidated: it could represent a direct effect of TNFα on airway smooth muscle [23] or be mediated by the release of the cysteinyl-leukotrienes LTC_4 and LTD_4 [24]. The local release of mediators from mast cells localized to the airway smooth muscle has recently been suggested to be important in the pathogenesis of airway hyperresponsiveness and bronchoconstriction in asthma [25]. TNFα induces histamine release from human mast cells directly [26] and participates in a positive autocrine loop that potentiates human mast cell cytokine secretion [27]; it is possible that TNFα is involved in mast cell/smooth muscle interaction and that this is particularly important in the development of airway hyperresponsiveness.

TNFα has a number of other actions which may be relevant to asthma: it is chemoattractant for neutrophils and monocytes [28]; it increases the cytotoxic effect of eosinophils on endothelial cells [29]; it is involved in activation and cytokine release by T cells [30]; and it increases epithelial expression of adhesion molecules such as ICAM-1 and V-CAM-1 [31] which play an important role is the conduction of T cells to the lung and in the subsequent development of airway hyperresponsiveness [32].

TNFα IN REFRACTORY ASTHMA

Around 10% of patients with asthma have refractory disease that cannot be controlled with traditional treatment. A better understanding of the mechanisms underlying refractory asthma is important as healthcare costs, morbidity and mortality are significant in this population of patients. The airway pathology of refractory asthma differs from mild-to-moderate asthma in that there is a more heterogeneous pattern of inflammatory response [33], with greater involvement of neutrophils [34], involvement of the distal lung [35] and increased airway remodelling [36]. In addition to its relevance to asthma in general, TNFα has a number of properties that might be relevant to refractory asthma, including: recruitment of neutrophils [37], induction of glucocorticoid resistance [38], myocyte proliferation [39] and stimulation of fibroblast growth and maturation to myofibroblasts by promoting TGFβ expression [40, 41]. Strong support for a role for TNFα in refractory asthma comes from the observation that TNFα expression in bronchial biopsies [42] and on peripheral blood mononuclear cells [43], and the concentration of TNFα in bronchoalveolar fluid [42] is increased in patients with refractory asthma when compared to patients with mild-to-moderate asthma and healthy controls. Moreover, inhibition of TNFα activity with etanercept is associated with a marked reduction in methacholine airway responsiveness, improved

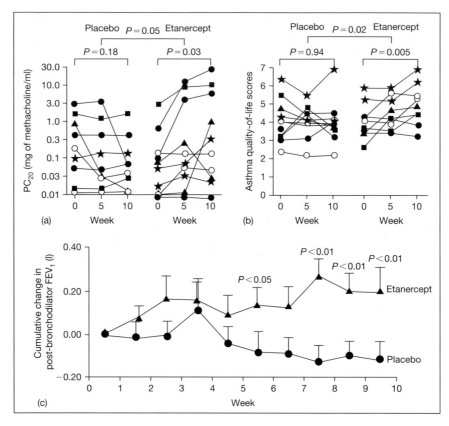

Figure 11.2 Concentration of inhaled methacholine causing a 20% decrease (PC_{20}) in the FEV_1 (a) and asthma quality-of-life scores (b) before, during, and after 10 weeks of etanercept or placebo and the cumulative mean (SEM) change in FEV_1 after the inhalation of 200 μg of sallbutamol each week during the 10-week treatment trial (c).

symptoms and quality of life scores and an increase in forced expiratory volume in 1 s (FEV_1) (Figure 11.2) [42, 43]. In one study, the beneficial effects of etanercept were related to the extent of upregulation of the TNFα axis, as reflected by peripheral blood mononuclear cell membrane TNFα expression [43]. The profile of action of etanercept in refractory asthma is interesting in that there is evidence of a marked improvement in airway function together with a reduction in induced sputum supernatant histamine concentration but little evidence of any other important anti-inflammatory effects. This suggests that the most important site of action of TNFα in refractory asthma is the airway smooth muscle and associated mast cells [25].

The data on the effects of TNFα blockade in refractory asthma is too preliminary to recommend it as a treatment. However, larger and longer clinical trials are underway and these should provide the necessary information on risk and benefit for clinicians to make an informed decision about the value of this therapy. These larger trials may identify clinical characteristics of patients who respond particularly well to the treatment. Potential explanations for TNFα upregulation include the coexistence of asthma with other inflammatory conditions associated with increased TNFα activity and genetic differences in the TNFα gene or genes associated with regulation of TNFα production [44]. A number of factors associated with TNFα upregulation including obesity [45], smoking [46] and endotoxin exposure [2] are also associated with more severe and corticosteroid-resistant asthma [34, 47, 48]. This raises the possibility that the coexistence of a high TNFα state with asthmatic airway inflammation may be important in the pathogenesis of refractory asthma. More work is needed on the mechanism of TNFα upregulation in refractory asthma.

SUMMARY

TNFα is a pleiotropic pro-inflammatory cytokine for which there is growing evidence for a role in asthma and refractory asthma in particular. Its effects are regulated both by local concentrations and cell surface receptor dynamics and it has recently become possible to modify TNFα activity using humanized monoclonal antibodies or recombinant soluble TNFα receptors. Investigation into the possibility of TNFα axis upregulation in refractory asthma and placebo-controlled trials of TNFα antagonism in this group of patients have begun and there is initial evidence of an important role for TNFα in refractory asthma.

REFERENCES

1. Coley WB. The treatment of malignant tumors by repeated inoculations of erysipelas. With a report of ten original cases. *Am J Med Sci* 1883; 105:487.
2. O'Malley WE, Achinstein B, Shear MJ. Journal of the National Cancer Institute, Vol. 29, 1962: action of bacterial polysaccharide on tumors. II. Damage of sarcoma 37 by serum of mice treated with Serratia marcescens polysaccharide, and induced tolerance. *Nutr Rev* 1988; 46:389–391.
3. Warren JS, Ward PA, Johnson KJ. Tumor necrosis factor: a plurifunctional mediator of acute inflammation. *Mod Pathol* 1988; 1:242–247.
4. Medzhitov R, Janeway C Jr. Innate immunity. *N Engl J Med* 2000; 343:338–344.
5. Kriegler M, Perez C, DeFay K, Albert I, Lu SD. A novel form of TNF/cachectin is a cell surface cytotoxic transmembrane protein: ramifications for the complex physiology of TNF. *Cell* 1988; 53: 45–53.
6. Zheng Y, Saftig P, Hartmann D, Blobel C. Evaluation of the contribution of different ADAMs to tumor necrosis factor alpha (TNFalpha) shedding and of the function of the TNFalpha ectodomain in ensuring selective stimulated shedding by the TNFalpha convertase (TACE/ADAM17). *J Biol Chem* 2004; 279:42898–42906.
7. Davis JM, Narachi MA, Alton NK, Arakawa T. Structure of human tumor necrosis factor alpha derived from recombinant DNA. *Biochemistry* 1987; 26:1322–1326.
8. Smith RA, Baglioni C. The active form of tumor necrosis factor is a trimer. *J Biol Chem* 1987; 262:6951–6954.
9. Brockhaus M, Schoenfeld HJ, Schlaeger EJ, Hunziker W, Lesslauer W, Loetscher H. Identification of two types of tumor necrosis factor receptors on human cell lines by monoclonal antibodies. *Proc Natl Acad Sci USA* 1990; 87:3127–3131.
10. Barnes PJ, Karin M. Nuclear factor-kappaB: a pivotal transcription factor in chronic inflammatory diseases. *N Engl J Med* 1997; 336:1066–1071.
11. Tracey KJ, Cerami A. Tumor necrosis factor: a pleiotropic cytokine and therapeutic target. *Annu Rev Med* 1994; 45:491–503.
12. Lantz M, Malik S, Slevin ML, Olsson I. Infusion of tumor necrosis factor (TNF) causes an increase in circulating TNF-binding protein in humans. *Cytokine* 1990; 2:402–406.
13. Leeuwenberg JF, Dentener MA, Buurman WA. Lipopolysaccharide LPS-mediated soluble TNF receptor release and TNF receptor expression by monocytes. Role of CD14, LPS binding protein, and bactericidal/permeability-increasing protein. *J Immunol* 1994; 152:5070–5076.
14. Leeuwenberg JF, Jeunhomme TM, Buurman WA. Slow release of soluble TNF receptors by monocytes in vitro. *J Immunol* 1994; 152:4036–4043.
15. McDermott MF, Aksentijevich I, Galon J *et al.* Germline mutations in the extracellular domains of the 55 kDa TNF receptor, TNFR1, define a family of dominantly inherited autoinflammatory syndromes. *Cell* 1999; 97:133–144.

16. Xanthoulea S, Pasparakis M, Kousteni S et al. Tumor necrosis factor (TNF) receptor shedding controls thresholds of innate immune activation that balance opposing TNF functions in infectious and inflammatory diseases. J Exp Med 2004; 200:367–376.

17. Choy EH, Panayi GS. Cytokine pathways and joint inflammation in rheumatoid arthritis. N Engl J Med 2001; 344:907–916.

18. Olsen NJ, Stein CM. New drugs for rheumatoid arthritis. N Engl J Med 2004; 350:2167–2179.

19. Ying S, Robinson DS, Varney V et al. TNF alpha mRNA expression in allergic inflammation. Clin Exp Allergy 1991; 21:745–750.

20. Bradding P, Roberts JA, Britten KM et al. Interleukin-4, -5, and -6 and tumor necrosis factor-alpha in normal and asthmatic airways: evidence for the human mast cell as a source of these cytokines. Am J Respir Cell Mol Biol 1994; 10:471–480.

21. Thomas PS, Yates DH, Barnes PJ. Tumor necrosis factor-alpha increases airway responsiveness and sputum neutrophilia in normal human subjects. Am J Respir Crit Care Med 1995; 152:76–80.

22. Thomas PS, Heywood G. Effects of inhaled tumour necrosis factor alpha in subjects with mild asthma. Thorax 2002; 57:774–778.

23. Adner M, Rose AC, Zhang Y et al. An assay to evaluate the long-term effects of inflammatory mediators on murine airway smooth muscle: evidence that TNFalpha up-regulates 5-HT(2A)-mediated contraction. Br J Pharmacol 2002; 137:971–982.

24. Huber M, Beutler B, Keppler D. Tumor necrosis factor alpha stimulates leukotriene production in vivo. Eur J Immunol 1988; 18:2085–2088.

25. Brightling CE, Bradding P, Symon FA, Holgate ST, Wardlaw AJ, Pavord ID. Mast-cell infiltration of airway smooth muscle in asthma. N Engl J Med 2002; 346:1699–1705.

26. van Overveld FJ, Jorens PG, Rampart M, de Backer W, Vermieire PA. Tumour necrosis factor stimulates human skin mast cells to release histamine and tryptase. Clin Exp Allergy 1991; 21:711–714.

27. Coward WR, Okayama Y, Sagara H, Wilson SJ, Holgate ST, Church MK. NF-kappa B and TNF-alpha: a positive autocrine loop in human lung mast cells? J Immunol 2002; 169:5287–5293.

28. Onda T, Nagakura T, Iikura Y. Asthmatic children and swimming training. 4. Neutrophil chemotactic activity in the supernatant of human lymphocytes and monocytes challenged with phytohemagglutinin and house dust mite allergen. Arerugi 1987; 36:299–305.

29. Slungaard A, Vercellotti GM, Walker G, Nelson RD, Jacob HS. Tumor necrosis factor alpha/cachectin stimulates eosinophil oxidant production and toxicity towards human endothelium. J Exp Med 1990; 171:2025–2041.

30. Scheurich P, Thoma B, Ucer U, Pfizenmaier K. Immunoregulatory activity of recombinant human tumor necrosis factor (TNF)-alpha: induction of TNF receptors on human T cells and TNF-alpha-mediated enhancement of T cell responses. J Immunol 1987; 138:1786–1790.

31. Lassalle P, Delneste Y, Gosset P, Tonnel AB, Capron A. Potential implication of endothelial cells in bronchial asthma. Int Arch Allergy Appl Immunol 1991; 94:233–238.

32. Walter MJ, Morton JD, Kajiwara N, Agapov E, Holtzman MJ. Viral induction of a chronic asthma phenotype and genetic segregation from the acute response. J Clin Invest 2002; 110:165–175.

33. American Thoracic Society. Proceedings of the ATS workshop on refractory asthma: current understanding, recommendations, and unanswered questions. Am J Respir Crit Care Med 2000; 162:2341–2351.

34. The ENFUMOSA cross-sectional European multicentre study of the clinical phenotype of chronic severe asthma. European Network for Understanding Mechanisms of Severe Asthma. Eur Respir J 2003; 22:470–477.

35. Berry MA, Hargadon B, Morgan A et al. Alveolar nitric oxide concentration in adults with asthma: evidence of distal lung inflammation in refractory asthma. Eur Respir J 2005; 25:986–991.

36. Busse W, Elias J, Sheppard D, Banks-Schlegel S. Airway remodeling and repair. Am J Respir Crit Care Med 1999; 160:1035–1042.

37. Thomas PS, Yates DH, Barnes PJ. Tumor necrosis factor-alpha increases airway responsiveness and sputum neutrophilia in normal human subjects. Am J Respir Crit Care Med 1995; 152:76–80.

38. Franchimont D, Martens H, Hagelstein MT et al. Tumor necrosis factor alpha decreases, and interleukin-10 increases, the sensitivity of human monocytes to dexamethasone: potential regulation of the glucocorticoid receptor. J Clin Endocrinol Metab 1999; 84:2834–2839.

39. Amrani Y, Panettieri RA Jr, Frossard N, Bronner C. Activation of the TNF alpha-p55 receptor induces myocyte proliferation and modulates agonist-evoked calcium transients in cultured human tracheal smooth muscle cells. Am J Respir Cell Mol Biol 1996; 15:55–63.

40. Sullivan DE, Ferris M, Pociask D, Brody AR. TNF-{alpha} induces TGF-{beta}1 expression in lung fibroblasts through the ERK pathway. *Am J Respir Cell Mol Biol* 2005; 32:342–349.

41. Desmouliere A, Geinoz A, Gabbiani F, Gabbiani G. Transforming growth factor-beta 1 induces alpha-smooth muscle actin expression in granulation tissue myofibroblasts and in quiescent and growing cultured fibroblasts. *J Cell Biol* 1993; 122:103–111.

42. Howarth PH, Babu KS, Arshad HS *et al*. Tumour necrosis factor (TNFalpha) as a novel therapeutic target in symptomatic corticosteroid dependent asthma. *Thorax* 2005; 60:1012–1018.

43. Berry MA, Hargadon B, Shelley M *et al*. Evidence of a role of tumor necrosis factor alpha in refractory asthma. *N Engl J Med* 2006; 354:697–708.

44. Li Kam Wa TC, Mansur AH, Britton J *et al*. Association between 308 tumour necrosis factor promoter polymorphism and bronchial hyperreactivity in asthma. *Clin Exp Allergy* 1999; 29:1204–1208.

45. Hotamisligil GS, Arner P, Caro JF, Atkinson RL, Spiegelman BM. Increased adipose tissue expression of tumor necrosis factor-alpha in human obesity and insulin resistance. *J Clin Invest* 1995; 95:2409–2415.

46. Churg A, Dai J, Tai H, Xie C, Wright JL. Tumor necrosis factor-alpha is central to acute cigarette smoke-induced inflammation and connective tissue breakdown. *Am J Respir Crit Care Med* 2002; 166:849–854.

47. Chaudhuri R, Livingston E, McMahon AD, Thomson L, Borland W, Thomson NC. Cigarette smoking impairs the therapeutic response to oral corticosteroids in chronic asthma. *Am J Respir Crit Care Med* 2003; 168:1308–1311.

48. Michel O, Ginanni R, Duchateau J, Vertongen F, Le Bon B, Sergysels R. Domestic endotoxin exposure and clinical severity of asthma. *Clin Exp Allergy* 1991; 21:441–448.

12

Are chemokines viable targets for asthma?

L. A. Murray, R. Schlenker-Herceg, A. M. Das

INTRODUCTION

Asthma is a disease process that has both genetic and environmental components contributing towards the initiation, progression and severity of the disease. There are approximately 15 million Americans currently diagnosed as having asthma. The worldwide prevalence appears to be increasing. Asthma manifests as a reversible airway obstruction, with patients having increased airway hyperresponsiveness (AHR) to specific and non-specific stimuli, as well as increased mucus production within the lung. Underlying the clinical symptoms is pronounced airway inflammation and remodelling, considered to be closely associated with disease pathology. The majority of asthmatics are classified as having mild-to-moderate disease, with current standard of care involving inhaled corticosteroids (ICS), β_2-adrenergic agonists and leukotriene receptor antagonists. However, approximately 5–10% of the asthmatic patients suffer from severe disease which is uncontrolled by standard therapy [1]. This subgroup of patients accounts for a majority of all the asthma-associated healthcare costs and represents a high unmet medical need [2]. At present it is not clear whether severe asthma is mild-to-moderate asthma progressing to severe asthma, or if it is a distinct disease [3].

Chemokines are a diverse collection of 'chemoattractant cytokines' that selectively recruit and activate various cell types by signalling through 7 transmembrane G protein-coupled receptors (reviewed by [4]). The chemokine family is classified into four main subgroups based on structural homology and the position of conserved cysteine residues [5]. The receptors are separated into subfamilies depending on the class of ligands [6]. To add to the complexity, multiple receptors can be expressed on the same cell type. Furthermore, certain chemokines are promiscuous in their binding and recent work has demonstrated that chemokines can behave as agonists as well as antagonists depending on the receptor the chemokine binds to [7, 8]. Since chemokines modulate the recruitment and activation of a variety of different cell types, they have been implicated in a variety of diseases including asthma [9]. A summary of chemokine receptor expression as well as chemokine production by cells associated with asthma is shown in Table 12.1.

Lynne A. Murray, PhD, Research Scientist, Department of Immunobiology, Centocor Research and Development, Radnor, Pennsylvania, USA

Rozsa Schlenker-Herceg, MD, Senior Director, Clinical Research, General Medicine, Centocor Research and Development, Radnor, Pennsylvania, USA

Anuk M. Das, PhD, Assistant Director, Department of Immunobiology, Centocor Research and Development, Radnor, Pennsylvania, USA

Table 12.1 Summary of major cell types shown to be involved in the pathology of asthma and their chemokine receptor expression and chemokine production profile

Cell type	Role/association with asthma	Chemokine receptor expression correlated with asthma	Chemokine production relevant to asthma
Epithelial cell	Goblet cell hyperplasia and metaplasia [107]	CCR3, CXCR3 [133, 134]	RANTES/CCL5, MCP4/CCL13, eotaxin/CCL11, eotaxin-2/CCL24, eotaxin-3/CCL26, IL-8/CXCL8 [55, 135, 136]
Eosinophil	Correlates with remodelling and exacerbations [28, 29]	CCR3, CCR1 [51]	
Neutrophil	Increased in severe asthma; correlates with exacerbations [26–28, 30–32]	CXCR2	IL-8/CXCL8 [135]
T cell	Increased in asthma; antibody isotype switching; cytokine production [30]	'Th2'-specific receptors: CCR3, CCR4, CCR8 [54]	
Mast cell	Histamine release inducing AHR [33, 34]	CCR3, CXCR3 [35, 36, 54]	Eotaxin/CCL11 [55]
Fibroblast/ myofibroblast	The extent of subepithelial fibrosis correlates with severity of asthma [61, 137–139]	CCR2 (Th2-derived fibroblasts) [73]	MCP1/CCL2, eotaxin/CCL11, IL-8/CXCL8 [135]
Smooth muscle cell	AHR [97]	CCR3, CCR2, CCR5, CCR8 [104, 105, 140]	RANTES/CCL5 [106]
Fibrocyte	Collagen production [83]	CCR2, CCR7, CXCR4 [87–89]	
Endothelial cells	Extent of angiogenesis correlates with severity [112, 113]	CCR2, CXCR2, CXCR3 [141–143]	Eotaxin/CCL11, IL-8/CXCL8 [55, 135]

TARGETING CHEMOKINES IN ASTHMA

TRANSLATIONAL MEDICINE AND THE USE OF ANIMAL MODELS TO STUDY ASTHMA

Studies using both clinical settings as well as animal models have garnered a great deal of insight into the central role that chemokines play in the variety of pathologies associated with allergic airway disease (AAD) and AHR (reviewed by [10]). Animal models have provided a great deal of insight into both the cell types involved in AAD, as well as identified key mediators critical to disease establishment and progression. Strategies of inducing AHR include antibody transfer, adoptive transfer of antigen-primed CD4[+] cells into naïve mice and allergen sensitization followed by pulmonary challenge (reviewed by [11]). However, this review will focus primarily on the role of chemokines in asthma determined through the administration of allergens to naïve mice. In these models, the immune system is primed to mount an allergic response to specific antigens.

Models of AAD induced by allergens generally utilize antigen-specific priming of the immune system through a local or systemic sensitization process. This is then followed by

Table 12.2 Summary of allergens commonly used in AAD models

Allergen type	Antigen
Intact protein	OVA (ovalbumin) CRA (cockroach antigen) HDM (house dust mite extract)
Peptide	Fel d 1 Der p 1
Fungal	*Aspergillus fumigatus*

Fel d 1 = Cat allergen; Der p 1 = house dust mite allergen.

pulmonary challenge of either the same or a related allergen. A summary of the most commonly used allergens is outlined in Table 12.2. As can be noted, there is significant diversity in choice of allergen. Furthermore, different investigators use different sensitization protocols, adjuvants and strains of mice, all of which have been shown to impact on the effectiveness of various therapeutics. Specific features of ovalbumin (OVA)-induced AAD have more recently rendered this antigen less favourable. Although OVA-induced AAD models have generated a vast wealth of knowledge around major cell types and mediators central to AAD, OVA-induced airway remodelling has some degree of resolution, mice become immunologically tolerant to OVA and the models require co-administration with adjuvants to ensure sufficient immune priming and thus sufficient detriment in lung function. Furthermore, OVA is not a commonly encountered environmental allergen, therefore more pathophysiological antigens are currently being used. These include cockroach antigen, house dust mite (HDM) extract and the fungal pathogen *Aspergillus fumigatus* (Table 12.2).

Some models of AAD elicit a more robust response. Depending on the particular hallmarks of AAD that investigators wish to evaluate, different animal models are used. For example, models using chronic repeated challenge with intranasal house dust mite results in an increase in AHR as well as a pronounced peribronchial eosinophilia, goblet cell hyperplasia and tissue remodelling [12]. In the HDM study, the investigators reported that this allergen induced a systemic Th2 response [12, 13]. In a fungal asthma model where the AAD pathologies were induced by *Aspergillus fumigatus*, an increase in remodelling and goblet cell hyperplasia was also reported, as with the HDM studies [14]. Furthermore, a persistent BAL eosinophilia was described, as was an increase in systemic immunoglobulin (Ig)E [14]. Therefore when conclusions are drawn from various AAD models, it is essential to compare directly all features of the model as well as the functional endpoints that are ultimately compared between studies.

CHEMOKINE MANIPULATION IN AAD MODELS

AAD models have demonstrated the timeframes of chemokine production during the onset and progression of AHR. The kinetics of production of chemokines has determined potential individual roles of chemokines in the various functional pathologies observed in the disease. For example, the kinetics of production of JE/CCL2 (a mouse orthologue of human MCP-1), eotaxin/CCL11, TARC/CCL17 and MDC/CCL22 correlated with the recruitment of specific leucocyte subsets expressing receptors for these chemokines [15–20]. However, it has been chemokine manipulation that has helped to determine potential redundancies in pathways. In animal models, specific receptors and ligands have been targeted through gene deletion as

Table 12.3 Effect of receptor blocking studies in AAD models by either receptor knockout mice or pharmacological intervention

Chemokine receptor	Therapeutic strategy targeting the receptor	Outcome
CCR1	Receptor knockout	Similar AHR, decreased subepithelial fibrosis [76]
CCR2	Receptor knockout	Increased eosinophilia, decreased IFNγ [144]; decreased AHR and inflammation [145]; no effect [146]; inhibits IL-13-induced impairment in lung function, inflammation and remodelling [22]
CCR3	Receptor knockout	No effect on mast cell recruitment [147]
CCR4	Receptor knockout	Decreased inflammation and AHR, no beneficial effect on subepithelial fibrosis [148]
CCR6	Receptor knockout	Decreased AHR and bronchial eosinophilia [56]
CCR7	Receptor knockout	Impaired antibody responses and altered secondary lymphoid organ morphology [149]
CCR8	Receptor knockout	Decreased Th2, decreased eosinophil recruitment [58]; no protection [59, 60]
CXCR2	Receptor knockout	Decreased AHR but increased B cells and serum IgE [150]
CXCR4	Receptor antagonist	Decreased lung tissue and BAL eosinophilia and AHR [151]; decreased inflammation and AHR [152]

Chemokine ligand	Therapeutic strategy targeting the ligand	Outcome
Eotaxin/CCL11	Antibody neutralization	Reduced eosinophilia [153]
Eotaxin/CCL11	Ligand knockout	Partial decrease in eosinophil recruitment [18]; no effect [57]
I309/CCL1	Antibody neutralization	Reduced eosinophil recruitment, no effect on Th2 cells; no effect on AHR [154]
JE/CCL2	Antibody neutralization	Decreased AHR, decreased pulmonary eosinophilia [17]
JE/CCL2	Ligand knockout	No Th2 cell generation [155]
MCP5/CCL12	Antibody neutralization	Decreased AHR and eosinophilia [17, 20]
MDC/CCL22	Antibody neutralization	Decreased AHR and pulmonary eosinophil number [16]
MIP1α/CCL3	Antibody neutralization	Decreased AHR and eosinophilia [17]
RANTES/CCL5	Mutated RANTES: receptor antagonist	Decreased pulmonary eosinophil number [17]
SDF1α/CXCL12	Antibody neutralization	Decreased lung tissue and BAL eosinophilia and AHR [151]

well as pharmacological intervention such as small molecule inhibitors or neutralizing antibody approaches. A summary of various animal models utilizing the different techniques of manipulating chemokine pathways during AAD models is shown in Table 12.3. Gene targeting is now a routine technique for studying the consequences of deleting either a single gene or multiple genes. Furthermore, site-specific over-expression of proteins of interest has also highlighted a role of mediators in driving disease pathology. The initial identification of specific mediators in human disease has helped to elucidate targets of interest to be over-expressed in animal models, thereby confirming a pathological role for these mediators in hallmarks of asthma. In particular, mice with lung-specific transgenic interleukin (IL)-13 expression had pathophysiological alterations in lung function, pulmonary inflammation and mucus metaplasia [21]. *In vivo*, lung-specific overexpression of interleukin (IL)-13 was also shown to induce subepithelial fibrosis in association with an increase in the levels of eotaxin/CCL11 and JE/CCL2 [21, 22]. Crossing these mice onto a CCR2-deficient background, CCR2 being the receptor for JE/CCL2, inhibits the subepithelial fibrosis and inflammation induced by IL-13 [22]. In contrast, mucus metaplasia was still evident in the IL-13 transgenic CCR2-deficient mice, indicating a CCR2-independent pathway induced by IL-13 [22].

CHEMOKINES AND HALLMARKS OF ASTHMA

To understand the potential for chemokine-directed therapeutics for asthma, it is important to understand the underlying pathophysiology of the disease, the cell types involved and also the expression of chemokines in asthma.

CHEMOKINES: CELL RECRUITMENT AND ACTIVATION IN ASTHMA

Even with significant corticosteroid use, increased numbers of inflammatory cells are found in the lungs of patients with severe asthma. Earlier reports have indicated that the amount of inflammation correlates with the extent of AHR [23]. Eosinophils, macrophages, mast cells and lymphocytes are inflammatory cell types associated with all severities of asthma [24–26]. However, increased numbers of neutrophils are only found in the lungs of patients with severe asthma [26–28] and eosinophil number has been shown to correlate with certain features of airway remodelling in asthmatics [28]. Moreover, in children with severe asthma, the presence of neutrophils as well as eosinophils has been correlated with exacerbations [29, 30–32]. Mast cells are relatively absent from the non-asthmatic lung, but elevated numbers have been found in the severe asthmatic lung [33]. Mast cell granules contain a variety of proteolytic enzymes and mediators such as histamine which directly affect bronchomotor tone [34]. Cross-linking of mast cell IgE receptors results in mast cell degranulation, thus releasing mediators that contribute to both AHR and inflammation. Mast cells express a variety of chemokines receptors including CCR3, CXCR1 and CXCR3 and thus may be actively recruited during inflammation-associated exacerbations of the asthmatic response [35, 36].

As has already been mentioned, chemokines play an important role in the recruitment of inflammatory cells into the lungs and the subsequent activation of both infiltrating and resident cells [9]. Chemokines bind to glycosaminoglycans (GAGs) on the endothelium thus providing a gradient along which leucocytes migrate [37]. The directed recruitment of leucocytes is mediated by the distinct expression of chemokine receptors (Table 12.1) and surface markers. The recruitment of leucocytes to tissue sites of inflammation, as occurs in the asthmatic lung, requires an orchestrated series of events that are mediated by adhesion molecules [38, 39]. Studies reporting neutralization of the chemokines eotaxin/CCL11, RANTES/CCL5, JE/CCL2, TARC/CCL17, SDF1α/CXCL12 or MDC/CCL22 or, chemokine receptors such as CXCR4 support the contribution of each of these molecules in inflammatory cell migration in models of AAD [15–20] and reviewed by [40]. Chemokines can increase the expression of adhesion molecules further facilitating recruitment of leucocytes. It has been suggested that the specific expression of chemokine receptors, as well as adhesion molecules, allows for more of a compartmentalization of leucocytes [41, 42]. Another function of chemokines is enhancing survival of leucocytes. For example, the chemokines eotaxin/CCL11 and IL-8/CXCL8, which are expressed at high levels in the lungs of severe asthmatics, can enhance eosinophil and neutrophil survival respectively [43, 44]. Indeed, increased eosinophil survival in the asthmatic lung has been reported [45]. Apoptosis of inflammatory cells serves to resolve inflammation and prevent damage to the host. Apoptotic neutrophils retain their granules and these apoptotic cells have been shown to be ultimately cleared in the lung by macrophages, fibroblasts and epithelial cells [46–50]. However, increased cell survival may result in a persistence of both neutrophils and eosinophils in the lung, thus prolonging the amount of time and potential damage these cells can perform in local tissue.

Numerous studies have correlated decreased eosinophil recruitment to the lung with an improvement in AHR. Chemokine receptor expression on eosinophils has been reported to be dependent on cell isolation technique, therefore suggesting that receptor expression may depend on cellular localization as well as differentiation state [51]. Eosinophils preferentially express CC chemokine receptors, including CCR3 and CCR1. However, elicited eosinophils express CCR1–CCR5, as detected by flow cytometry, and receptor functionality has been demonstrated with *in vitro* chemotaxis experiments [51]. Interestingly, CCR3 is also expressed on mast cells and type 2 T helper cells (Th2) [52–54]. Eotaxin/CCL11, a CCR3 ligand, is produced during allergic reactions by a number of cell types including epithelial cells, endothelial cells, mast cells and alveolar macrophages [55]. Due to the pleiotropic nature of eotaxin/CCL11 and how this particular chemokine is involved in the functions of a number of cell types associated with asthma, an anti-eotaxin/CCL11 monoclonal antibody is in clinical trials for asthma (Table 12.4). However, as described above, the role of other chemokines in recruiting eosinophils cannot be discounted due to eosinophils expressing other chemokine receptors [51]. For example, CCR6-deficient mice have decreased airway resistance which correlated with decreased pulmonary eosinophilia and decreased IL-5 in an AAD model [56].

With a strong role being hypothesized for eotaxin inducing eosinophil recruitment, this led to the hypothesis that eotaxin knockout mice would be protected in AAD models. In one study, there was a slight reduction in eosinophil recruitment and in another study there was no impact on eosinophil migration [18, 57]. However, in both studies, there was no benefit in lung function [18, 57]. This highlights the functional redundancy of chemokines, in that neutralization of one chemokine is not sufficient at inhibiting pulmonary eosinophil recruitment in mouse models of AAD. Another example where interpretation of potentially beneficial therapeutic outcomes varies depending on the model has been observed with CCR8. In one study using CCR8 KO mice, there was decreased Th2 response with decreased eosinophil recruitment to the lung [58]. However, in two further studies, no protection was conferred in CCR8 KO mice with eosinophil number not being impacted by gene deletion [59, 60]. It is important to note that none of the studies reported any physiological benefit, with all cohorts of mice having comparably impaired lung function.

CHEMOKINES: RESIDENT CELL ACTIVATION

Another hallmark of asthma is subepithelial fibrosis with increased thickness of the lamina reticularis underneath the basement membrane, and altered composition of the extracellular matrix [61–63]. There are multiple underlying mechanisms associated with subepithelial fibrosis including eosinophil and fibrocyte accumulation [64]; activation and proliferation of fibroblasts; and deposition of extracellular matrix proteins by myofibroblasts [63].

Fibroblast/Myofibroblast in Subepithelial Fibrosis

An increase in subepithelial basement membrane thickness has been associated with an increase in transforming growth factor β (TGFβ)-positive cells and fibroblasts, suggesting an environment or milieu conducive for collagen generation [65–67]. Profibrotic cytokines such as TGFβ, IL-4 and IL-13, have been demonstrated to induce differentiation of fibroblasts to myofibroblasts [68, 69]. There is a significant increase in myofibroblast numbers in the lung following allergen challenge [70]. An increase in the number of myofibroblasts in the mucosa of asthmatics has been shown to correlate with subepithelial collagen deposition [71]. Moreover, myofibroblast hyperplasia is evident in patients with chronic asthma

Table 12.4 Chemokine-directed therapies currently in development that could have efficacy in asthma (adapted from [156])

Chemokine pathway targeted	Compound	Company	Therapeutic strategy	Current reported indications	Status
MCP1: CCR2	ABN-912	Novartis	mAb to ligand	Inflammation, atherosclerosis, RA, MS	Phase 1/2
	MLN-1202	Millenium	mAb to receptor		Phase 2
	INCB-3284	Incyte	Small molecule receptor antagonist		Phase 1/2
Eotaxin: CCR3	CAT-213	Cambridge Antibody Technology	mAb to ligand	Asthma, allergy, allergic rhinitis	Phase 2
	766994	Glaxo SmithKline	Small molecule receptor antagonist		Phase 2
CCR4	IC-487892	ICOS & Array Biopharma	Small molecule receptor antagonist	Inflammation, allergy	Pre-clinical
IL-8: CXCR2	ABX-IL-8	Abgenix	mAb to ligand	RA, psoriasis, COPD	Phase 2 stopped due to failure to show efficacy in psoriasis
	BKT-RP3	Biokine Therapeutics	Peptide inhibitors of IL-8/CXCL8	Oncology	Pre-clinical
	SB-656933	Glaxo SmithKline	Small molecule receptor antagonist	COPD	Phase 1
SDF1: CXCR4	CTCE-9908	Chemokine Therapeutics	Peptide inhibitors of SDF1α/CXCL12	Oncology	Phase 1
	CS-3955	Kureha Chemical Industry and Sankyo	Small molecule receptor antagonist	HIV	Pre-clinincal

COPD = Chronic obstructive pulmonary disease; mAb = monoclonal antibody; MS = multiple sclerosis; RA = rheumatoid arthritis.

[71]. Indeed, the contribution of myofibroblasts to collagen generation has been shown with colocalization of myofibroblast α-smooth muscle actin with procollagen I (mRNA) by *in situ* hybridization [72]. Myofibroblasts have also been shown to be significant sources of MCP-1/CCL2 and TGFβ [72], thus indicating that this cell type may also play an important role in directing the inflammatory processes involved in asthma. Interestingly, MCP-1/ CCL2 can induce the generation of TGFβ from macrophages and fibroblasts, thus feeding back to fibroblasts and contributing to *de novo* collagen generation [73–75]. Moreover, the Th2-associated cytokines IL-4 and IL-13, together with TGFβ, have been shown to induce eotaxin/CCL11 production from human airway fibroblasts *in vitro* [67, 69], thus potentiating the eosinophilia observed in the lungs of asthmatics. Further, mice deficient in CCR1

receptor (which binds the chemokine ligands RANTES/CCL5, MIP-1α/CCL3 and MCP-3/CCL7) were shown to have a similar degree of airway inflammation and AHR in a murine model of chronic fungal airway disease, but less subepithelial fibrosis in comparison to wild type controls [76]. Due to the generation of chemokines such as MCP-1/CCL2, RANTES/CCL5, and eotaxin/CCL11 by fibroblasts [67, 73, 77, 78], fibroblasts may play an active role in recruiting inflammatory cells such as eosinophils and mast cells. Fibroblasts also generate matrix metalloproteinases (MMPs) which break down collagen thereby maintaining homeostasis of the subepithelial basement membrane. Interestingly, another function of MMPs is the cleavage of chemokines which are bound to GAGs [79]. This increased the local concentration, as well as potentially increasing the biological activity of chemokines [79, 80]. Isolating pulmonary fibroblasts from Th1-type biased or Th2-type granulomas has determined a clear phenotypic difference in receptor expression between the two fibroblast cell types. Pulmonary fibroblasts isolated from a Th2 fibrotic environment express increased levels of JE/CCL2 and its receptor CCR2. These fibroblasts also express increased levels of procollagen mRNA when stimulated with JE/CCL2, in comparison to Th1 environment-derived fibroblasts [73].

More recently, circulating collagen I^+ cells have been identified in bronchial mucosa of allergic asthma patients [81, 82]. These circulating collagen I^+ cells, or 'fibrocytes' were initially described at sites of wound repair [83]. However, it has recently been postulated that an over-exuberant recruitment of these cells to sites of pulmonary injury contributes to the aberrant deposition of collagen which ultimately induces pathologic fibrosis [82–86]. Furthermore, fibrocytes express a variety of chemokine receptors including CCR2, CXCR4 and CCR7 and inhibition of the respective chemokine ligands inhibits fibrocyte recruitment and ultimately reduces collagen deposition [87–90].

As technologies advance, the precise composition of cellular infiltrates, the extent of subepithelial fibrosis and the impact this has on hyperresponsiveness of asthmatic patients will be further clarified. As has been alluded to, in this particular aspect of asthma, chemokines not only recruit effector cells but directly affect collagen deposition. Therefore, targeting this family of mediators may lead to a beneficial decrease in subepithelial fibrosis which contributes to the pathology of asthma.

Airway Remodelling: Smooth Muscle Hypertrophy

Airway smooth muscle (ASM) mass is increased in both fatal and non-fatal asthma, with initial findings dating back to 1971 [91, 92] and reviewed by [61, 93]. The increase in ASM mass was localized to major bronchi, however it can also be increased in peripheral airways, as has been observed in sudden fatal asthma patients [94]. Interestingly, this specific anatomical increase in airway thickness was not observed in asthmatics who died from non-asthmatic causes [95]. A three–four-fold increase in ASM mass has been described in asthmatics [96]. This increase alone may be the causative factor in the increase in bronchomotor tone and bronchoconstrictor force observed in these patients [97]. Taken together this suggests that augmented ASM mass correlates with a poor outcome.

ASM from asthmatics has a higher proliferative capacity compared to ASM from normal subjects [98]. The increase in ASM may be due to proliferation induced by inflammatory mediators such as thromboxane, IL-6 and endothelin-1 [99–101]. Moreover, reactive oxygen species have been shown to contribute to ASM proliferation [102, 103]. Therefore the presence of neutrophils in the asthmatic lung *via* chemokine-mediated recruitment due to either increased severity of asthma or during exacerbations of disease, may result in the generation of reactive oxygen species and a mitogenic environment.

ASM expresses a variety of chemokine receptors, which have all been shown to be functional. Eotaxin/CCL11 induces migration of ASM *in vitro via* signalling through CCR3, however has no effect on proliferation [104]. The potential role of chemokines directly inducing

ASM proliferation has yet to be reported. However, it is interesting to note that MCP-1/CCL2 can cause the proliferation of vascular smooth muscle cells [105]. ASM cells are potent generators of chemokines such as RANTES/CCL5, and depending on the presence of either Th1 or Th2 cytokines, may modulate the inflammatory component of the disease [106].

Airway Remodelling: Mucus Gland Hypertrophy

Goblet cells are found within the epithelium of the upper and lower respiratory tracts. These cells produce a variety of mucins, and mucus is formed when mucins combine with other lipid glycoproteins. Excess mucus secretion occurs because of an increase in mucin gene expression and/or goblet cell hyperplasia [107]. An increase in mucin gene expression has been observed in asthmatics [108] and this increased mucus production can compromize airway calibre [109]. Again, neutrophils present due to, e.g. exacerbations, may be playing a central role in this pathophysiological change as neutrophil elastase has been shown to stimulate mucus cell metaplasia [110]. Furthermore, neutrophils release tumour necrosis factor α (TNFα) which increases epidermal growth factor receptor (EGFR) expression on epithelial cells and this has been shown to directly effect mucus production [111]. Finally, the role of another potential chemokine pathway was demonstrated using an AAD model in CCR1-deficient mice. Mice deficient in CCR1 have decreased numbers of goblet cells in comparison to wild-type mice in a murine model of allergic asthma [76]. In the IL-13 transgenic mice, mucus production was CCR2-independent [22]. Therefore, crossing IL-13 transgenic mice onto a CCR1-deficient background may result in decreased mucus production.

Airway Remodelling: Angiogenesis

Histopathological changes in fatal asthma have shown dilated, congested blood vessels [112, 113]. Interestingly, vascular changes often occur early in the disease process [114] and studies have suggested that the extent of angiogenesis parallels the severity of asthma [115]. There is a pronounced increase in airway thickness in asthma, therefore an increase in vascularization may be required to support the increase in asthmatic tissue mass. Furthermore, aberrant angiogenesis may be induced by hypoxia due to impaired gas exchange in the lungs of asthmatics. Chemokines, in particular CXC chemokines have been shown to regulate the angiogenic balance in the lung and are induced in hypoxaemic conditions [116]. Increased angiogenesis in asthmatics has also been shown to be associated with the chemokine SDF1α/CXCL12 [117]. However, the extent and function of angiogenesis and whether angiogenesis is a major contributing factor to disease severity remain to be elucidated. Increased angiogenesis in the bronchial vasculature in asthma may contribute to the increased interstitial oedema due to microvasculature leakage. Also, an increase in vessel number may increase leucocyte infiltration into the lung, thus perpetuating the inflammatory cascade in the lung.

THERAPEUTIC OPTIONS

As recommended by international guidelines, the cornerstone of the clinical management of asthma is inhaled corticosteroids (ICS) that are generally combined with long-acting inhaled β_2-agonists (LABA). Beyond high-dose ICS, LABA and other long-term controllers (theophyllin, leukotriene modifier), it is not clear what the 'next step' medication should be for patients with severe asthma. Usually, continuous oral corticosteroids (OCS) are added in order to control the disease. Based on the pathophysiology discussed above, more specific, targeted anti-inflammatory therapies may have a role in the treatment of asthma.

Specific targeting of IgE with an anti-IgE antibody represents a new, effective approach to the treatment of allergic asthma, including severe asthma. Following administration of omalizumab, a humanized mAb against IgE, reduction of serum-free IgE, downregulation of IgE receptors, reduction of submucosal eosinophils were accompanied by decreased AHR and reduced skin test reactivity [118–120]. Clinically, omalizumab reduces the number of asthma exacerbations, asthma symptoms, the need for ICS and rescue medication, and improves asthma-related quality of life [121–124]. Inhibiting TNFα has a dramatic effect in chronic inflammatory diseases such as rheumatoid arthritis and Crohn's disease. Small clinical trials suggest that TNFα levels are increased in severe asthmatics and blocking TNFα may have beneficial effects. Addition of etanercept, a soluble TNFα receptor, to background ICS and OCS improved AHR, lung function and quality of life in subjects with severe asthma [125, 126].

The two therapeutics described above are large molecule monoclonal antibodies. As has been examined in this review, the majority of murine AAD studies modulating chemokine pathways have used neutralizing antibodies. Advantages of antibody-based therapeutics include extended half-life and relative specificity of neutralization, as small molecules are often cleared rapidly and may have off-target effects. The current route of administration of antibody-based therapies is often intravenous. However, advances in intrapulmonary delivery techniques may provide even greater therapeutic benefits.

The strategy of targeting chemokine ligands or receptors is dependent on the chosen pathway. Due to the promiscuity of chemokines, targeting one ligand instead of one receptor may be sufficient to block multiple pathologies. This was hypothesized for eotaxin, but as minimal protection was conferred in eotaxin knockout mice, the hypothesis has since needed reviziting [18, 57]. If a specific chemokine receptor mediates multiple pathologies associated with asthma then perhaps this approach is desirable. For example, CCR2 mediates multiple IL-13-dependent pathologies, so the specific targeting of CCR2 may be attractive. Another chemokine receptor that is attractive for targeting in asthma is CXCR2 due to the role of this receptor in both recruiting and activating neutrophils. A list of chemokine-specific therapeutics currently in development that may have cross-efficacy in asthma is outlined in Table 19.4. One thing that is interesting to note is how certain compounds are targeting several disease indications. This highlights the pleiotropic nature of chemokines, with specific chemokines having a pathologic role in numerous pathologies. This may also be due to overlapping pathologies within diseases. For example, both allergic rhinitis and asthma have a pronounced eosinophilic component and therefore inhibiting eosinophil recruitment may be beneficial for both patient groups. Another interesting feature of chemokine-based therapies includes the nature of inhibition. As outlined in Table 12.4, chemokines are amenable to small molecule antagonists as well as large molecule compounds. These two features have made chemokine-based therapies attractive to numerous pharmaceutical companies as they can combine cross-therapeutic biological rationale and expertise with advancing technological platforms in the development of novel compounds.

Another area that must be considered when evaluating therapeutic strategies for asthma is the reliability of animal models in reflecting human disease. The AAD models all reproduce specific hallmarks of human disease, however asthma may be a disease of much longer duration, which slowly stabilizes and progresses and thus cannot be accurately mimicked in short-term animal models. One example of how translational studies and animal models have not been reflected in clinical experience was with anti-IL-5. IL-5 is a cytokine known to be central to eosinophil recruitment, activation, maturation and survival [127, 128]. In a monkey model of AAD, anti-IL-5 completely inhibited pulmonary eosinophilia and AHR [129]. However, clinically, a neutralizing antibody to IL-5, mepolizumab, reduced the number of eosinophils in the airways and also impacted subepithelial fibrosis. Critically, though, lung function in the asthmatic patients was not improved [130, 131]. No clinical benefit was also observed in another anti-IL-5 study in severe asthmatics [132]. One of the hypotheses as to why anti-IL-5 failed to demonstrate clinical efficacy is that there was an incomplete inhibition of eosinophil numbers in the lungs [131] and this may not have been observed in the animal models as the recruitment of these cells types is induced in a very short time-frame; in asthma however a more persistent eosinophilia is present. Also, the pulmonary architecture varies between species so the targeting of pathogenic cells may be amenable in animal models in comparison to targeting specific anatomical locations in established, chronic lung disease, as exists in the asthmatic lung.

SUMMARY

Therapies directed at chemokines provide options for regulating underlying inflammation. However, due to the pleiotropic effect of chemokines, intervention of chemokines may not only control underlying inflammation, but have a more broad spectrum effect on pathologies, such as regulating mucus hyperplasia or bronchomotor control. Animal models have not always correlated with clinical efficacy, however the use of these models has added greatly to our understanding of the disease and also highlighted the importance of chemokines at driving various pathologies. Asthma is a complex multifactorial disease with several pathological pathways. As shown with IL-13 transgenic mice bred on a CCR2-deficient background, there is overlap in pathways, however not all of the pathways converge through the same downstream mediators. Also, specific targeting of one pro-inflammatory mediator may be insufficient for asthma, as demonstrated with the disappointment of anti-IL-5 in asthma. Therefore, future work utilizing neutralization of multiple pathways may provide more sufficient therapeutic regimens.

REFERENCES

1. Barnes P, Woolcock A. Difficult asthma. *Eur Respir J* 1998; 12:1209–1218.
2. Barnes P, Jonsson B, Klim J. The costs of asthma. *Eur Respir J* 1996; 9:636–642.
3. Wenzel SE, Busse WW, Banks-Schlegel S et al. A different disease, many diseases or mild asthma gone bad? Challenges of severe asthma. *Eur Respir J* 2003; 22:397–398.
4. Luster AD. Chemokines–chemotactic cytokines that mediate inflammation. *N Engl J Med* 1998; 338:436–445.
5. Zlotnik A, Yoshie O. Chemokines: a new classification system and their role in immunity. *Immunity* 2000; 12:121–127.
6. Murphy PM, Baggiolini M, Charo IF et al. International union of pharmacology. XXII. Nomenclature for chemokine receptors. *Pharmacol Rev* 2000; 52:145–176.
7. Petkovic V, Moghini C, Paoletti S, Uguccioni M, Gerber B. I-TAC/CXCL11 is a natural antagonist for CCR5. *J Leukoc Biol* 2004; 76:701–708.
8. Xanthou G, Duchesnes CE, Williams TJ, Pease JE. CCR3 functional responses are regulated by both CXCR3 and its ligands CXCL9, CXCL10 and CXCL11. *Eur J Immunol* 2003; 33:2241–2250.
9. Schwarz MK, Wells TN. New therapeutics that modulate chemokine networks. *Nat Rev Drug Discov* 2002; 1:347–358.
10. D'Ambrosio D, Mariani M, Panina-Bordignon P, Sinigaglia F. Chemokines and their receptors guiding T lymphocyte recruitment in lung inflammation. *Am J Respir Crit Care Med* 2001; 164:1266–1275.
11. Lloyd CM, Gonzalo JA, Coyle AJ, Gutierrez-Ramos JC. Mouse models of allergic airway disease. *Adv Immunol* 2001; 77:263–295.
12. Johnson JR, Wiley RE, Fattouh R et al. Continuous exposure to house dust mite elicits chronic airway inflammation and structural remodeling. *Am J Respir Crit Care Med* 2004; 169:378–385.
13. Cates EC, Fattouh R, Wattie J et al. Intranasal exposure of mice to house dust mite elicits allergic airway inflammation via a GM-CSF-mediated mechanism. *J Immunol* 2004; 173:6384–6392.
14. Hogaboam CM, Blease K, Mehrad B et al. Chronic airway hyperreactivity, goblet cell hyperplasia, and peribronchial fibrosis during allergic airway disease induced by Aspergillus fumigatus. *Am J Pathol* 2000; 156:723–732.
15. Lloyd CM, Delaney T, Nguyen T et al. CC chemokine receptor (CCR)3/eotaxin is followed by CCR4/monocyte-derived chemokine in mediating pulmonary T helper lymphocyte type 2 recruitment after serial antigen challenge in vivo. *J Exp Med* 2000; 191:265–274.

16. Gonzalo JA, Pan Y, Lloyd CM *et al*. Mouse monocyte-derived chemokine is involved in airway hyperreactivity and lung inflammation. *J Immunol* 1999; 163:403–411.
17. Gonzalo JA, Lloyd CM, Wen D *et al*. The coordinated action of CC chemokines in the lung orchestrates allergic inflammation and airway hyperresponsiveness. *J Exp Med* 1998; 188:157–167.
18. Rothenberg ME, MacLean JA, Pearlman E, Luster AD, Leder P. Targeted disruption of the chemokine eotaxin partially reduces antigen-induced tissue eosinophilia. *J Exp Med* 1997; 185:785–790.
19. Lamkhioued B, Renzi PM, Abi-Younes S *et al*. Increased expression of eotaxin in bronchoalveolar lavage and airways of asthmatics contributes to the chemotaxis of eosinophils to the site of inflammation. *J Immunol* 1997; 159:4593–4601.
20. Jia GQ, Gonzalo JA, Lloyd C *et al*. Distinct expression and function of the novel mouse chemokine monocyte chemotactic protein-5 in lung allergic inflammation. *J Exp Med* 1996; 184:1939–1951.
21. Zhu Z, Homer RJ, Wang Z *et al*. Pulmonary expression of interleukin-13 causes inflammation, mucus hypersecretion, subepithelial fibrosis, physiologic abnormalities, and eotaxin production. *J Clin Invest* 1999; 103:779–788.
22. Zhu Z, Ma B, Zheng T *et al*. IL-13-induced chemokine responses in the lung: role of CCR2 in the pathogenesis of IL-13-induced inflammation and remodeling. *J Immunol* 2002; 168:2953–2962.
23. Virchow JC Jr, Kroegel C, Hage U, Kortsik C, Matthys H, Werner P. Comparison of sputum-ECP levels in bronchial asthma and chronic bronchitis. *Allergy* 1993; 48(suppl):112–118; discussion 143–145.
24. Kallenbach J, Baynes R, Fine B, Dajee D, Bezwoda W. Persistent neutrophil activation in mild asthma. *J Allergy Clin Immunol* 1992; 90:272–274.
25. Jatakanon A, Uasuf C, Maziak W, Lim S, Chung KF, Barnes PJ. Neutrophilic inflammation in severe persistent asthma. *Am J Respir Crit Care Med* 1999; 160(pt 1):1532–1539.
26. Lamblin C, Gosset P, Tillie-Leblond I *et al*. Bronchial neutrophilia in patients with noninfectious status asthmaticus. *Am J Respir Crit Care Med* 1998; 157:394–402.
27. Wenzel SE, Szefler SJ, Leung DY, Sloan SI, Rex MD, Martin RJ. Bronchoscopic evaluation of severe asthma. Persistent inflammation associated with high dose glucocorticoids. *Am J Respir Crit Care Med* 1997; 156(pt 1):737–743.
28. Wenzel SE, Schwartz LB, Langmack EL *et al*. Evidence that severe asthma can be divided pathologically into two inflammatory subtypes with distinct physiologic and clinical characteristics. *Am J Respir Crit Care Med* 1999; 160:1001–1008.
29. de Blic J, Tillie-Leblond I, Tonnel AB, Jaubert F, Scheinmann P, Gosset P. Difficult asthma in children: an analysis of airway inflammation. *J Allergy Clin Immunol* 2004; 113:94–100.
30. Azzawi M, Johnston PW, Majumdar S, Kay AB, Jeffery PK. T lymphocytes and activated eosinophils in airway mucosa in fatal asthma and cystic fibrosis. *Am Rev Respir Dis* 1992; 145:1477–1482.
31. Sur S, Crotty TB, Kephart GM *et al*. Sudden-onset fatal asthma. A distinct entity with few eosinophils and relatively more neutrophils in the airway submucosa? *Am Rev Respir Dis* 1993; 148:713–719.
32. Carroll N, Carello S, Cooke C, James A. Airway structure and inflammatory cells in fatal attacks of asthma. *Eur Respir J* 1996; 9:709–715.
33. Balzar S, Chu HW, Strand M, Wenzel S. Relationship of small airway chymase-positive mast cells and lung function in severe asthma. *Am J Respir Crit Care Med* 2005; 171:431–439.
34. Holgate ST. The role of mast cells and basophils in inflammation. *Clin Exp Allergy* 2000; 30(suppl 1): 28–32.
35. Price KS, Friend DS, Mellor EA, De Jesus N, Watts GF, Boyce JA. CC chemokine receptor 3 mobilizes to the surface of human mast cells and potentiates immunoglobulin E-dependent generation of interleukin 13. *Am J Respir Cell Mol Biol* 2003; 28:420–427.
36. Brightling CE, Ammit AJ, Kaur D *et al*. The CXCL10/CXCR3 axis mediates human lung mast cell migration to asthmatic airway smooth muscle. *Am J Respir Crit Care Med* 2005; 171:1103–1108.
37. Middleton J, Patterson AM, Gardner L, Schmutz C, Ashton BA. Leukocyte extravasation: chemokine transport and presentation by the endothelium. *Blood* 2002; 100:3853–3860.
38. Butcher EC. Leukocyte-endothelial cell recognition: three (or more) steps to specificity and diversity. *Cell* 1991; 67:1033–1036.
39. Springer TA. Traffic signals for lymphocyte recirculation and leukocyte emigration: the multistep paradigm. *Cell* 1994; 76:301–314.
40. Lukacs NW. Role of chemokines in the pathogenesis of asthma. *Nat Rev Immunol* 2001; 1:108–116.
41. Campbell JJ, Hedrick J, Zlotnik A, Siani MA, Thompson DA, Butcher EC. Chemokines and the arrest of lymphocytes rolling under flow conditions. *Science* 1998; 279:381–384.

42. Kunkel EJ, Boisvert J, Murphy K *et al*. Expression of the chemokine receptors CCR4, CCR5, and CXCR3 by human tissue-infiltrating lymphocytes. *Am J Pathol* 2002; 160:347–355.

43. Sampson AP. The role of eosinophils and neutrophils in inflammation. *Clin Exp Allergy* 2000; 30(suppl 1): 22–27.

44. Shinagawa K, Trifilieff A, Anderson GP. Involvement of CCR3 reactive chemokines in eosinophil survival. *Int Arch Allergy Immunol* 2003; 130:150–157.

45. Woolley KL, Gibson PG, Carty K, Wilson AJ, Twaddell SH, Woolley MJ. Eosinophil apoptosis and the resolution of airway inflammation in asthma. *Am J Respir Crit Care Med* 1996; 154:237–243.

46. Hall SE, Savill JS, Henson PM, Haslett C. Apoptotic neutrophils are phagocytosed by fibroblasts with participation of the fibroblast vitronectin receptor and involvement of a mannose/fucose-specific lectin. *J Immunol* 1994; 153:3218–3227.

47. Savill J, Smith J, Sarraf C, Ren Y, Abbott F, Rees A. Glomerular mesangial cells and inflammatory macrophages ingest neutrophils undergoing apoptosis. *Kidney Int* 1992; 42:924–936.

48. Savill JS, Henson PM, Haslett C. Phagocytosis of aged human neutrophils by macrophages is mediated by a novel 'charge-sensitive' recognition mechanism. *J Clin Invest* 1989; 84:1518–1527.

49. Haslett C. Granulocyte apoptosis and its role in the resolution and control of lung inflammation. *Am J Respir Crit Care Med* 1999; 160(pt 2):S5–S11.

50. Haslett C. Resolution of acute inflammation and the role of apoptosis in the tissue fate of granulocytes. *Clin Sci (Lond)* 1992; 83:639–648.

51. Lukacs NW, Oliveira SH, Hogaboam CM. Chemokines and asthma: redundancy of function or a coordinated effort? *J Clin Invest* 1999; 104:995–999.

52. Sallusto F, Mackay CR, Lanzavecchia A. Selective expression of the eotaxin receptor CCR3 by human T helper 2 cells. *Science* 1997; 277:2005–2007.

53. Brightling CE, Bradding P, Symon FA, Holgate ST, Wardlaw AJ, Pavord ID. Mast-cell infiltration of airway smooth muscle in asthma. *N Engl J Med* 2002; 346:1699–1705.

54. Ochi H, Hirani WM, Yuan Q, Friend DS, Austen KF, Boyce JA. T helper cell type 2 cytokine-mediated comitogenic responses and CCR3 expression during differentiation of human mast cells in vitro. *J Exp Med* 1999; 190:267–280.

55. Ying S, Robinson DS, Meng Q *et al*. Enhanced expression of eotaxin and CCR3 mRNA and protein in atopic asthma. Association with airway hyperresponsiveness and predominant co-localization of eotaxin mRNA to bronchial epithelial and endothelial cells. *Eur J Immunol* 1997; 27:3507–3516.

56. Lukacs NW, Prosser DM, Wiekowski M, Lira SA, Cook DN. Requirement for the chemokine receptor CCR6 in allergic pulmonary inflammation. *J Exp Med* 2001; 194:551–555.

57. Yang Y, Loy J, Ryseck RP, Carrasco D, Bravo R. Antigen-induced eosinophilic lung inflammation develops in mice deficient in chemokine eotaxin. *Blood* 1998; 92:3912–3923.

58. Chensue SW, Lukacs NW, Yang TY *et al*. Aberrant in vivo T helper type 2 cell response and impaired eosinophil recruitment in CC chemokine receptor 8 knockout mice. *J Exp Med* 2001; 193:573–584.

59. Goya I, Villares R, Zaballos A *et al*. Absence of CCR8 does not impair the response to ovalbumin-induced allergic airway disease. *J Immunol* 2003; 170:2138–2146.

60. Chung CD, Kuo F, Kumer J *et al*. CCR8 is not essential for the development of inflammation in a mouse model of allergic airway disease. *J Immunol* 2003; 170:581–587.

61. Bousquet J, Jeffery PK, Busse WW, Johnson M, Vignola AM. Asthma. From bronchoconstriction to airways inflammation and remodeling. *Am J Respir Crit Care Med* 2000; 161:1720–1745.

62. Laitinen A, Altraja A, Kampe M, Linden M, Virtanen I, Laitinen LA. Tenascin is increased in airway basement membrane of asthmatics and decreased by an inhaled steroid. *Am J Respir Crit Care Med* 1997; 156(pt 1):951–958.

63. Hoshino M, Nakamura Y, Sim J, Shimojo J, Isogai S. Bronchial subepithelial fibrosis and expression of matrix metalloproteinase-9 in asthmatic airway inflammation. *J Allergy Clin Immunol* 1998; 102:783–788.

64. Blyth DI, Wharton TF, Pedrick MS, Savage TJ, Sanjar S. Airway subepithelial fibrosis in a murine model of atopic asthma: suppression by dexamethasone or anti-interleukin-5 antibody. *Am J Respir Cell Mol Biol* 2000; 23:241–246.

65. Minshall EM, Hogg JC, Hamid QA. Cytokine mRNA expression in asthma is not restricted to the large airways. *J Allergy Clin Immunol* 1998; 101:386–390.

66. Wenzel S. Severe/fatal asthma. *Chest* 2003; 123(suppl):405S–410S.

67. Wenzel SE, Trudeau JB, Barnes S *et al*. TGF-beta and IL-13 synergistically increase eotaxin-1 production in human airway fibroblasts. *J Immunol* 2002; 169:4613–4619.

68. Desmouliere A, Geinoz A, Gabbiani F, Gabbiani G. Transforming growth factor-beta 1 induces alpha-smooth muscle actin expression in granulation tissue myofibroblasts and in quiescent and growing cultured fibroblasts. *J Cell Biol* 1993; 122:103–111.

69. Doucet C, Brouty-Boye D, Pottin-Clemenceau C, Jasmin C, Canonica GW, Azzarone B. IL-4 and IL-13 specifically increase adhesion molecule and inflammatory cytokine expression in human lung fibroblasts. *Int Immunol* 1998; 10:1421–1433.

70. Gizycki MJ, Adelroth E, Rogers AV, O'Byrne PM, Jeffery PK. Myofibroblast involvement in the allergen-induced late response in mild atopic asthma. *Am J Respir Cell Mol Biol* 1997; 16:664–673.

71. Brewster CE, Howarth PH, Djukanovic R, Wilson J, Holgate ST, Roche WR. Myofibroblasts and subepithelial fibrosis in bronchial asthma. *Am J Respir Cell Mol Biol* 1990; 3:507–511.

72. Zhang K, Rekhter MD, Gordon D, Phan SH. Myofibroblasts and their role in lung collagen gene expression during pulmonary fibrosis. A combined immunohistochemical and in situ hybridization study. *Am J Pathol* 1994; 145:114–125.

73. Hogaboam CM, Bone-Larson CL, Lipinski S *et al.* Differential monocyte chemoattractant protein-1 and chemokine receptor 2 expression by murine lung fibroblasts derived from Th1- and Th2-type pulmonary granuloma models. *J Immunol* 1999; 163:2193–2201.

74. Smith RE, Strieter RM, Phan SH, Kunkel SL. C-C chemokines: novel mediators of the profibrotic inflammatory response to bleomycin challenge. *Am J Respir Cell Mol Biol* 1996; 15:693–702.

75. Gharaee-Kermani M, Denholm EM, Phan SH. Costimulation of fibroblast collagen and transforming growth factor beta1 gene expression by monocyte chemoattractant protein-1 via specific receptors. *J Biol Chem* 1996; 271:17779–17784.

76. Blease K, Mehrad B, Standiford TJ *et al.* Airway remodeling is absent in CCR1−/− mice during chronic fungal allergic airway disease. *J Immunol* 2000; 165:1564–1572.

77. Teran LM, Mochizuki M, Bartels J *et al.* Th1- and Th2-type cytokines regulate the expression and production of eotaxin and RANTES by human lung fibroblasts. *Am J Respir Cell Mol Biol* 1999; 20:777–786.

78. Chibana K, Ishii Y, Asakura T, Fukuda T. Up-regulation of cysteinyl leukotriene 1 receptor by IL-13 enables human lung fibroblasts to respond to leukotriene C4 and produce eotaxin. *J Immunol* 2003; 170:4290–4295.

79. Li Q, Park PW, Wilson CL, Parks WC. Matrilysin shedding of syndecan-1 regulates chemokine mobilization and transepithelial efflux of neutrophils in acute lung injury. *Cell* 2002; 111:635–646.

80. Van den Steen PE, Proost P, Wuyts A, Van Damme J, Opdenakker G. Neutrophil gelatinase B potentiates interleukin-8 tenfold by aminoterminal processing, whereas it degrades CTAP-III, PF-4, and GRO-alpha and leaves RANTES and MCP-2 intact. *Blood* 2000; 96:2673–2681.

81. Epperly MW, Guo H, Gretton JE, Greenberger JS. Bone marrow origin of myofibroblasts in irradiation pulmonary fibrosis. *Am J Respir Cell Mol Biol* 2003; 29:213–224.

82. Schmidt M, Sun G, Stacey MA, Mori L, Mattoli S. Identification of circulating fibrocytes as precursors of bronchial myofibroblasts in asthma. *J Immunol* 2003; 171:380–389.

83. Bucala R, Spiegel LA, Chesney J, Hogan M, Cerami A. Circulating fibrocytes define a new leukocyte subpopulation that mediates tissue repair. *Mol Med* 1994; 1:71–81.

84. Abe R, Donnelly SC, Peng T, Bucala R, Metz CN. Peripheral blood fibrocytes: differentiation pathway and migration to wound sites. *J Immunol* 2001; 166:7556–7562.

85. Chesney J, Bucala R. Peripheral blood fibrocytes: mesenchymal precursor cells and the pathogenesis of fibrosis. *Curr Rheumatol Rep* 2000; 2:501–505.

86. Chesney J, Metz C, Stavitsky AB, Bacher M, Bucala R. Regulated production of type I collagen and inflammatory cytokines by peripheral blood fibrocytes. *J Immunol* 1998; 160:419–425.

87. Hashimoto N, Jin H, Liu T, Chensue SW, Phan SH. Bone marrow-derived progenitor cells in pulmonary fibrosis. *J Clin Invest* 2004; 113:243–252.

88. Moore BB, Murray L, Das A, Wilke CA, Herrygers AB, Toews GB. The role of CCL12 in the recruitment of fibrocytes and lung fibrosis. *Am J Respir Cell Mol Biol* 2006; 35:175–181.

89. Phillips RJ, Burdick MD, Hong K *et al.* Circulating fibrocytes traffic to the lungs in response to CXCL12 and mediate fibrosis. *J Clin Invest* 2004; 114:438–446.

90. Moore BB, Kolodsick JE, Thannickal VJ *et al.* CCR2-mediated recruitment of fibrocytes to the alveolar space after fibrotic injury. *Am J Pathol* 2005; 166:675–684.

91. Takizawa T, Thurlbeck WM. Muscle and mucous gland size in the major bronchi of patients with chronic bronchitis, asthma, and asthmatic bronchitis. *Am Rev Respir Dis* 1971; 104:331–336.

92. Dunnill MS. The pathology of asthma. *Ciba Found Study Group* 1971; 38:35–46.

93. Pare PD, Bai TR, Roberts CR. The structural and functional consequences of chronic allergic inflammation of the airways. *Ciba Found Symp* 1997; 206:71–86; discussion 86–89, 106–110.

94. Saetta M, Di Stefano A, Rosina C, Thiene G, Fabbri LM. Quantitative structural analysis of peripheral airways and arteries in sudden fatal asthma. *Am Rev Respir Dis* 1991; 143:138–143.

95. Sobonya RE. Quantitative structural alterations in long standing allergic asthma. *Am Rev Respir Dis* 1984; 130:289–292.

96. Hogg JC. Pathology of asthma. *J Allergy Clin Immunol* 1993; 92(pt 1):1–5.

97. Knox AJ. Airway re-modelling in asthma: role of airway smooth muscle. *Clin Sci (Lond)* 1994; 86:647–652.

98. Johnson PR, Roth M, Tamm M *et al*. Airway smooth muscle cell proliferation is increased in asthma. *Am J Respir Crit Care Med* 2001; 164:474–477.

99. Noveral JP, Grunstein MM. Role and mechanism of thromboxane-induced proliferation of cultured airway smooth muscle cells. *Am J Physiol* 1992; 263(pt 1):L555–L561.

100. Stewart AG, Grigoriadis G, Harris T. Mitogenic actions of endothelin-1 and epidermal growth factor in cultured airway smooth muscle. *Clin Exp Pharmacol Physiol* 1994; 21:277–285.

101. De S, Zelazny ET, Souhrada JF, Souhrada M. IL-1 beta and IL-6 induce hyperplasia and hypertrophy of cultured guinea pig airway smooth muscle cells. *J Appl Physiol* 1995; 78:1555–1563.

102. Brar SS, Kennedy TP, Sturrock AB *et al*. NADPH oxidase promotes NF-kappaB activation and proliferation in human airway smooth muscle. *Am J Physiol Lung Cell Mol Physiol* 2002; 282:L782–L795.

103. Brar SS, Kennedy TP, Whorton AR, Murphy TM, Chitano P, Hoidal JR. Requirement for reactive oxygen species in serum-induced and platelet-derived growth factor-induced growth of airway smooth muscle. *J Biol Chem* 1999; 274:20017–20026.

104. Kodali RB, Kim WJ, Galaria II *et al*. CCL11 (Eotaxin) induces CCR3-dependent smooth muscle cell migration. *Arterioscler Thromb Vasc Biol* 2004; 24:1211–1216.

105. Viedt C, Vogel J, Athanasiou T *et al*. Monocyte chemoattractant protein-1 induces proliferation and interleukin-6 production in human smooth muscle cells by differential activation of nuclear factor-kappaB and activator protein-1. *Arterioscler Thromb Vasc Biol* 2002; 22:914–920.

106. John M, Hirst SJ, Jose PJ *et al*. Human airway smooth muscle cells express and release RANTES in response to T helper 1 cytokines: regulation by T helper 2 cytokines and corticosteroids. *J Immunol* 1997; 158:1841–1847.

107. Fahy JV. Goblet cell and mucin gene abnormalities in asthma. *Chest* 2002; 122(suppl):320S–326S.

108. Ordonez CL, Khashayar R, Wong HH *et al*. Mild and moderate asthma is associated with airway goblet cell hyperplasia and abnormalities in mucin gene expression. *Am J Respir Crit Care Med* 2001; 163:517–523.

109. Sidebotham HJ, Roche WR. Asthma deaths; persistent and preventable mortality. *Histopathology* 2003; 43:105–117.

110. Voynow JA, Fischer BM, Malarkey DE *et al*. Neutrophil elastase induces mucus cell metaplasia in mouse lung. *Am J Physiol Lung Cell Mol Physiol* 2004; 287:L1293–L1302.

111. Kim S, Nadel JA. Role of neutrophils in mucus hypersecretion in COPD and implications for therapy. *Treat Respir Med* 2004; 3:147–159.

112. Dunnill MS. The pathology of asthma, with special reference to changes in the bronchial mucosa. *J Clin Pathol* 1960; 13:27–33.

113. Walzer I, Frost TT. Death occurring in bronchial asthma; a report of five cases. *J Allergy* 1952; 23:204–214.

114. Orsida BE, Li X, Hickey B, Thien F, Wilson JW, Walters EH. Vascularity in asthmatic airways: relation to inhaled steroid dose. *Thorax* 1999; 54:289–295.

115. Vrugt B, Wilson S, Bron A, Holgate ST, Djukanovic R, Aalbers R. Bronchial angiogenesis in severe glucocorticoid-dependent asthma. *Eur Respir J* 2000; 15:1014–1021.

116. Strieter RM, Burdick MD, Gomperts BN, Belperio JA, Keane MP. CXC chemokines in angiogenesis. *Cytokine Growth Factor Rev* 2005; 16:593–609.

117. Hoshino M, Aoike N, Takahashi M, Nakamura Y, Nakagawa T. Increased immunoreactivity of stromal cell-derived factor-1 and angiogenesis in asthma. *Eur Respir J* 2003; 21:804–809.

118. MacGlashan DW Jr, Bochner BS, Adelman DC *et al*. Down-regulation of Fc(epsilon)RI expression on human basophils during in vivo treatment of atopic patients with anti-IgE antibody. *J Immunol* 1997; 158:1438–1445.

119. Djukanovic R, Wilson SJ, Kraft M *et al*. Effects of treatment with anti-immunoglobulin E antibody omalizumab on airway inflammation in allergic asthma. *Am J Respir Crit Care Med* 2004; 170:583–593.

120. Fahy JV, Fleming HE, Wong HH *et al*. The effect of an anti-IgE monoclonal antibody on the early- and late-phase responses to allergen inhalation in asthmatic subjects. *Am J Respir Crit Care Med* 1997; 155:1828–1834.

121. Soler M, Matz J, Townley R *et al*. The anti-IgE antibody omalizumab reduces exacerbations and steroid requirement in allergic asthmatics. *Eur Respir J* 2001; 18:254–261.

122. Buhl R, Hanf G, Soler M *et al*. The anti-IgE antibody omalizumab improves asthma-related quality of life in patients with allergic asthma. *Eur Respir J* 2002; 20:1088–1094.

123. Buhl R, Soler M, Matz J *et al*. Omalizumab provides long-term control in patients with moderate-to-severe allergic asthma. *Eur Respir J* 2002; 20:73–78.

124. Busse W, Corren J, Lanier BQ *et al*. Omalizumab, anti-IgE recombinant humanized monoclonal antibody, for the treatment of severe allergic asthma. *J Allergy Clin Immunol* 2001; 108:184–190.

125. Howarth PH, Babu KS, Arshad HS *et al*. Tumour necrosis factor (TNFalpha) as a novel therapeutic target in symptomatic corticosteroid dependent asthma. *Thorax* 2005; 60:1012–1018.

126. Berry MA, Hargadon B, Shelley M *et al*. Evidence of a role of tumor necrosis factor alpha in refractory asthma. *N Engl J Med* 2006; 354:697–708.

127. Clutterbuck EJ, Hirst EM, Sanderson CJ. Human interleukin-5 (IL-5) regulates the production of eosinophils in human bone marrow cultures: comparison and interaction with IL-1, IL-3, IL-6, and GMCSF. *Blood* 1989; 73:1504–1512.

128. Yamaguchi Y, Hayashi Y, Sugama Y *et al*. Highly purified murine interleukin 5 (IL-5) stimulates eosinophil function and prolongs in vitro survival. IL-5 as an eosinophil chemotactic factor. *J Exp Med* 1988; 167:1737–1742.

129. Mauser PJ, Pitman AM, Fernandez X *et al*. Effects of an antibody to interleukin-5 in a monkey model of asthma. *Am J Respir Crit Care Med* 1995; 152:467–472.

130. Leckie MJ, ten Brinke A, Khan J *et al*. Effects of an interleukin-5 blocking monoclonal antibody on eosinophils, airway hyperresponsiveness, and the late asthmatic response. *Lancet* 2000; 356:2144–2148.

131. Flood-Page P, Menzies-Gow A, Phipps S *et al*. Anti-IL-5 treatment reduces deposition of ECM proteins in the bronchial subepithelial basement membrane of mild atopic asthmatics. *J Clin Invest* 2003; 112:1029–1036.

132. Kips JC, O'Connor BJ, Langley SJ *et al*. Effect of SCH55700, a humanized anti-human interleukin-5 antibody, in severe persistent asthma: a pilot study. *Am J Respir Crit Care Med* 2003; 167:1655–1659.

133. Stellato C, Brummet ME, Plitt JR *et al*. Expression of the C-C chemokine receptor CCR3 in human airway epithelial cells. *J Immunol* 2001; 166:1457–1461.

134. Kelsen SG, Aksoy MO, Yang Y *et al*. The chemokine receptor CXCR3 and its splice variant are expressed in human airway epithelial cells. *Am J Physiol Lung Cell Mol Physiol* 2004; 287:L584–L591.

135. Strieter RM, Lukacs NW, Standiford TJ, Kunkel SL. Cytokines. 2. Cytokines and lung inflammation: mechanisms of neutrophil recruitment to the lung. *Thorax* 1993; 48:765–769.

136. Heiman AS, Abonyo BO, Darling-Reed SF, Alexander MS. Cytokine-stimulated human lung alveolar epithelial cells release eotaxin-2 (CCL24) and eotaxin-3 (CCL26). *J Interferon Cytokine Res* 2005; 25:82–91.

137. Cohn L, Elias JA, Chupp GL. Asthma: mechanisms of disease persistence and progression. *Annu Rev Immunol* 2004; 22:789–815.

138. Chetta A, Foresi A, Del Donno M *et al*. Bronchial responsiveness to distilled water and methacholine and its relationship to inflammation and remodeling of the airways in asthma. *Am J Respir Crit Care Med* 1996; 153:910–917.

139. Boulet L, Belanger M, Carrier G. Airway responsiveness and bronchial-wall thickness in asthma with or without fixed airflow obstruction. *Am J Respir Crit Care Med* 1995; 152:865–871.

140. Schecter AD, Calderon TM, Berman AB *et al*. Human vascular smooth muscle cells possess functional CCR5. *J Biol Chem* 2000; 275:5466–5471.

141. Strieter RM, Belperio JA, Keane MP. CXC chemokines in angiogenesis related to pulmonary fibrosis. *Chest* 2002; 122(suppl):298S–301S.

142. Salcedo R, Ponce ML, Young HA *et al*. Human endothelial cells express CCR2 and respond to MCP-1: direct role of MCP-1 in angiogenesis and tumor progression. *Blood* 2000; 96:34–40.

143. Lasagni L, Francalanci M, Annunziato F *et al*. An alternatively spliced variant of CXCR3 mediates the inhibition of endothelial cell growth induced by IP-10, Mig, and I-TAC, and acts as functional receptor for platelet factor 4. *J Exp Med* 2003; 197:1537–1549.

144. Traynor TR, Kuziel WA, Toews GB, Huffnagle GB. CCR2 expression determines T1 versus T2 polarization during pulmonary Cryptococcus neoformans infection. *J Immunol* 2000; 164:2021–2027.

145. Campbell EM, Charo IF, Kunkel SL *et al.* Monocyte chemoattractant protein-1 mediates cockroach allergen-induced bronchial hyperreactivity in normal but not CCR2−/− mice: the role of mast cells. *J Immunol* 1999; 163:2160–2167.

146. MacLean JA, De Sanctis GT, Ackerman KG *et al.* CC chemokine receptor-2 is not essential for the development of antigen-induced pulmonary eosinophilia and airway hyperresponsiveness. *J Immunol* 2000; 165:6568–6575.

147. Ma W, Bryce PJ, Humbles AA *et al.* CCR3 is essential for skin eosinophilia and airway hyperresponsiveness in a murine model of allergic skin inflammation. *J Clin Invest* 2002; 109:621–628.

148. Schuh JM, Power CA, Proudfoot AE, Kunkel SL, Lukacs NW, Hogaboam CM. Airway hyperresponsiveness, but not airway remodeling, is attenuated during chronic pulmonary allergic responses to Aspergillus in CCR4−/− mice. *FASEB J* 2002; 16:1313–1315.

149. Forster R, Schubel A, Breitfeld D *et al.* CCR7 coordinates the primary immune response by establishing functional microenvironments in secondary lymphoid organs. *Cell* 1999; 99:23–33.

150. De Sanctis GT, MacLean JA, Qin S *et al.* Interleukin-8 receptor modulates IgE production and B-cell expansion and trafficking in allergen-induced pulmonary inflammation. *J Clin Invest* 1999; 103:507–515.

151. Gonzalo JA, Lloyd CM, Peled A, Delaney T, Coyle AJ, Gutierrez-Ramos JC. Critical involvement of the chemotactic axis CXCR4/stromal cell-derived factor-1 alpha in the inflammatory component of allergic airway disease. *J Immunol* 2000; 165:499–508.

152. Lukacs NW, Berlin A, Schols D, Skerlj RT, Bridger GJ. AMD3100, a CxCR4 antagonist, attenuates allergic lung inflammation and airway hyperreactivity. *Am J Pathol* 2002; 160:1353–1360.

153. Gonzalo JA, Lloyd CM, Kremer L *et al.* Eosinophil recruitment to the lung in a murine model of allergic inflammation. The role of T cells, chemokines, and adhesion receptors. *J Clin Invest* 1996; 98:2332–2345.

154. Bishop B, Lloyd CM. CC chemokine ligand 1 promotes recruitment of eosinophils but not Th2 cells during the development of allergic airways disease. *J Immunol* 2003; 170:4810–4817.

155. Gu L, Tseng S, Horner RM, Tam C, Loda M, Rollins BJ. Control of TH2 polarization by the chemokine monocyte chemoattractant protein-1. *Nature* 2000; 404:407–411.

156. Murray LA, Syed F, Li L, Griswold DE, Das AM. Role of chemokines in severe asthma. *Curr Drug Targets* 2006; 7:579–588.

13

Antagonism of the chemokine receptor CCR3 as a potential therapeutic treatment for asthma

E. Wise, J. E. Pease

INTRODUCTION

The incidence of allergic disease such as asthma and atopic dermatitis in the Western world is rising. Such diseases arise due to an undesirable type-2 response to an otherwise inno-cuous antigen (or allergen) and are characterized by an increase in the number of inflam-matory cells within the affected tissue, e.g. eosinophils, T helper (Th)2 lymphocytes, basophils and mast cells. These cells mediate the inflammatory response *via* the release of mediators such as bioactive lipids, cytokines and charged granular proteins, contributing to the pathology of allergic disease. The specific recruitment of inflammatory cells to the site of an allergic response is mediated by the local production of *chemo*attractant cyto*kines* or chemokines, which act on chemokine receptors expressed on the surface of these cells. Several chemokines and their receptors have been implicated in the pathogenesis of allergic disease; this chapter will focus upon the role of the eosinophil and the selective recruitment of this cell. This is achieved primarily by interactions between the eotaxin family of chemokines and the cell surface receptor CCR3.

THE IMPORTANCE OF THE EOSINOPHIL IN ALLERGIC DISEASE

The accumulation of eosinophils within the bronchial wall is a characteristic feature of asthma [1]. Once recruited, eosinophils are capable of releasing bioactive lipids such as LTC_4 that induce bronchoconstriction and mucus hypersecretion. Eosinophils can also induce tis-sue damage by the release of granule proteins such as major basic protein, eosinophil cationic protein and eosinophil peroxidase, a function which relates to their traditionally perceived role of protecting the host against parasitic worms. Eosinophil activation and granule release is thought to play a significant role in the underlying bronchial hyper-reactivity that is a hallmark of human asthma [2, 3].

An additional, long-term consequence of allergic inflammation is the associated structural changes in the tissue. In diseases such as asthma, this manifests itself as airway remodelling, the hallmarks of which include subepithelial fibrosis, myofibroblast accumulation, airway smooth muscle hyperplasia and hypertrophy, mucous gland and goblet cell hyperplasia accompanied by disruption of the epithelium layer [4]. The exact molecular mechanisms

Emma Wise, BSc, PhD, Research Associate, Leukocyte Biology Section, National Heart and Lung Institute, Faculty of Medicine, Imperial College London, UK

James Edward Pease, BSc, PhD, Reader in Leukocyte Biology, Leukocyte Biology Section, National Heart and Lung Institute, Faculty of Medicine, Imperial College London, UK

involved remain to be elucidated, but eosinophils have been implicated in the process since they are known to be sources for a range of profibrotic factors such as transforming growth factor β (TGFβ) and fibroblast growth factor-2 (FGF-2) [5].

SELECTIVE RECRUITMENT OF LEUCOCYTES BY THE EOTAXIN FAMILY OF CHEMOKINES

Selective leucocyte recruitment in both inflammatory and homeostatic processes is governed by chemokines. These are a family of small basic proteins, which, in humans, number more than forty. Chemokines act on distinct subsets of leucocytes *via* specific G protein-coupled receptors (GPCRs) expressed on the cell surface [6]. Together, the chemokines and their receptors govern multiple aspects of host defence and inflammation, including leucocyte trafficking, haematopoiesis, and angiogenesis [7–9]. The family can be divided into two major subsets by examination of conserved amino-terminal cysteine residues. The CXC class have a single amino acid interposed between these cysteines and are mainly active on neutrophils and T lymphocytes, whilst in the CC class the cysteines are adjacent and the chemokines typically are attractants for monocytes, basophils, eosinophils and lymphocytes, but not neutrophils.

The first predominantly eosinophil-selective chemoattractant was isolated following the protein purification of bronchoalveolar lavage (BAL) fluid taken from allergen-challenged, sensitized guinea pigs [10]. It was appropriately named 'eotaxin' as it was found to specifically recruit eosinophils when intradermally injected into naïve recipients [10]. Protein sequencing revealed it to be a member of the growing CC family of chemokines. The cDNA encoding eotaxin was subsequently cloned [11], followed by the identification of human [12], murine [13] and rat [14] orthologues. Following a meeting of the chemokine community in 1999, the nomenclature of chemokines was standardized and eotaxin is now also known as CCL11 [7]. This chemokine is expressed by many cells [15–25] (Figure 13.1, Table 13.1) and its generation within the lung appears to be dependent upon the presence of

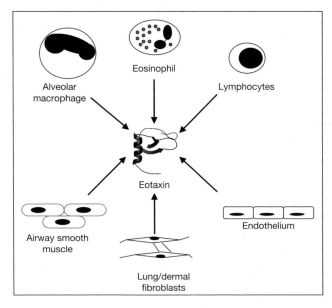

Figure 13.1 Eotaxin/CCL11 is produced by a variety of cells. These include both structural cells such as endothelial and smooth muscle cells and also those of the immune system, such as macrophages and lymphocytes.

Table 13.1 The Eotaxin family of chemokines

Colloquial name	Systematic name	Chromosomal location	Produced by	References
Eotaxin-1	CCL11	17q21.1–21.2	Endothelial cells	[15]
			Epithelial cells	[15]
			Asthmatic bronchial epithelium	[16]
			IL-4 and IL-13 treated BEAS-2B cells	[17]
			Alveolar macrophages	[18, 19]
			A549 alveolar epithelial cells	[20]
			Lung fibroblasts	[22]
			Dermal fibroblasts	[21]
			Airway smooth muscle cells	[24]
			Eosinophils	[19]
			Lymphocytes	[19]
			Keratinocytes	[25]
Eotaxin-2 (MPIF-2)	CCL24	7q11.23	Nasal endothelium and epithelium	[34]
			Bronchial epithelial cells	[16, 18]
			Asthmatic bronchial epithelium	[16]
			A549 alveolar epithelial cells	[20]
			HaCAT keratinocyte line	[35]
			Monocytes	[36]
Eotaxin-3	CCL26	7q11.23	IL-4-treated HUVEC cells	[37]
			IL-4, IL-13 treated airway smooth muscle cells	[38]
			IL-4 and IL-13 treated BEAS-2B cells	[17]
			A549 alveolar epithelial cells	[20]
			Asthmatic bronchial epithelium	[16]
			Intestinal epithelial cells	[39]
			HaCAT keratinocyte line	[35]

The colloquial and systematic names are shown, together with the chromosomal locations of the relative genes and the cell types reported to produce each chemokine.

T lymphocytes [26]. A combination of the cytokines tumour necrosis factor α (TNFα) and interleukin (IL)-4 has been demonstrated to induce transcription of the CCL11 gene in lung fibroblasts [22] and human airway epithelial cells [23]. In the latter cells, this induction has been shown to be mediated *via* the transcription factors nuclear factor-κB (NF-κB) and STAT-6, respectively with the CCL11 gene promoter containing overlapping consensus binding sites [27]. IL-13, which has been shown to play a prominent role in the aetiology of bronchial hyperreactivity, also appears to act, at least in part, by promoting CCL11 generation [28–30].

The eotaxin family of chemokines also comprises two other members, namely eotaxin-2/CCL24 and eotaxin-3/CCL26 which along with CCL11 selectively bind the chemokine receptor known as CCR3 (Table 13.1). However, despite their similarities in name and their specificity for CCR3, CCL24 and CCL26 have limited identity with CCL11 at the amino acid level (39% and 37%, respectively). In keeping with this, CCL24 and CCL26 are found in a different chromosomal location to CCL11 located on chromosome 7q11.23 in contrast to CCL11, which is found on chromosome 17q11.2 [31, 32]. Since CCL24 and CCL26 are located within a region of ~40 kilobases it has been hypothesized that they evolved by gene duplication from a common ancestor, perhaps independently of CCL11 [32]. In contrast, studies

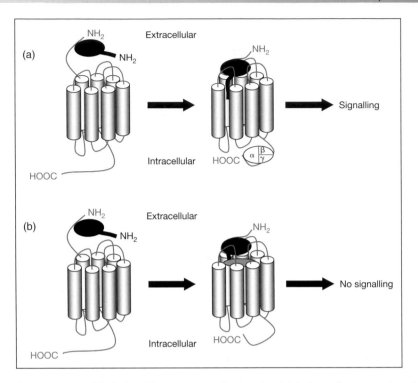

Figure 13.2 The two-step model of chemokine receptor activation. Panel (a) shows the proposed mechanism by which a chemokine receptor is activated by its chemokine. The chemokine (black) is tethered to the chemokine receptor *via* the receptor N-terminus. This tethering facilitates the activation of the receptor by insertion of the chemokine N-terminus in an intrahelical pocket, inducing a conformational change which recruits heterotrimeric G proteins to the intracellular domains of the receptor and results in intracellular signalling. Panel (b) shows the same schematic, but in the presence of a small molecule receptor antagonist (grey disc) which binds to a similar intrahelical pocket to that of the chemokine N-terminus, thereby inhibiting receptor activation.

of the murine genome have only revealed two eotaxin genes, corresponding to CCL11 and CCL24 [33]. As is the case with CCL11, CCL24 and CCL26 are produced by a variety of structural cells and leucocytes [16, 17, 20, 34–39] (Table 13.1).

THE EOTAXIN RECEPTOR, CCR3

Members of the eotaxin family of chemokines exert their effects *via* a GPCR named CCR3, which was independently identified and characterized in 1996, by several labs [40–42]. CCR3 is expressed on the surface of eosinophils [40], Th2 cells [43], basophils [44] and mast cells [45], key players in the process of allergic inflammation. Like other GPCRs, CCR3 contains 7 trans-membrane spanning helical domains and signals predominantly *via* pertussis-sensitive $G_{\alpha i}$ subunits. It is noteworthy that although the eotaxins are highly selective for CCR3 activation, CCR3 itself is highly promiscuous and can be activated by a range of CC chemokines including CCL8/monocycte chemoattractant protein (MCP)-2, CCL7/MCP-3, CCL13/MCP-4 and CCL5/RANTES [46].

It has been established using chimeric CCR3/CCR1 constructs that CCL11 binding and receptor activation occur *via* a two-step model [47] as demonstrated for other chemokine:receptor interactions and illustrated in Figure 13.2(a) [48]. According to this model, the first step comprises a high-affinity interaction between the core residues of the chemokine and the N-terminus of the receptor. Interactions between the N-terminus of the chemokine and the remaining extracellular domains of the receptor backbone are then able to occur. It has been hypothesized that these latter interactions induce conformational changes within the receptor resulting in G protein recruitment and receptor signalling. Highly conserved between chemokine receptors is an aspartate/arginine/tyrosine motif at the cytoplasmic end of the third transmembrane helix, which is thought to hold GPCRs in an inactive conformation in the absence of ligand serving as an 'ionic lock' [49]. Mutation of this domain within CCR3 is poorly tolerated, suggestive of an important function.

FUNCTIONAL CONSEQUENCES OF EOTAXIN/CCL11 SIGNALLING

CCL11-induced signalling in eosinophils is known to trigger chemotaxis *via* the formation of stress fibres and focal adhesions, the release of reactive oxygen species (or respiratory burst) and degranulation and release of cationic granular proteins. Whilst G protein signalling has been shown to be important for these functions, other signalling molecules and pathways play their part. Eosinophil chemotaxis has been shown to be dependent on the mitogen-activated protein kinases (MAPK) p42 and p44 [50], p38 MAPK, ERK2 [51] and the p21 G proteins RhoA and Rock which are important for their ability to induce actin polymerization and the formation of focal adhesions [52]. RhoA, Rock along with protein C kinase, tyrosine kinase and PI3K are also necessary for eosinophil respiratory burst [52, 53]. Similarly, eotaxin-induced eosinophil degranulation has been demonstrated to be dependent on p38 MAPK and ERK2 [51].

THE IMPORTANCE OF EOTAXIN/CCL11 IN EOSINOPHIL MOBILIZATION AND MIGRATION AS BORNE OUT BY *IN VIVO* EXPERIMENTATION

The importance of both CCL11 and CCR3 in both homeostasis and allergic inflammation has been supported by animal models of disease, principally employing the guinea pig and the mouse. In a guinea pig model of allergic inflammation, CCL11 levels in airway tissue and BAL were found to correlate with eosinophil recruitment [54]. Administration to mice of a CCL11 neutralizing antibody resulted in a transient reduction in lung eosinophilia and associated bronchial hyperresponsiveness following allergen challenge with ovalbumin with neutralization of CCL5, CCL12 and CCL2 having similar effects upon eosinophil trafficking in the lung interstitium, suggestive of a coordinated effort involving several chemokines and leucocyte subsets [55]. A subsequent study by the same group examined the role of CCL11 in the recruitment of Th2 lymphocytes in allergic airways disease using an adoptive transfer approach [56] and found that CCL11 was involved in the early phase of Th2 lymphocyte recruitment with the CCR4 ligand CCL22 the principal chemokine involved in the later phase recruitment.

Mice deficient in CCL11 were subsequently employed to further dissect the role of the chemokine in allergic inflammation. Genetic differences between animal strains can lead to conflicting reports in the literature, e.g. BALB/c mice deficient in CCL11 showed a reduction in ovalbumin-induced lung eosinophilia [57]. In contrast, CCL11-deficient mice of the outbred ICR strain exhibited no difference in allergen-driven recruitment of eosinophils to the lung [58]. Whilst CCL11 undeniably has an important role in eosinophil chemotaxis, it has also been shown to act in concert with the important eosinophil survival factor IL-5, promoting eosinophil recruitment from the microcirculation [59] and eosinophil mobilization from the bone marrow [60, 61]. Thus, CCL11 along with other cytokines may further contribute to eosinophilia.

The pivotal role of CCR3 in eosinophil migration has been ably demonstrated by the finding of reduced eosinophil numbers in the airways of intraperitoneally (i.p.) sensitized CCR3-deficient mice, following allergic challenge [62]. Upon closer investigation it was determined that this phenomenon was not due to defective recruitment of eosinophils (since the lung vasculature was full of eosinophils in challenged mice), but rather to a defect in migration from the vasculature into the lung parenchyma. Intriguingly, CCR3$^{-/-}$ mice had elevated airway hyperresponsiveness (AHR) to methacholine upon allergen challenge which was attributed to the increased numbers of intraepithelial mast cells within the trachea. In contrast, a model of allergic skin inflammation using skin sensitization, carried out by the same group, showed that CCR3 was critical for eosinophil migration into the skin and lungs and found that CCR3-deficient mice have reduced AHR responses upon methacholine and allergen challenge [63]. The differences between the differential AHR observed in both models are unclear but were attributed to the different routes of immunization used for allergen sensitization, namely the intraperitoneal route in the former study and the intradermal route in the latter.

Both CCR3 and CCL11 are also important in constitutive eosinophil homing to the gut and consequent homeostasis, as mice deficient in either ligand or receptor show reduced eosinophil numbers in the gut [57, 62]. This is in contrast to CCL24-deficient mice which have been reported to have normal base-line eosinophil levels in the gastrointestinal tract [64].

EOTAXINS IN HUMAN DISEASE

An array of evidence from both *in vitro* and *in vivo* human studies supports the hypotheses derived from animal models, implicating eotaxins in the pathogenesis of allergic disease. CCL11-producing cells have been detected in the sputum of asthmatics 24 h after the inhalation of allergen [64]. These CCL11 positive cells upon closer analysis were found to be mostly macrophages, eosinophils, epithelial cells and lymphocytes. Similarly, cells expressing both CCL11 and CCL24 mRNA and protein have been found in the submucosa and epithelium of bronchial biopsies in asthmatic patients [15, 18, 66]. Likewise, CCL26 has been shown to be produced by airway smooth muscle cells [38].

The eotaxins have been reported to induce eosinophil chemotaxis *in vitro* with CCL26 being an order of magnitude less potent than CCL11 and CCL24 [32, 67]. However, recent work has begun to shed light on the differential roles of this chemokine family in inducing eosinophil migration. In atopic subjects CCL11 mRNA and protein expression was shown to peak at 6 h after intradermal allergen challenge and was found to correlate with early eosinophil infiltration whereas CCL24 mRNA expression was maximal at 24 h and correlated with late infiltrating eosinophils [66]. The role of CCL26 in eosinophil recruitment *in vivo* remains to be elucidated; mRNA for this chemokine has been shown to be upregulated in bronchial biopsies from asthmatics 24 h after challenge [68]. Furthermore, a recent microarray study of patients with eosinophilic oesophagitis has revealed that the CCL26 transcript is the most highly induced mRNA in oesophageal samples from sufferers of this condition when compared to healthy controls [69]. Thus, it would be intriguing to study the expression of this chemokine *in vivo* after allergic challenge and its relationship with eosinophilia and disease.

SELECTIVE ANTAGONISM OF CCR3

For many pharmaceutical companies, CCR3 has been the immediate focus of drug development aimed at treating allergic disease. The expression of the receptor on the surface of cells with a pivotal role in allergic inflammation such as eosinophils, mast cells, Th2 lymphocytes and basophils [40–44, 70], coupled with the abundance of data detailing elevated levels of its ligands in allergic disease, makes for the compelling hypothesis that targeting CCR3 would reduce leucocyte recruitment to inflamed tissues. In the Western world where asthma prevails but parasitic infections are relatively rare, specific blockade of eosinophil recruitment would be anticipated to be without major side-effects.

SMALL MOLECULE ANTAGONISTS OF CCR3

Initial proof-of-principle studies supported the notion that selective CCR3 blockade was feasible, employing blocking monoclonal antibodies raised against human, guinea pig and macaque orthologues of CCR3. These were demonstrated to inhibit CCR3 function both *in vitro* and *in vivo* [46, 71, 72]. Like all other chemokine receptors described to date, CCR3 is a member of the superfamily of GPCRs. Approximately 50% of currently prescribed drugs act at these receptors [73]. Consequently, these targets are deemed to be highly 'druggable' by small molecules, and a potent, well-tolerated small molecule antagonist of CCR3 is a highly desirable, potential therapeutic.

The first small molecule antagonist of CCR3 to be described in the scientific press was UCB 35625 (a trans-isomer of BANYU J113863) which also possesses sub-nanomolar inhibitory activity at the closely-related chemokine receptor, CCR1 [74, 75]. This molecule was a potent inhibitor of eosinophil shape change responses in the gated autofluorescence/forward scatter assay [76], which ourselves and others have used as a convenient means of characterizing eosinophil responses to chemoattractatants [72, 77]. Closely following these reports was the description of two small molecules named SB-297006 and SB-328437 discovered by scientists at SmithKlineBeecham [78]. These two molecules also had low-nanomolar activity at CCR3 and unlike UCB 35625 had little cross-reactivity at CCR1. The bi-specificity of UCB 35625 led us to postulate that the molecule interacts with the highly conserved transmembrane helices of both CCR1 and CCR3, a hypothesis that was supported by subsequent receptor mutagenesis and molecular modelling [79]. The antagonist is believed to dock within an intrahelical pocket which impedes the ability of the chemokine to induce a conformation change in the chemokine receptor required for subsequent intracellular signalling (Figure 13.2(b)).

High-throughput screening of chemical libraries in biotechnology/pharmaceutical companies led to the discovery of several small molecule antagonists of CCR3 with *in vitro* activities typically in the low nanomolar range [74, 75, 77, 78, 80–97] (Figure 13.3 and Table 13.2). In many cases, the further development of small molecules was halted following the publication of data from clinical trials with monoclonal antibodies directed against IL-5 [98, 99]. Neutralization of IL-5 resulted in a dramatic decrease in blood eosinophil levels, presumably by inhibiting IL-5-mediated release from the bone marrow, with little improvement of lung function, bringing into question the role of eosinophils in mediating the symptoms of asthma. Consequently, many in the pharmaceutical industry lost interest in targeting CCR3.

Subsequently, critiques of these studies have challenged trial size and study design [100–102] and more recent studies elucidating the role of the eosinophil in airway remodelling have rekindled interest in CCR3 as a therapeutic target. Deletion of the murine (IL)-5 gene was observed to suppress both lung eosinophilia and tissue remodelling, with a decrease in the growth factor TGFβ_1 [103], correlating with clinical data in which anti-IL-5 blockade resulted in a reduction in the numbers of airway eosinophils expressing mRNA for TGFβ_1 and in the deposition of extracellular matrix proteins in the reticular basement membrane of bronchial biopsies [104]. The recent generation of mice deficient in eosinophils has allowed the role of the cell to be probed further, with data derived from allergen challenge implicating the eosinophil in both airway remodelling [105] and airway hyperresponsiveness [106]. Thus, the notion that CCR3 antagonists might be of benefit in the treatment of asthma is again in vogue.

In addition, the expression of CCR3 on both mature human mast cells and their progenitors [70, 107] suggests that antagonism of this receptor might also prove beneficial in modulating mast cell trafficking and therefore allergic responses. It should be noted, however, that results obtained *in vivo* with CCR3 gene-deleted mice have so far been contradictory in this respect. For example, following infection of CCR3-deficient mice with the nematode *Trichinella spiralis*,

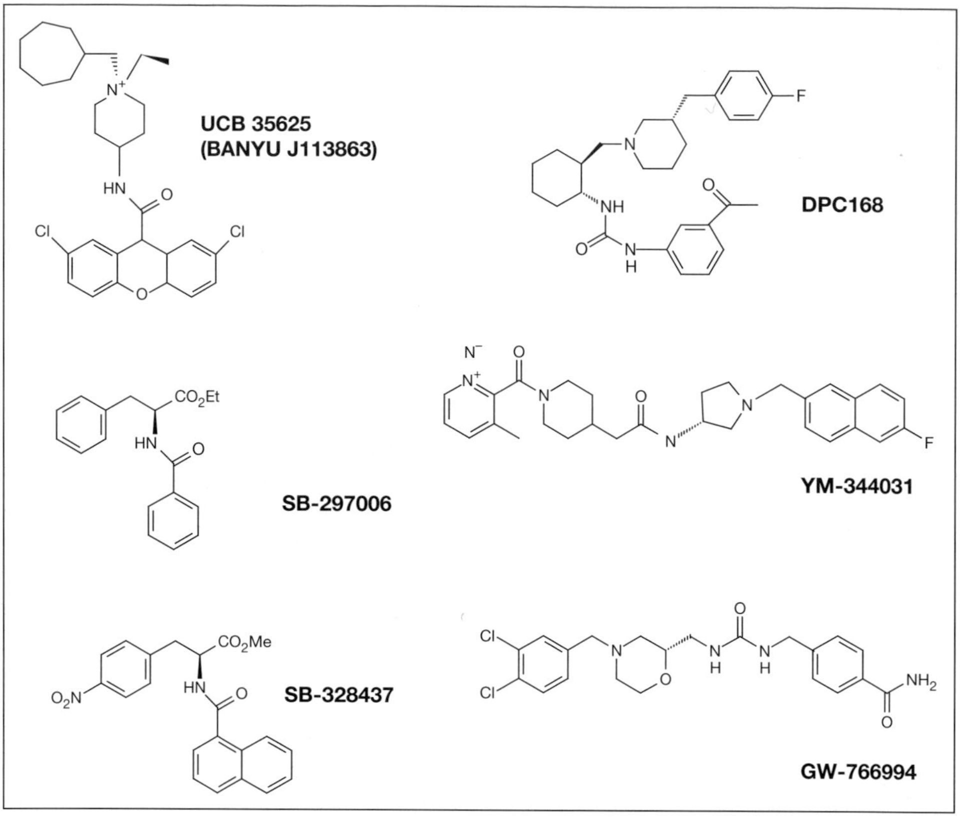

Figure 13.3 A selection of small molecule CCR3 antagonists described in the literature. The chemical structure together with the name of the compound are shown. Further details of the compounds can be found in the main text and in Table 13.2.

a normal mast cell hyperplasia in both the jejunum and caecum was reported, which correlated with unimpaired worm expulsion [108]. In contrast, when sensitized intraperitoneally with ovalbumin and challenged with aerosolized ovalbumin, the same CCR3-deficient mice had increased numbers of tracheal intraepithelial mast cells and an increased hyperresponsiveness compared to wild type mice [62]. This suggests that, in the mouse at least, eosinophils and mast cells have distinct requirements for CCR3 in terms of tissue trafficking.

SUMMARY

Although our knowledge of the chemokine family has greatly enhanced the understanding of the mechanisms underlying allergic reactions, converting this knowledge into effective therapy for allergic diseases still presents major challenges for the future. Before the successful progression of small molecule antagonists into clinical trials, much depends upon the ability of these molecules to be appropriate tools for the *in vivo* blockade of CCR3 in well-established rodent models of allergic inflammation. Since most small molecule antagonists are initially discovered by screens of chemical libraries against the human receptor, the ability of these molecules to cross the species barrier is crucial. Surprisingly, despite significant homology between human and rodent chemokine receptors, this often remains a rate-limiting step. Consequently, despite several publications describing the *in vitro* efficacy

Table 13.2 Small molecule antagonists of CCR3 described in the literature

Company	Antagonist	In vitro data	In vivo data	References
Abbott Laboratories	A-122057 A-122058	Inhibition of CCL11 binding with IC_{50} values of 600 and 975 nM, respectively	Oral dosage of 10 mg/kg, caused a reduction in CCL11-induced peritoneal eosinophilia	[80]
Banyu Pharmaceutical Co. Ltd.	Compound X	Inhibition of CCL11 binding to CCR3 CHO transfectants (IC_{50} = 2.3 nM)	None published to date	[81]
Banyu Pharmaceutical Co. Ltd.	2b/BANYU I	Inhibitor of CCL11 induced Ca^{2+} increases in eosinophils (IC_{50} = 27 nM). Reported 820-fold selectivity for CCR3 over CCR1 receptors. Later characterized as an inverse agonist by scientists at Schering-Plough	None published to date	[83, 84]
Banyu Pharmaceutical Co. Ltd.	J113863/ UCB 35625	Bi-specific antagonist of both hCCR1 and hCCR3 with nanomolar potencies, although is unable to displace ligand at similar concentrations	None published to date	[74, 75]
Boehringer Ingelheim	4a	Inhibition of CCL11 binding (K_i = 110 nM)	None published to date	[85]
Bristol-Myers Squibb	DPC 168	Inhibition of CCL11-induced chemotaxis at hCCR3 (IC_{50} = 10–60 pM) and mCCR3 (IC_{50} = 41 nM)	Dose-dependent reduction of eosinophil recruitment into the lungs of mice in a model of allergic airway inflammation. Entered into phase I clinical trials	[97]
Bristol-Myers Squibb	45	IC_{50} values of 0.7, 0.8 and 0.4 nM in binding, calcium flux and chemotaxis assays respectively	None published to date	[87]
Bristol-Myers Squibb	87	IC_{50} values of 8 and 20 nM in binding and chemotaxis assays respectively	None published to date	[88]

Table 13.2 (continued)

Company	Antagonist	In vitro data	In vivo data	References
GlaxoSmithKline	SB-297006 SB-328437	Inhibition of CCL11 binding to eosinophils. IC_{50} = 39 nM for SB-297006 and 4 nM for SB-328437)	Failure to antagonize the binding of murine or guinea pig CCL11 to corresponding CCR3 orthologues at concentrations up to 10 000 times the IC_{50} for inhibiting human CCR3, precluding in vivo studies	[78]
GlaxoSmithKline	Phenylalanine derivatives	Low nanomolar antagonists of CCR3 binding and chemotaxis	None published to date	[89, 90]
GlaxoSmithKline	GW-766994	None published	Described as having good selectivity, good PK properties in the rat and dog and no significant P450 inhibition. Subsequently entered clinical development	[91]
GlaxoSmithKline	GW-701897B	None published	Prevention of antigen-induced clustering of eosinophils along the vagus nerves and hyper-responsive to vagal stimulation following antigen inhalation in a guinea pig model of airway inflammation	[92]

Company	Compound		Reference
Schering-Plough	4i	Inhibitor of intracellular calcium release (IC_{50} = 215 nM) and of chemotaxis of CCR3 transfectants (IC_{50} = 136 nM)	Very low AUC of 264 ng h/ml at 3 mpk (i.v.) in a rat pharmacokinetic study, precluding advancement into in vivo studies	[93]
Schering-Plough	14n	Inhibitor of CCL11 binding (K_i = 3.5 nM) and human eosinophil chemotaxis (IC_{50} = 160 nM)	Reasonable AUC of 1341 ng h/ml at 10 mpk po in a rat pharmacokinetic study, although lower affinity for the rat receptor (K_i = 2981 nM) resulted in significant challenges with in vivo profiling. Produced an undesired 85% inhibition at 1 mM in the hERG voltage clamp assay precluding further advancement	[94]
Roche Biosciences	RO1164875/608 RO116-9132/238 RO320-2947/001 RO330-0802/001	Low inhibition of CCL11 induced chemotaxis at low nanomolar concentrations	None published to date	[77]
Yamanouchi Pharmaceutical Co.	YM-344031	Inhibition of chemotaxis of human CCR3-expressing cell (IC_{50} = 19.9 nM)	Oral administration to macaques (1–10 mg/kg) significantly inhibited CCL11-induced eosinophil shape change in whole blood. Oral administration to mice (100 mg/kg) prevented both immediate- and late-phase allergic skin reactions	[95]

Table 13.2 (continued)

Company	Antagonist	In vitro data	In vivo data	References
Yamanouchi Pharmaceutical Co.	YM-355179	Inhibtion of intracellular Ca^{2+} influx, chemotaxis, and eosinophil degranulation (Respective IC_{50} values of 8.0, 24, and 29 nM)	Oral administration of YM-355179 (1 mg/kg) inhibited CCL11-induced shape change of whole blood eosinophils in macaques. Intravenous injection of YM-355179 (1 mg/kg) also inhibited eosinophil infiltration into macaque airways following segmental bronchoprovocation with CCL11	[96]

Data describing the reported efficacy of the compounds *in vitro* and *in vivo* is also shown.

of CCR3-specific antagonists, descriptions of their efficacy *in vivo* lag well behind. The small molecule CCR3 antagonist A-122058 (Abbott Laboratories) has been reported to be efficacious in reducing the number of eosinophils in a mouse peritoneal model of eosinophil recruitment following injection with CCL11 [80]. Likewise, the Yamanouchi Pharmaceutical Company have recently described compounds with efficacy in a murine model of cutaneous inflammation [95] and in a macaque model of eosinophil recruitment to the lung following bronchoprovocation with CCL11 [96].

To date, the only small molecule antagonist reported to be in a phase II trial is the compound GW-766994 from GlaxoSmithKline, but no details have been published regarding its efficacy in an allergic asthma and rhinitis study [109]. This follows on from the recent reports of the efficacy of the GlaxoSmithKline compound GW-701897B in reducing vagally-mediated bronchoconstriction in antigen-challenged guinea pigs [92]. An important point is the fact that chemokine antagonists, like many small molecules targeting GPCRs, appear to function by binding to the transmembrane helices. Since these regions are often highly conserved between different receptors, unsurprisingly, some of these compounds have activity at additional receptors [79]. One example of this is the compound UCB 35625, which antagonizes both CCR1 and CCR3 [74]. Data from our laboratory suggest that whilst all individuals express CCR3 on their eosinophils, in around 15–20% of individuals CCR1 is also expressed at high levels [110, 111] rendering the eosinophils of these individuals highly responsive to both CCL11 and CCL3, supporting the hypothesis that the CCR1:CCL3 axis has the potential to recruit eosinophils in allergic disorders affecting a significant proportion of the population. Indeed, expression of CCL3 in the lungs of human asthmatics is well-documented [33, 112, 113]. It might be envisaged that targeting of multiple chemokine receptors with small molecule antagonists may provide a more efficacious therapy for the future treatment of allergic disease.

ACKNOWLEDGEMENTS

The authors are grateful to the Wellcome Trust for funding our research in this area and to Professor Tim Williams for critical reading of this manuscript.

REFERENCES

1. Gleich GJ. Mechanisms of eosinophil-associated inflammation. *J Allergy Clin Immunol* 2000; 105:651–663.
2. Flavahan NA, Slifman NR, Gleich GJ, Vanhoutte PM. Human eosinophil major basic protein causes hyperreactivity of respiratory smooth muscle. Role of the epithelium. *Am Rev Respir Dis* 1988; 138:685–688.
3. Venge P, Dahl R, Fredens K, Peterson CG. Epithelial injury by human eosinophils. *Am Rev Respir Dis* 1988; 138(pt 2):S54–S57.
4. Kay AB, Phipps S, Robinson DS. A role for eosinophils in airway remodelling in asthma. *Trends Immunol* 2004; 25:477–482.
5. Wong DT, Elovic A, Matossian K *et al*. Eosinophils from patients with blood eosinophilia express transforming growth factor beta 1. *Blood* 1991; 78:2702–2707.
6. Rot A, Von Andrian UH. Chemokines in innate and adaptive host defense: basic chemokinese grammar for immune cells. *Annu Rev Immunol* 2004; 22:891–928.
7. Zlotnik A, Yoshie O. Chemokines: a new classification system and their role in immunity. *Immunity* 2000; 12:121–127.
8. Murphy PM, Baggiolini M, Charo IF *et al*. International union of pharmacology. XXII. Nomenclature for chemokine receptors. *Pharmacol Rev* 2000; 52:145–176.
9. Murphy PM. International Union of Pharmacology. XXX. Update on chemokine receptor nomenclature. *Pharmacol Rev* 2002; 54:227–229.
10. Jose PJ, Griffiths-Johnson DA, Collins PD *et al*. Eotaxin: a potent eosinophil chemoattractant cytokine detected in a guinea-pig model of allergic airways inflammation. *J Exp Med* 1994; 179:881–887.
11. Jose PJ, Adcock IM, Griffiths-Johnson DA *et al*. Eotaxin: cloning of an eosinophil chemoattractant cytokine and increased mRNA expression in allergen-challenged guinea-pig lungs. *Biochem Biophys Res Commun* 1994; 205:788–794.

12. Ponath PD, Qin S, Ringler DJ *et al*. Cloning of the human eosinophil chemoattractant, eotaxin. Expression, receptor binding and functional properties suggest a mechanism for the selective recruitment of eosinophils. *J Clin Invest* 1996; 97:604–612.

13. Rothenberg ME, Luster AD, Leder P. Murine eotaxin: an eosinophil chemoattractant inducible in endothelial cells and in interleukin 4-induced tumor suppression. *Proc Natl Acad Sci USA* 1995; 92:8960–8964.

14. Williams CMM, Newton DJ, Wilson SA, Williams TJ, Coleman JW, Flanagan BF. Conserved structure and tissue expression of rat eotaxin. *Immunogenetics* 1998; 47:178–180.

15. Ying S, Robinson DS, Meng Q *et al*. Enhanced expression of eotaxin and CCR3 mRNA and protein in atopic asthma. Association with airway hyperresponsiveness and predominant co-localization of eotaxin mRNA to bronchial epithelial and endothelial cells. *Eur J Immunol* 1997; 27:3507–3516.

16. Komiya A, Nagase H, Yamada H *et al*. Concerted expression of eotaxin-1, eotaxin-2, and eotaxin-3 in human bronchial epithelial cells. *Cell Immunol* 2003; 225:91–100.

17. Kobayashi I, Yamamoto S, Nishi N *et al*. Regulatory mechanisms of Th2 cytokine-induced eotaxin-3 production in bronchial epithelial cells: possible role of interleukin 4 receptor and nuclear factor-kappaB. *Ann Allergy Asthma Immunol* 2004; 93:390–397.

18. Ying S, Meng Q, Zeibecoglou K *et al*. Eosinophil chemotactic chemokines (eotaxin, eotaxin-2, RANTES, monocyte chemoattractant protein-3 (MCP-3), and MCP-4), and C-C chemokine receptor 3 expression in bronchial biopsies from atopic and nonatopic (intrinsic) asthmatics. *J Immunol* 1999; 163:6321–6329.

19. Zeibecoglou K, Macfarlane AJ, Ying S *et al*. Increases in eotaxin-positive cells in induced sputum from atopic asthmatic subjects after inhalational allergen challenge. *Allergy* 1999; 54:730–735.

20. Abonyo BO, Alexander MS, Heiman AS. Autoregulation of CCL26 synthesis and secretion in A549 cells: a possible mechanism by which alveolar epithelial cells modulate airway inflammation. *Am J Physiol Lung Cell Mol Physiol* 2005; 289:L478–L488.

21. Miyamasu M, Yamaguchi M, Nakajima T *et al*. Th1-derived cytokine IFN-gamma is a potent inhibitor of eotaxin synthesis in vitro. *Int Immunol* 1999; 11:1001–1004.

22. Teran LM, Mochizuki M, Bartels J *et al*. Th1- and Th2-type cytokines regulate the expression and production of eotaxin and RANTES by human lung fibroblasts. *Am J Respir Cell Mol Biol* 1999; 20:777–786.

23. Stellato C, Matsukura S, Fal A *et al*. Differential regulation of epithelial-derived C-C chemokine expression by IL-4 and the glucocorticoid budesonide. *J Immunol* 1999; 163:5624–5632.

24. Ghaffar O, Hamid Q, Renzi PM *et al*. Constitutive and cytokine-stimulated expression of eotaxin by human airway smooth muscle cells. *Am J Respir Crit Care Med* 1999; 159:1933–1942.

25. Fukagawa K, Nakajima T, Saito H *et al*. IL-4 induces eotaxin production in corneal keratocytes but not in epithelial cells. *Int Arch Allergy Immunol* 2000; 121:144–150.

26. MacLean JA, Ownbey R, Luster AD. T cell-dependent regulation of eotaxin in antigen-induced pulmonary eosinophilia. *J Exp Med* 1996; 184:1461–1469.

27. Matsukura S, Stellato C, Plitt JR *et al*. Activation of eotaxin gene transcription by NF-kappa B and STAT6 in human airway epithelial cells. *J Immunol* 1999; 163:6876–6883.

28. Wills-Karp M, Luyimbazi J, Xu X *et al*. Interleukin-13: central mediator of allergic asthma [see comments]. *Science* 1998; 282:2258–2261.

29. Zhu Z, Homer RJ, Wang Z *et al*. Pulmonary expression of interleukin-13 causes inflammation, mucus hypersecretion, subepithelial fibrosis, physiologic abnormalities, and eotaxin production. *J Clin Invest* 1999; 103:779–788.

30. Li L, Xia Y, Nguyen A *et al*. Effects of Th2 cytokines on chemokine expression in the lung: IL-13 potently induces eotaxin expression by airway epithelial cells. *J Immunol* 1999; 162:2477–2487.

31. Nomiyama H, Osborne LR, Imai T *et al*. Assignment of the human CC chemokine MPIF-2/eotaxin-2 (SCYA24) to chromosome 7q11.23. *Genomics* 1998; 49:339–340.

32. Kitaura M, Suzuki N, Imai T *et al*. Molecular cloning of a novel human CC chemokine (Eotaxin-3) that is a functional ligand of CC chemokine receptor 3. *J Biol Chem* 1999; 274:27975–27980.

33. Zimmermann N, Hogan SP, Mishra A *et al*. Murine eotaxin-2: a constitutive eosinophil chemokine induced by allergen challenge and IL-4 overexpression. *J Immunol* 2000; 165:5839–5846.

34. Schaefer D, Meyer JE, Pods R *et al*. Endothelial and epithelial expression of eotaxin-2 (CCL24) in nasal polyps. *Int Arch Allergy Immunol* 2006; 140:205–214.

35. Kagami S, Saeki H, Komine M *et al*. Interleukin-4 and interleukin-13 enhance CCL26 production in a human keratinocyte cell line, HaCaT cells. *Clin Exp Immunol* 2005; 141:459–466.

36. Watanabe K, Jose PJ, Rankin SM. Eotaxin-2 generation is differentially regulated by lipopolysaccharide and IL-4 in monocytes and macrophages. *J Immunol* 2002; 168:1911–1918.

37. Shinkai A, Yoshisue H, Koike M *et al*. A novel human CC chemokine, eotaxin-3, which is expressed in IL-4-stimulated vascular endothelial cells, exhibits potent activity toward eosinophils. *J Immunol* 1999; 163:1602–1610.

38. Zuyderduyn S, Hiemstra PS, Rabe KF. TGF-beta differentially regulates TH2 cytokine-induced eotaxin and eotaxin-3 release by human airway smooth muscle cells. *J Allergy Clin Immunol* 2004; 114:791–798.

39. Blanchard C, Durual S, Estienne M, Emami S, Vasseur S, Cuber JC. Eotaxin-3/CCL26 gene expression in intestinal epithelial cells is up-regulated by interleukin-4 and interleukin-13 via the signal transducer and activator of transcription 6. *Int J Biochem Cell Biol* 2005; 37:2559–2573.

40. Ponath PD, Qin S, Post TW *et al*. Molecular cloning and characterization of a human eotaxin receptor expressed selectively on eosinophils. *J Exp Med* 1996; 183:2437–2448.

41. Daugherty BL, Siciliano SJ, DeMartino J, Malkowitz L, Sirontino A, Springer MS. Cloning, expression and characterization of the human eosinophil eotaxin receptor. *J Exp Med* 1996; 183:2349–2354.

42. Kitaura M, Nakajima T, Imai T *et al*. Molecular cloning of human eotaxin, an eosinophil-selective CC chemokine, and identification of a specific eosinophil eotaxin receptor, CC chemokine receptor 3. *J Biol Chem* 1996; 271:7725–7730.

43. Sallusto F, Mackay CR, Lanzavecchia A. Selective expression of the eotaxin receptor CCR3 by human T helper 2 cells. *Science* 1997; 277:2005–2007.

44. Uguccioni M, Mackay CR, Ochensberger B *et al*. High expression of the chemokine receptor CCR3 in human blood basophils. Role in activation by eotaxin, MCP-4, and other chemokines. *J Clin Invest* 1997; 100:1137–1143.

45. Romagnani P, De Paulis A, Beltrame C *et al*. Tryptase-chymase double-positive human mast cells express the eotaxin receptor CCR3 and are attracted by CCR3-binding chemokines. *Am J Pathol* 1999; 155:1195–1204.

46. Heath H, Qin S, Wu L *et al*. Chemokine receptor usage by human eosinophils. The importance of CCR3 demonstrated using an antagonistic monoclonal antibody. *J Clin Invest* 1997; 99:178–184.

47. Pease JE, Wang J, Ponath PD, Murphy PM. The N-terminal extracellular segments of the chemokine receptors CCR1 and CCR3 are determinants for MIP-1α and eotaxin binding, respectively, but a second domain is essential for receptor activation. *J Biol Chem* 1998; 273:19972–19976.

48. Monteclaro FS, Charo IF. The amino-terminal extracellular domain of the MCP-1 receptor, but not the RANTES/MIP-1alpha receptor, confers chemokine selectivity. Evidence for a two-step mechanism for MCP-1 receptor activation. *J Biol Chem* 1996; 271:19084–19092.

49. Ballesteros JA, Jensen AD, Liapakis G *et al*. Activation of the beta 2-adrenergic receptor involves disruption of an ionic lock between the cytoplasmic ends of transmembrane segments 3 and 6. *J Biol Chem* 2001; 276:29171–29177.

50. Boehme SA, Sullivan SK, Crowe PD *et al*. Activation of mitogen-activated protein kinase regulates eotaxin-induced eosinophil migration. *J Immunol* 1999; 163:1611–1618.

51. Kampen GT, Stafford S, Adachi T *et al*. Eotaxin induces degranulation and chemotaxis of eosinophils through the activation of ERK2 and p38 mitogen-activated protein kinases. *Blood* 2000; 95:1911–1917.

52. Adachi T, Vita R, Sannohe S *et al*. The functional role of rho and rho-associated coiled-coil forming protein kinase in eotaxin signaling of eosinophils. *J Immunol* 2001; 167:4609–4615.

53. Elsner J, Hochstetter R, Kimmig D, Kapp A. Human eotaxin represents a potent activator of the respiratory burst of human eosinophils. *Eur J Immunol* 1996; 26:1919–1925.

54. Humbles AA, Conroy DM, Marleau S *et al*. Kinetics of eotaxin generation and its relationship to eosinophil accumulation in allergic airways disease: analysis in a guinea pig model *in vivo*. *J Exp Med* 1997; 186:601–612.

55. Gonzalo J-A, Lloyd CM, Wen D *et al*. The coordinated action of CC chemokines in the lung orchestrates allergic inflammation and airways hyperresponsiveness. *J Exp Med* 1998; 188:157–167.

56. Lloyd CM, Delaney T, Nguyen T *et al*. CC chemokine receptor (CCR)3/eotaxin is followed by CCR4/monocyte-derived chemokine in mediating pulmonary T helper lymphocyte type 2 recruitment after serial antigen challenge *in vivo*. *J Exp Med* 2000; 191:265–273.

57. Rothenberg ME, MacLean JA, Pearlman E, Luster AD, Leder P. Targeted disruption of the chemokine eotaxin partially reduces antigen-induced tissue eosinophilia. *J Exp Med* 1997; 185:785–790.

58. Yang Y, Loy J, Ryseck RP, Carrasco D, Bravo R. Antigen-induced eosinophilic lung inflammation develops in mice deficient in chemokine eotaxin. *Blood* 1998; 92:3912–3923.

59. Collins PD, Marleau S, Griffiths-Johnson DA, Jose PJ, Williams TJ. Co-operation between interleukin-5 and the chemokine eotaxin to induce eosinophil accumulation *in vivo*. *J Exp Med* 1995; 182:1169–1174.

60. Palframan RT, Collins PD, Severs NJ, Rothery S, Williams TJ, Rankin SM. Mechanisms of acute eosinophil mobilization from the bone marrow stimulated by interleukin 5: the role of specific adhesion molecules and phosphatidylinositol 3-kinase. *J Exp Med* 1998; 188:1621–1632.

61. Palframan RT, Collins PD, Williams TJ, Rankin SM. Eotaxin induces a rapid release of eosinophils and their progenitors from the bone marrow. *Blood* 1998; 91:2240–2248.

62. Humbles AA, Lu B, Friend DS *et al*. The murine CCR3 receptor regulates both the role of eosinophils and mast cells in allergen-induced airway inflammation and hyperresponsiveness. *Proc Natl Acad Sci USA* 2002; 99:1479–1484.

63. Ma W, Bryce PJ, Humbles AA *et al*. CCR3 is essential for skin eosinophilia and airway hyperresponsiveness in a murine model of allergic skin inflammation. *J Clin Invest* 2002; 109:621–628.

64. Pope SM, Fulkerson PC, Blanchard C *et al*. Identification of a cooperative mechanism involving interleukin-13 and eotaxin-2 in experimental allergic lung inflammation. *J Biol Chem* 2005; 280: 13952–13961.

65. Menzies-Gow A, Ying S, Sabroe I *et al*. Eotaxin (CCL11) and eotaxin-2 (CCL24) induce recruitment of eosinophils, basophils, neutrophils, and macrophages as well as features of early- and late-phase allergic reactions following cutaneous injection in human atopic and nonatopic volunteers. *J Immunol* 2002; 169:2712–2718.

66. Ying S, Robinson DS, Meng Q *et al*. C-C chemokines in allergen-induced late-phase cutaneous responses in atopic subjects: association of eotaxin with early 6-hour eosinophils, and of eotaxin-2 and monocyte chemoattractant protein-4 with the later 24-hour tissue eosinophilia, and relationship to basophils and other C-C chemokines (Monocyte chemoattractant protein-3 and RANTES). *J Immunol* 1999; 163:3976–3984.

67. Duchesnes CE, Murphy PM, Williams TJ, Pease JE. Alanine scanning mutagenesis of the chemokine receptor CCR3 reveals distinct extracellular residues involved in recognition of the eotaxin family of chemokines. *Mol Immunol* 2006; 43:1221–1231.

68. Berkman N, Ohnona S, Chung FK, Breuer R. Eotaxin-3 but not eotaxin gene expression is upregulated in asthmatics 24 hours after allergen challenge. *Am J Respir Cell Mol Biol* 2001; 24:682–687.

69. Blanchard C, Wang N, Stringer KF *et al*. Eotaxin-3 and a uniquely conserved gene-expression profile in eosinophilic esophagitis. *J Clin Invest* 2006; 116:536–547.

70. Ochi H, Hirani WM, Yuan Q, Friend DS, Austen KF, Boyce JA. T helper cell type 2 cytokine-mediated comitogenic responses and CCR3 expression during differentiation of human mast cells in vitro. *J Exp Med* 1999; 190:267–280.

71. Sabroe I, Conroy DM, Gerard NP *et al*. Cloning and characterization of the guinea pig eosinophil eotaxin receptor, CCR3: blockade using a monoclonal antibody in vivo. *J Immunol* 1998; 161:6139–6147.

72. Zhang L, Soares MP, Guan Y *et al*. Functional expression and characterization of macaque C-C chemokine receptor 3 (CCR3) and generation of potent antagonistic anti-macaque CCR3 monoclonal antibodies. *J Biol Chem* 2002; 277:33799–33810.

73. Fredriksson R, Lagerstrom MC, Lundin LG, Schioth HB. The G-protein-coupled receptors in the human genome form five main families. Phylogenetic analysis, paralogon groups, and fingerprints. *Mol Pharmacol* 2003; 63:1256–1272.

74. Sabroe I, Peck MJ, Jan Van Keulen B *et al*. A small molecule antagonist of the chemokine receptors CCR1 and CCR3: potent inhibition of Eosinophil function and CCR3-mediated HIV-1 entry. *J Biol Chem* 2000; 275:25985–25992.

75. Naya A, Sagara Y, Ohwaki K *et al*. Design, synthesis, and discovery of a novel CCR1 antagonist. *J Med Chem* 2001; 44:1429–1435.

76. Sabroe I, Hartnell A, Jopling LA *et al*. Differential regulation of eosinophil chemokine signaling via CCR3 and non-CCR3 pathways. *J Immunol* 1999; 162:2946–2955.

77. Bryan SA, Jose PJ, Topping JR *et al*. Responses of leukocytes to chemokines in whole blood and their antagonism by novel CC-chemokine receptor 3 antagonists. *Am J Respir Crit Care Med* 2002; 165: 1602–1609.

78. White JR, Lee JM, Dede K *et al*. Identification of potent, selective non-peptide CCR3 antagonist that inhibits eotaxin-1, eotaxin-2 and MCP-4 induced eosinophil migration. *J Biol Chem* 2000; 275: 36626–36631.

79. de Mendonca FL, da Fonseca PC, Phillips RM, Saldanha JW, Williams TJ, Pease JE. Site-directed mutagenesis of CC chemokine receptor 1 reveals the mechanism of action of UCB 35625, a small molecule chemokine receptor antagonist. *J Biol Chem* 2005; 280:4808–4816.

80. Warrior U, McKeegan EM, Rottinghaus SM et al. Identification and characterization of novel antagonists of the CCR3 receptor. *J Biomol Screen* 2003; 8:324–331.
81. Saeki T, Ohwaki K, Naya A et al. Identification of a potent and nonpeptidyl CCR3 antagonist. *Biochem Biophys Res Commun* 2001; 281:779–782.
82. Naya A, Kobayashi K, Ishikawa M et al. Discovery of a novel CCR3 selective antagonist. *Bioorg Med Chem Lett* 2001; 11:1219–1223.
83. Wan Y, Jakway JP, Qiu H et al. Identification of full, partial and inverse CC chemokine receptor 3 agonists using [35S]GTPgammaS binding. *Eur J Pharmacol* 2002; 456:1–10.
84. Naya A, Kobayashi K, Ishikawa M et al. Structure-activity relationships of 2-(benzothiazolylthio) acetamide class of CCR3 selective antagonist. *Chem Pharm Bull (Tokyo)* 2003; 51:697–701.
85. Anderskewitz R, Bauer R, Bodenbach G et al. Pyrrolidinohydroquinazolines – a novel class of CCR3 modulators. *Bioorg Med Chem Lett* 2005; 15:669–673.
86. De Lucca GV, Kim UT, Johnson C et al. Discovery and structure-activity relationship of N-(ureidoalkyl)-benzyl-piperidines as potent small molecule CC chemokine receptor-3 (CCR3) antagonists. *J Med Chem* 2002; 45:3794–3804.
87. Varnes JG, Gardner DS, Santella JB 3rd et al. Discovery of N-propylurea 3-benzylpiperidines as selective CC chemokine receptor-3 (CCR3) antagonists. *Bioorg Med Chem Lett* 2004; 14:1645–1649.
88. Wacker DA, Santella JB 3rd, Gardner DS et al. CCR3 antagonists: a potential new therapy for the treatment of asthma. Discovery and structure-activity relationships. *Bioorg Med Chem Lett* 2002; 12:1785–1789.
89. Dhanak D, Christmann LT, Darcy MG et al. Discovery of potent and selective phenylalanine derived CCR3 antagonists. Part 1. *Bioorg Med Chem Lett* 2001; 11:1441–1444.
90. Dhanak D, Christmann LT, Darcy MG et al. Discovery of potent and selective phenylalanine derived CCR3 receptor antagonists. Part 2. *Bioorg Med Chem Lett* 2001; 11:1445–1450.
91. Hodgson S, Charlton S, Warne P. Chemokines and drug discovery. *Drug News Perspect* 2004; 17:335–338.
92. Fryer AD, Stein LH, Nie Z et al. Neuronal eotaxin and the effects of CCR3 antagonist on airway hyperreactivity and M2 receptor dysfunction. *J Clin Invest* 2006; 116:228–236.
93. Ting PC, Umland SP, Aslanian R et al. The synthesis of substituted bipiperidine amide compounds as CCR3 ligands: antagonists versus agonists. *Bioorg Med Chem Lett* 2005; 15:3020–3023.
94. Ting PC, Lee JF, Wu J et al. The synthesis of substituted bipiperidine amide compounds as CCR3 antagonists. *Bioorg Med Chem Lett* 2005; 15:1375–1378.
95. Suzuki K, Morokata T, Morihira K et al. In vitro and in vivo characterization of a novel CCR3 antagonist, YM-344031. *Biochem Biophys Res Commun* 2006; 339:1217–1223.
96. Morokata T, Suzuki K, Masunaga Y et al. A novel, selective, and orally available antagonist for CC chemokine receptor 3. *J Pharmacol Exp Ther* 2006; 317:244–250.
97. De Lucca GV, Kim UT, Vargo BJ et al. Discovery of CC chemokine receptor-3 (CCR3) antagonists with picomolar potency. *J Med Chem* 2005; 48:2194–2211.
98. Kips JC, O'Connor BJ, Langley SJ et al. Effect of SCH55700, a humanized anti-human interleukin-5 antibody, in severe persistent asthma: a pilot study. *Am J Respir Crit Care Med* 2003; 167:1655–1659.
99. Leckie MJ, ten Brinke A, Khan J et al. Effects of an interleukin-5 blocking monoclonal antibody on eosinophils, airway hyper-responsiveness, and the late asthmatic response. *Lancet* 2000; 356:2144–2148.
100. O'Byrne PM, Inman MD, Parameswaran K. The trials and tribulations of IL-5, eosinophils, and allergic asthma. *J Allergy Clin Immunol* 2001; 108:503–508.
101. Kay AB, Menzies-Gow A. Eosinophils and interleukin-5: the debate continues. *Am J Respir Crit Care Med* 2003; 167:1586–1587.
102. Erin EM, Williams TJ, Barnes PJ, Hansel TT. Eotaxin receptor (CCR3) antagonism in asthma and allergic disease. *Curr Drug Targets Inflamm Allergy* 2002; 1:201–214.
103. Cho JY, Miller M, Baek KJ et al. Inhibition of airway remodeling in IL-5-deficient mice. *J Clin Invest* 2004; 113:551–560.
104. Flood-Page P, Menzies-Gow A, Phipps S et al. Anti-IL-5 treatment reduces deposition of ECM proteins in the bronchial subepithelial basement membrane of mild atopic asthmatics. *J Clin Invest* 2003; 112:1029–1036.
105. Humbles AA, Lloyd CM, McMillan SJ et al. A critical role for eosinophils in allergic airways remodeling. *Science* 2004; 305:1776–1779.
106. Lee JJ, Dimina D, Macias MP et al. Defining a link with asthma in mice congenitally deficient in eosinophils. *Science* 2004; 305:1773–1776.

107. Brightling CE, Ammit AJ, Kaur D *et al*. The CXCL10/CXCR3 axis mediates human lung mast cell migration to asthmatic airway smooth muscle. *Am J Respir Crit Care Med* 2005; 171:1103–1108.
108. Gurish MF, Humbles A, Tao H *et al*. CCR3 is required for tissue eosinophilia and larval cytotoxicity after infection with Trichinella spiralis. *J Immunol* 2002; 168:5730–5736.
109. GSK Annual Report 2004 http://www.gsk.com/investors/reps04/20F-2004.pdf; 2004.
110. Phillips R, Stubbs VELS, Henson MR, Williams TJ, Pease JE, Sabroe I. Variations in eosinophil chemokine responses: an investigation of CCR1 and CCR3 function, expression in atopy, and identification of a functional CCR1 promoter. *J Immunol* 2003; 170:6190–6201.
111. Alam R, York J, Boyars M *et al*. Increased MCP-1, RANTES, and MIP-1alpha in bronchoalveolar lavage fluid of allergic asthmatic patients. *Am J Respir Crit Care Med* 1996; 153(pt 1):1398–1404.
112. Tillie-Leblond I, Hammad H, Desurmont S *et al*. CC chemokines and interleukin-5 in bronchial lavage fluid from patients with status asthmaticus. Potential implication in eosinophil recruitment. *Am J Respir Crit Care Med* 2000; 162(pt 1):586–592.
113. Holgate ST, Bodey KS, Janezic A, Frew AJ, Kaplan AP, Teran LM. Release of RANTES, MIP-1 alpha, and MCP-1 into asthmatic airways following endobronchial allergen challenge. *Am J Respir Crit Care Med* 1997; 156:1377–1383.

Abbreviations

ACTH	adrenocorticotropic hormone
AP-1	activator/activating protein-1
APC	antigen-presenting cells
AQLQ	Asthma Quality of Life Questionnaire
Arg	arginine
ASM	airway smooth muscle
AUC	area under the [plasma] concentration time surve
BAL	bronchoalveolar lavage
BALF	bronchoalveolar lavage fluid
BCG	Bacillus Calmette Guerin
BDP	beclomethasone dipropionate
bEGF	fibroblast growth factor
β_2-AR	β_2-adrenergic receptor
BMP	beclomethasone monopropionate
bpm	beats per minute
BUP	Bupropion hydrochloride
cAMP	cyclic adenosine monophosphate
CD	corticosteroid-dependent
CFC	chlorofluorocarbon
cGMP	cyclic guanosine monophosphate
COPD	chronic obstructive pulmonary disease
COX	cyclo-oxygenase
CpG	Cytosine-Guanine
CR	corticosteroid-resistant
CREB	cAMP responsive element
CS	corticosteroid sensitive
Cys	cysteine
CysLT	cysteinyl leukotriene
DNA	deoxyribonucleic acid
DPI	dry powder inhaler
DS	discriminative stimulus
EC_{50}	the molar concentration of an agonist that produces 50% of the maximum possible response for that agonist
ECP	eosinophilic cationic protein
ED	emergency department
ED_{80}	the effective dose of a substance required to give 80% of the maximum biological response to that substance
EFS	electrical field stimulation
ENFUMOSA	European Network for Understanding Mechanisms of Severe Asthma
ETS	environmental tobacco smoke

FB	formoterol + budesonide
FEF	forced expiratory flow
FeNO	exhaled nitric oxide
FEV_1	forced expiratory volume in one second
FP	fluticasone propionate
FVC	forced vital capacity
GCS	glucocorticoids
GINA	Global Initiative for Asthma
Gln	glutamine
Glu	glutamic acid
Gly	glycine
GM-CSF	granulocyte-macrophage colony-stimulating factor
GR	glucocorticosteroid receptor
GRE	glucocorticosteroid receptor element
GRK2	G protein-coupled receptor kinase-2
HAT	histone acetyltransferase
HDAC	histone de-acetylase
HFA MDI	hydrofluorocarbon metered-dose inhaler
HLA-DR	human leucocyte antigen DR genes
HPA	hypothalamic–pituitary–adrenocortical
HSP	heat shock protein
HYD	hydrocortisone
IC_{50}	the molar concentration of an antagonist that produces 50% of the maximum possible inhibitory response for that antagonist
ICAM-1	intercellular adhesion molecule-1
ICS	inhaled corticosteroid
Ig	immunoglobulin
IKK	IκB kinase
IL	interleukin
INNOVATE	Investigation of Omalizumab in severe Asthma TrEatment
IκBα	inhibitor κB alpha
JAK	Janus kinase
JNK	Jun N-terminal kinase
LABA	long-acting β-agonist
LBD	ligand binding domain
LPS	lipopolysaccharide
LRTI	lower respiratory tract infection
LT	leukotriene
LTRA	leukotriene receptor antagonist
LXR	liver X receptor
MAPK	mitogen-activated protein kinase
MBL	mannose-binding lectin
MCH	metacholine
MCP	monocyte chemotactic protein
MF	mometasone furoate
MKP-1	MAPK phosphatase 1
NANC	non-adrenergic non-cholinergic
NF-κB	nuclear factor-κB
NF-λB	nuclear factor-λB
NHR	nuclear hormone receptor
NIPPV	non-invasive positive-pressure ventilation
NK	natural killer

NOS	nitric oxide synthase
NOS2	inducible nitric oxide synthase
ODN	oligodeoxynucleotide
OPG	osteoprotegerin
PaO_2	partial pressure of oxygen in the arterial blood
PBMC	peripheral blood mononuclear cell
PC_{20}	provocative concentration of a substance that causes a 20% fall in FEV_1
pD_2	potency
PDE	phoshodiesterase
PEF	peak expiratory flow
PEFR	peak expiratory flow rate
PFT	pulmonary function test
PGD_2	prostaglandin D_2
PGE_2	prostaglandin E_2
PKA	protein kinase A
PKC	protein kinase C
pMDI	pressurized meter dose inhaler
POMC	pro-opiomelanocort
PPAR	peroxisome proliferator-activated receptor
PR	pulse rate
QoL	quality of life
RANKL	receptor activator of NF-κB
RANTES	Regulated on Activation, Normal T-cell Expressed and Secreted
RSV	respiratory syncytial virus
RT-PCR	reverse transcription polymerise chain reaction
SAR	seasonal allergic rhinitis
SCF	stem cell factor
SCID	severe combined immunodeficiency
SIT	(allergen)-specific immunotherapy
SLIT	sublingual immunotherapy
SMART	Symbicort® Maintenance and Reliever Medication
SNP	single nucleotide polymorphism
SpO_2	arterial oxygen saturation measured by pulse oximetry
SRS-A	slow-releasing substances of anaphylaxis
STAT	signal transduction-activated transcription factors
TAT	tyrosine aminotransferase
TCC	total cell count
TENOR	The Epidemiology and Natural History of Asthma: Outcomes and Treatment Regimens study
TGFβ	tansforming growth factor β
Th2	T helper 2
TLR	toll-like receptor
TNF	tumour necrosis factor alpha α
Treg	regulatory T cells

Index